INTRODUCTION TO SYNDEMICS

INTRODUCTION TO SYNDEMICS

A Critical Systems Approach to Public and Community Health

MERRILL SINGER

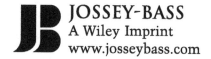

JOSSEY-BASS
A Wiley Imprint
www.josseybass.com

Published by Jossey-Bass

A Wiley Imprint

989 Market Street, San Francisco, CA 94103-1741—www.josseybass.com

Jossey-Bass books and products are available through most bookstores. To contact Jossey-Bass directly call our Customer Care Department within the U.S. at 800-956-7739, outside the U.S. at 317-572-3986, or fax 317-572-4002.

Jossey-Bass also publishes its books in a variety of electronic formats. Some content that appears in print may not be available in electronic books.

Library of Congress Cataloging-in-Publication Data
Singer, Merrill.
    Introduction to syndemics : a critical systems approach to public and community health/ Merrill Singer. — 1st ed.
        p. ; cm.
    Includes bibliographical references and index.
    ISBN   978-0-470-47203-3 (pbk.)
        1. Epidemics.   2. Social medicine.   3. Poor—Health and hygiene.   I. Title.
        [DNLM: 1. Health Status Disparities.   2. Ecology.   3. Healthcare Disparities.
    4. Social Medicine.   5. Systems Theory.   WA 300.1 S617i 2009]
    RA652.S56 2009
    362.1—dc22

                                                                    2009008869

FIRST EDITION
PB Printing   10 9 8 7 6 5 4 3 2

This book is devoted to my colleagues in the United States, Canada, New Zealand, and elsewhere who have taken an interest in and contributed to the body of work on syndemics. This book is dedicated to Bruce Gould, associate dean for primary care medicine, University of Connecticut Health Center, a role model, friend, and physician.

CONTENTS

PART THREE
SOCIETY, HISTORY, AND THE ENVIRONMENT   121

PART FOUR
APPLICATIONS OF THE SYNDEMIC PERSPECTIVE   197

PREFACE

In ancient Greek the term μέθοδος (*methodos*) was used to refer to the pursuit of knowledge and the approach taken for conducting such inquiry. Although the opening syllable conveys the notion of being in the midst of something (*metha*), the remainder of the word (*odos*) refers to an approach or journey. This book, the product of a personal and professional journey that began over twenty-five years ago, provides an introduction to the emergent concept of *syndemics*, which I developed as part of an ongoing effort to rethink the public health and social scientific understanding of disease so that it focused attention on the multifaceted interactions that occur among the health of a community, political and economic structures, and the encompassing physical and social environment. This reconceptualization developed specifically out of many years of work on the health challenges associated with social disparity, especially in the context of the human immunodeficiency virus and the acquired immunodeficiency syndrome (HIV/AIDS) epidemic (Singer, 1994; Singer & Snipes, 1992).

Employed for over twenty-five years as an applied medical anthropology researcher in a community-based, direct service, and research organization located in a primarily Latino and African American inner-city neighborhood, I was made painfully and daily aware of the many health problems caused by being poor and marginalized in American society. Poverty is well known to bring about regular exposure to diverse biological stressors, including social discrimination, food insufficiency and malnutrition, diverse infectious pathogens, toxic substances in the living and working environment, and climatic extremes owing to inadequacies of clothing and shelter. As summarized by the Prevention Institute (2002), "The chief underlying cause of health disparities is increasingly understood to be social and economic inequality; i.e., social bias and institutional racism, limited education, poverty, and related environmental conditions that either directly produce ill health or promote unhealthy behaviors that lead to poor health" (p. 3). More pointedly, Harvard public health researcher Nancy Krieger, who has produced an impressive body of work on these issues, asserts: "Social inequality kills. It deprives individuals and communities of a healthy start in life, increases their burden of disability and disease, and brings early death. Poverty and discrimination, inadequate medical care, and violation of human rights all act as powerful social determinants of who lives and who dies, at what age, and with what degree of suffering" (2005, p. 15).

Generally speaking, in short, health and wealth go hand in hand, and as a result the poor have worse health than the more affluent social groups. Consequently, many of the people and my coworkers and I studied and provided with health and social support services suffered from multiple diseases and multiple social problems, making it difficult often to know where to begin in addressing their myriad needs. Although the historical tendency has been to start with a specific health problem (consider for example the traditional argument in the substance abuse treatment field that you have to concentrate initially on a person's substance abuse issues before addressing his or her other challenges), over the years it became increasingly apparent to me that to be effective in creating change a new, more holistic way of thinking was needed about health and illness in *health disparity populations*.

Rather than starting with the *part* (with this disease or that social condition), why not look at the *whole* (the full array of the health and social problems suffered by an individual or a community) and assess the nature of the interconnections among the parts, including the intricate ways in which they promote and reinforce each other and thereby create a complex and burdensome web of entwined health and social problems? With the emergence of HIV/AIDS and its rapid spread among the inner-city poor (a process that was occurring while the assumption among public health officials was that HIV/AIDS was a disease limited primarily to multipartnered gay men), it became apparent that studying this disease and responding to it with public health initiatives as though it were separate from other diseases and conditions also prevalent in the community was a distortion. Indeed, it became clear that even the public health term *epidemic*, which had quickly come to be used to describe the sudden spread of HIV/AIDS, did not sufficiently describe the growing (and several decades later still intense) inner-city HIV/AIDS crisis, which involved the transmission of this disease in close conjunction with a set of other health conditions (such as tuberculosis [TB], sexually transmitted diseases [STDs], hepatitis, cirrhosis, infant mortality, drug abuse, suicide, homicide, and so forth), all of which were intertwined and strongly influenced and sustained by broader political, economic, and social factors. In this process of rethinking the concept of syndemics was born. From the syndemics perspective, contemporary threats to the health of the poor, including violence, substance abuse, malnutrition, and HIV/AIDS, are not *concurrent* epidemics in that they are not completely separable phenomena. Rather they emerge among the poor as closely intertwined threads in the often tattered fabric of their daily lives.

A syndemic, in short, involves a set of enmeshed and mutually enhancing health problems that, *working together* in a context of noxious social and physical conditions, can significantly affect the overall disease burden and health status of a population. For example, in the Multicenter AIDS Cohort Study conducted between 1994 and 2000, Thio et al. (2002) divided the individuals in their research sample into four groups: those with HIV only, those with hepatitis B only, those with both HIV and hepatitis B, and those who were free of either disease. These researchers found that liver disease–related deaths were highest in the dually infected subgroup and were especially high in those with low CD4 cell counts (a sign of advanced HIV infection). Men infected with hepatitis B and HIV were seventeen times more likely to die of liver disease than were those infected with just hepatitis B. Similarly, in January 2004, the World Health Organization (WHO) announced its decision to support expanded collaboration between tuberculosis and HIV/AIDS programs in order to curb the growing spread of TB and HIV coinfection. The new WHO policy guidelines defined the public health activities needed to address what the WHO referred to as "the dual epidemic of TB and HIV." According to WHO director-general Lee Jong-wook, "TB/HIV is a deadly combination and needs to be tackled with an approach treating the whole person" (WHO, 2004b, p. 1).

Defined as *the concentration and deleterious interaction of two or more diseases or other health conditions in a population, especially as a consequence of social inequity and the unjust exercise of power,* syndemics appear to have played an important role in human disease history (and hence in human history generally), are having a significant impact on diverse populations currently, and are likely to have consequential influence on the emergent health profile of the twenty-first century. As a result the syndemics concept is receiving a growing level of attention in the field of public health, among social scientists concerned with health, and also in other disciplines that focus on the health effects of social and environmental conditions.

In the various fields in which a syndemic understanding of disease has garnered interest, it is generally recognized that the traditional biomedical approach to disease, an approach that dominated thinking about health throughout the twentieth century, resulted from an effort to diagnostically isolate, closely study, and therapeutically treat individual cases of disease, as if each disease were a distinct entity that existed in nature separate from other diseases and independent of the biosocial contexts in which it was found. This approach proved useful in its time in focusing medical attention on the immediate causes and biological expressions of disease (seen as any harmful change that interferes with the normal form, structure, or function of the body or any of its parts or systems) and contributed to the emergence of diverse pharmaceutical, surgical, and other biomedical treatments for specific diseases, some of which have been enormously successful, especially for acute conditions.

Similarly, "research protocols, prevention programs, policy interventions, and other aspects of public health practice have focused on one disease at a time, leaving other health problems to be addressed by parallel enterprises" (Syndemics Prevention Network, 2005d). This traditional approach is seen, for example, in public health textbooks. To take but one instance, Kathryn Jacobsen's (2008) very thorough epidemiological introduction to global health includes a chapter titled "HIV/AIDS, Malaria, and TB." Each of these diseases is discussed in a separate section, with a clear description of the disease and its causes, its geographical distribution, and the strategies for its prevention and treatment. The section on AIDS discusses it as a source of opportunistic infections by other pathogens, and the section on TB notes that people "with HIV infection are more likely to develop active TB disease than people without HIV infection" and that "TB is a leading cause of death in people with AIDS" (p. 163). Moreover, the book's discussion of influenza mentions the *antigenic shift* that occurs when "two different influenza viruses attack the same cell and the genetic material from both recombines to form a new type of influenza" (p. 175). Finally, in a discussion of the immune system, the book notes that "poor nutrition . . . can . . . cause immune system suppression and lead to other diseases" (p. 29). Even though there are these fleeting references to syndemic processes and consequences, overall the volume is guided by a conventional, one-disease-at-a-time orientation. Although promoting an appreciation of the complexities and unique features of each disease, this approach cannot offer an equally developed appreciation of the fact that in the real world a disease does not usually exist in isolation from other diseases and disorders and that synergistic interactions have considerable effect on disease course and consequence. Moreover, these interactions may play a critical role in treatment and outcome. A telling example of this is the account provided by Watt, Jongsakul, and Suttinot (2003) of a Thai woman patient who "presented with leptospirosis [a bacterial disease that can result in renal failure] and was treated appropriately with high-dose intravenous penicillin. Her condition deteriorated rapidly, however, and she died with adult respiratory distress syndrome, the most common cause of death from *O. tsutsugamushi* infection [also known as scrub typhus]. Perhaps a fatal outcome could have been avoided had antibiotics active against scrub typhus been administered. A mixed infection should be considered in patients with either leptospirosis or scrub typhus who are responding poorly to treatment" (p. 90).

Finally, the traditional biomedical approach tends to pay little attention to the fact that the social environments of people with diseases are critical to understanding the clustering and spread of diseases within and between populations, disease expression through bodily signs and symptoms, and the added burden of intertwined diseases at the individual and population levels.

The purpose of this book, then, is to draw attention to the developing field of *syndemic theory and research* and to provide a framework for the analysis of disease interactions, including their origins and the threat they present to human life and well-being, and for the prevention of damaging disease interactions by addressing underlying social and environmental causes. As Julie Gerberding (2005), the former head of the Centers for Disease Control and Prevention (CDC), has stated, the "application of complex systems theories or syndemic science to health protection challenges is in its infancy" (p. 1405). Nonetheless, it is the CDC's position that this line of attack represents a "promising new frontier for public health action in response to the critical challenges of our time" (Leischow & Milstein, 2006, p. 405). Further, the CDC has heralded the syndemic orientation as offering an approach for "establishing new theories of change, new alliances among interest groups, new funding policies, and new levels of achievement in protecting the public's health" (Syndemics Prevention Network, 2005a).

Syndemic theory extends the work of other health researchers who have long recognized the critical importance of disease interaction in a social context. In an important series of papers on health in New York City, for example, Rodrick Wallace and Deborah Wallace (Wallace, 1988, 1990; Wallace & Wallace, 1998) drew attention to the "synergism of plagues" produced by public policies designed to restrict municipal services in low-income neighborhoods as a way of getting people to move away, thus freeing up the land for profitable economic development. The tragic result was a mass movement of people to new (also poor) areas, overcrowding, and an unraveling of community relationships and support structures, as well as a set of linked epidemics of tuberculosis, measles, substance abuse, AIDS, low-weight births, and street violence. Examining these health issues by separating them, overlooking the ways in which they are intimately linked and mutually enhancing, and ignoring the underlying social and biological processes involved in their development and expression does not lead to insight born of fine-grained analysis. Rather it distorts on-the-ground and in-the-body realities and obscures the nature of the connections between the health of physical bodies and the health of social bodies. The syndemics perspective is intended to capture, analyze, and respond to these complex realities. As an approach to addressing community health issues, it "complements single-issue prevention strategies that may be effective in controlling discrete problems but often are mismatched to the goal of improving community health in its widest sense" (Syndemics Prevention Network, 2005a).

The appeal of this new conception is seen in the rising number of recent scholarly publications in public health, biomedicine, and dentistry (for example, Freudenberg, Fahs, Galea, & Greenberg, 2006; Hein & Small, 2007; Milstein, 2008), biology (for example, Herring & Sattenspiel, 2007), and the health-related social sciences (for example, Marshall, 2005; Singer, 2006a; Singer & Clair, 2003; Singer, Erickson, et al., 2006) that have adopted a syndemic approach. It is being used in accounting for health patterns and developing community-based prevention initiatives (as seen, for example, in the work on diabetes prevention among Native Americans by Bachar et al., 2006). There are efforts under way within the CDC to build a national syndemics prevention strategy and online prevention community (see Syndemics Prevention Network, 2008a). Moreover, the concept is appearing in national (see, for example, National Institutes of Health, Office of AIDS Research, 2006) and international health reports (for example, Laserson & Wells, 2007). It is being discussed at international health conferences (for example, by Prince Charles in a speech at the 2006 Enhancing the Healing Environment conference, St James's Palace, London), in dictionaries and encyclopedias (for example, Easton, 2004; MacQueen, 2002; Milstein, 2005; Ragsdale, 2008; Singer, 2004a, 2008), in book chapters (for example, Nichter, 2008; Singer, 2009; Stall, Friedman, & Catania, 2007), in the mass media (for example, Specter, 2005), in student graduate theses (for example, Erstad, 2006), and in the classroom (American Association of Public Health Physicians, 2006).

In light of the growing evidence for and recognition of the utility of the syndemics concept across various health disciplines, another way to state the purpose of this book is that it marks the coming of age of the syndemics *methodos* by assembling, assessing, and amplifying the key components of this approach to understanding and addressing human health as an intricate biosocial process.

THE AUTHOR

Merrill Singer, a cultural and medical anthropologist who earned his PhD degree from the University of Utah, holds a dual appointment as senior research scientist at the Center for Health, Intervention, and Prevention and professor of anthropology at the University of Connecticut. Additionally, he is affiliated with the Center for Interdisciplinary Research on AIDS (CIRA) at Yale University. He has authored, coauthored, or edited twenty books and over two hundred articles and book chapters on health and social issues. Active in the building of social science of health theory, the development of methods in qualitative health research, and the use of research in the development of community-based health promotion and intervention, he has been the recipient of the Rudolph Virchow Award from the Critical Anthropology of Health Caucus of the Society for Medical Anthropology, the George Foster Practicing Medical Anthropology Award from the Society for Medical Anthropology, the AIDS and Anthropology Prize Paper award from the AIDS and Anthropology Research Group, and the Prize for Distinguished Achievement in the Critical Study of North America from the Society for the Anthropology of North America. Since 1984 he has been the principal investigator on a continuous series of basic and applied federally funded health studies, and he has carried out health research in the United States, Brazil, China, and Haiti.

ACKNOWLEDGMENTS

This book is the product of work stretching well over a decade, and it has benefited from the inputs, insights, and support of many colleagues who warrant my gratitude and heartfelt appreciation, including Elizabeth Toledo, with whom I had my first conversations and coauthored my first conference presentation about syndemics; Jeremy Lauer, Larry Sawchuk, and Alan Swedlund, who read and commented on sections of the book; the Wenner-Gren Foundation, which provided a forum for the development of some of the ideas presented here, and also the participants in the foundation's symposium "Plagues: Models and Metaphors in the Human 'Struggle' with Disease," who offered their feedback; the School of Advanced Research (SAR) and Paul Farmer, Linda Whiteford, and Barbara Rylko-Bauer, who were the organizers of the SAR symposium "Global Health in the Time of Violence," as well as all participants in the symposium who provided feedback on my syndemics and violence presentation at the symposium; Petra Rethmann and Ann Herring of McMaster University, Mary-Ellen Kelm, Craig Janes, and Kitty Corbett of Simon Frasier University, Alan and Josie Smart and Melanie Rock of the University of Calgary, Hans Baer of the University of Melbourne, and Judith Littlefield of Auckland University, who facilitated my visits to their respective universities to give presentations on syndemics and related topics; Al Mata, who facilitated my first publication on syndemics; Scott Clair and Pam Erickson, who collaborated on earlier publications that helped to advance my thinking about syndemics, and again, Pam Erickson, who supportively endured the demands that finishing a book imposes on an author and those nearby.

INTRODUCTION TO SYNDEMICS

PART

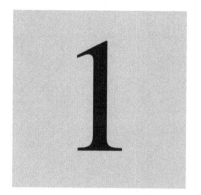

INTRODUCING KEY CONCEPTS IN SYNDEMICS

Chapter One, "Learning from Lichen: Reconceptualizing Health and Disease," which makes up Part One of this book, introduces the reader to the concept of syndemics and to the biosocial syndemic perspective on human health. Examining the syndemic perspective in a historical context, it describes the developing recognition that health and illness are shaped by multiple and complex factors, and it shows how the identification and study of syndemics has grown out of these far-reaching shifts in the ways that we conceptualize disease.

LEARNING FROM LICHEN

Reconceptualizing Health and Disease

After studying this chapter, you should be able to

- Locate the syndemic perspective within the evolutionary history of the scientific understanding of disease, including dilemmas encountered in meeting Robert Koch's criteria when attempting to determine the cause of an infectious disease.

- Understand the syndemic approach as one that supersedes two limitations of conventional biomedical approaches to disease—reductionism and mind-body dualism.

- Recognize the fundamental importance of biosocial interconnections and relationships in syndemics theory.

- Explain why syndemics were often not recognized in the past.

- Explain how the consideration of social factors, such as social disparity, differentiates syndemic processes from the biomedical conception of comorbidity and also differentiates syndemics among humans from synergistic disease inter-actions among animals.

ON NOT PLANTING CUT FLOWERS: THE WEIGHT OF HISTORY

It was just a few decades ago, in the 1970s, that medical anthropology, the source discipline for the syndemics concept, was a new field. George Foster and Barbara Anderson, in laying out an analytical approach to health-related issues for this new field, suggested a structural division of medical systems into two components: a *disease theory* system and a *health care* system, defining the first component as the "beliefs about the nature of health [and] the causes of illness" that prevail within a particular medical system (Foster & Anderson, 1978, p. 37). It is these beliefs that I am concerned with here.

The historical pathway leading to the contemporary biomedical and public health understanding of disease causation is both long and intricate (Richardson, 1991). On the one hand it is part of the larger historical course leading from prescientific to scientific modes of thought, and on the other hand it runs from simple to more complex scientific understandings of what disease is and how it develops within bodies, within populations, and within social and environmental contexts. The syndemic orientation, although recent in expression, is in fact an outgrowth of the new way of thinking about the causes of sickness that emerged and caught hold in the mid-1800s in a process commonly referred to as *the rise of germ theory*. This approach led first to the biomedical and public health conception of the nature of both contagious and noncontagious diseases (and more recently to reexamination of the assumed differences between these two broad categories of disease). This point then—the transition to a modern biological understanding of disease—is the starting place for examining the syndemic perspective, in that, as noted by historian Daniel Boorstin, trying to understand the present or plan for the future without a sense of the past is like trying to plant cut flowers (McCullogh, 2005).

GERM THEORY AND THE BIOMEDICAL CONCEPTION OF DISEASE

A critical moment in the evolution of biomedicine occurred during the mid-nineteenth century. During this epoch the healing system that was to evolve into modern biomedicine underwent a profound transformation, as detailed in the following sections.

Health as Balance

Prior to the mid-nineteenth century and dating back to the era of ancient Greece, physicians commonly understood health in terms of the balance among bodily fluids known as **humors.** Most prominent among ancient Greek physicians was Hippocrates (circa 460–370 B.C.), a man often credited in the West with being the father of medicine. Rejecting the notion of disease as a divine punishment for violations of spiritual laws—a disease theory that long predates ancient Greece yet lives on in the modern world (as seen, for example, in some religious interpretations of the HIV/AIDS epidemic as God's punishment of a sinful world)—Hippocrates and his peers believed that certain human moods, emotions, and behaviors were directly under the influence of blood, yellow bile, black bile, and phlegm (and that these humors were, in turn, linked to the four elements of fire, air, water, and earth in the natural environment). When these four humors were not in balance (a state called *dyscrasia,* or "bad mixture"), a person fell ill and remained so unless balance was restored through medical intervention. As Erickson (2008) notes, Hippocrates rationalized disease, thereby laying the foundation for the "biomedical understanding that diseases—both individual . . . and epidemic . . . are natural processes not supernatural punishments" (p. 25).

The humoral notion of disease causation was elaborated further by another ancient physician, Galen (circa 131–200 A.D.), who stressed that understanding of disease must be based on experiential awareness of human anatomy and physiology. (Owing to a government ban on human dissection, Galen gathered his own knowledge of human anatomy, sometimes inaccurately, from examining the corpses of pigs, primates, and other animals.) Galen's influence spread throughout the Western and Arab worlds and remained a factor in medical approaches to healing through the mid-1800s. As Hays (2000) observes, "Bleedings and purges . . . remained the order of the day for the early nineteenth century physician, however much he might have forsworn allegiance to Galenic humors" (p. 216).

Pollution Theory

Also important in historical thinking about disease causation, and reflective of the naturalistic and environmental understanding found in humoral theory, was the theory about the effects of *miasma*, or pollution theory. This understanding viewed toxic vapors given off by decomposing organic matter in the environment as the cause of many diseases. One such disease was malaria, believed to be caused by poisonous and foul-smelling environmental vapors arising from bodies of water found at low elevations and filled with particles of decomposed matter. This led European colonists in Africa, for example, to settle at high attitudes, a strategy that proved effective because it located the homes and offices of colonial administrators above the normal (temperature-sensitive) breeding elevation of mosquitoes, the real **vectors** of malarial infection. (Global warming and the resulting breeding of mosquitoes at ever higher elevations would make such a practice less effective today.)

Cholera in London   From 1831 to 1833 and again from 1848 to 1849, London, then the most populous city in the world, experienced several epidemics of cholera. The name *cholera* is derived from the Greek term for bile and reflects that this water-borne disease was originally conceptualized as resulting from an imbalance of humors. However, in mid-nineteenth-century London, William Farr, a doctor who served as the assistant commissioner for the 1851 city census, asserted that cholera was transmitted by bad air and, in London, specifically by a noxious concentration of *miasmata* (a non-living entity of organic origin) found along the banks of the Thames (at that time a heavily polluted industrial river). During this era there was no understanding that a single disease could produce multiple symptoms, and thus the diarrhea caused by a cholera infection was seen as a totally different disease from the cholera itself (and not, as it was found to be many decades later, an adaptive strategy that creates an intestinal alkalinity favorable to *Vibrio cholerae,* the immediate causative agent of cholera). When a major cholera epidemic again broke out in London, in 1854, Farr was appointed by the General Board of Health to the Committee for Scientific Enquiries in Relation to the Cholera Epidemic. Although not as severe as the epidemic of 1849, the 1854 epidemic—during which about 11,000 Londoners succumbed (Winterton, 1980)—was especially devastating in the Broad Street area of the Soho district, where the death toll reached three times the rate in London as a whole.

Snow on Broad Street   In addition to being the site of numerous cowsheds, animal slaughterhouses, grease-boiling pots, overcrowded working-class dwellings, and decaying sewers, Soho was home to the now infamous Broad Street pump. John Snow, a physician who had initially gained fame in 1846 by successfully administering the anesthesia chloroform to Queen Victoria during the births of Prince Leopold and Princess Beatrice, claimed that this public water station was the source of the local outbreak and that some kind of living entity in the water, an unseen germ of some sort spread by fecal contamination, was the cause. Snow was convinced the pump was a primary source of infection because the surrounding area was so hard hit during the outbreak. Between August 31 and September 10, over 500 people who lived on or near Broad Street (now renamed Broadwick Street) died of cholera (and ultimately 616 people in Soho were victims of the epidemic). People were fleeing the neighborhood in terror. Snow lived nearby, and he began interviewing the family members of those who had died, thereby inventing field epidemiology in the process. Using addresses that Farr had provided (despite his disagreement with Snow's perspective on disease causation), it was not long before Snow realized that families who drew their water from the Broad Street pump were the hardest hit and that most of the deaths were among people who lived only a short distance from the pump. He also found that not one of the seventy workers at the nearby Broad Street brewery had gotten sick; these workers were given free beer everyday and consequently never drank water from the pump.

This sociogeographical patterning of disease cases, Snow concluded, could not be explained by miasma theory. To prove his case he even tried examining samples of water from the pump under a microscope, although not one powerful enough for him to see the microbes they contained. Nonetheless he was convinced by his other findings that the germs were there and the cause of the illness and death occurring around him. He consequently self-published a report for distribution to fellow physicians and friends, followed by an essay published in the *London Medical Gazette* (Summers, 1989). Meanwhile, William Budd, in Bristol, England, who would later gain medical fame by demonstrating that typhoid fever was a waterborne pathogenic disease, had reached a conclusion somewhat similar to Snow's and published his view in a book a month after Snow's essay appeared. The difference was that Budd thought the agent of cholera was a fungus, which he and a group of fellow physicians believed they had observed in the stools of cholera patients, a view that was soon discredited.

Contested Understandings The initial response of health officials to Snow's assertion is reflected in the tone of the summary of it developed by John Simon, a physician who served as the head medical officer of London at the time: "This doctrine is, that cholera propagates itself by a 'morbid matter' which, passing from one patient in his evacuations, is accidentally swallowed by other persons as a pollution of food or water; that an increase of the swallowed germ of the disease takes place in the interior of the stomach and bowels, giving rise to the essential actions of cholera, as at first a local derangement; and that the morbid matter of cholera having the property of reproducing its own kind must necessarily have some sort of structure, most likely that of a cell" (quoted in Frerichs, 2001). Although Simon plainly understood Snow's theory, lacking direct evidence of the cell in question he found the argument, so to speak, hard to swallow, and rejected the relevance of germ theory to the cholera epidemic.

Similarly, despite Snow's national stature, the Committee for Scientific Enquiries, under Farr's influence, eventually concluded that "[a]fter careful inquiry, we see no reason to adopt [the belief that the Broad Street pump was to blame for the outbreak]. We do not feel it established that the water was contaminated in the manner alleged [by Snow]; nor is there before us any sufficient evidence to show whether inhabitants of that district, drinking from that well, suffered in proportion more than other inhabitants of the district who drank from other sources" (Eyler, 1979, p. 118).

Instead, cleaving to miasma theory, the committee concluded that "on the whole evidence, it seems impossible to doubt that the influences, which determine in mass the geographical distribution of cholera in London, belong less to the water than to the air." Indeed, the committee went so far as to scold those who followed Snow in accepting the germ theory of disease: "Many of the public believe that everything we eat and drink teems with life, and that even our bodies abound with minute living and parasitic productions. This is a vulgar error and the notion is as disgusting as it is erroneous" (quoted in Winterton, 1980, p. 17).

Another well-known proponent of the miasmatic theory at the time (although like others working in medicine she later embraced germ theory) was Florence Nightingale, who had gained an international reputation as a devoted nurse during the Crimean War (no mean accomplishment given the opposition to female nurses caring for wounded male soldiers). Because of her belief in miasma theory (and her statistical calculations showing that seven times as many British soldiers died from diseases contracted in the hospital as died from wounds received on the battlefield), she campaigned for the reform of hospitals, insisting that they be regularly cleaned and scoured until sanitary and fresh smelling. During the 1854 cholera epidemic, while serving as superintendent at the Institute for the Care of Sick Gentlewomen, in Upper Harley Street, London, Nightingale also volunteered at Middlesex Hospital, which received many of the victims of the epidemic. Of the 278 cases of cholera treated at the hospital, 123 died—a fatality rate of 53 percent—including one of the hospital's nurses (Johnson, 2006). Yet to Nightingale's mind's eye what was occurring was not the transmission of living, disease-causing microorganisms but rather the emergence of impurities from foul environments. This view also led her to write about her experience with another disease (in a footnote in the pamphlet "Notes on Nursing for the Labouring Classes"), "I have seen with my eyes and smelt with my nose smallpox growing up in first specimens, whether in closed rooms, or in overcrowded wards, where it could not by any possibility have been 'caught' but must have begun" (quoted in Penner, 2004, p. 92).

Ending the Epidemic   Although the Committee for Scientific Enquiries was later to reach its conclusion that the cause of the cholera epidemic was bad air, when the members of the London Board of Governors heard Snow's argument, they ordered the closing of the Broad Street pump, and the epidemic soon faded away. Consequently, although no one in London had seen the germ involved in the development of cholera, the 1854 epidemic ultimately gave considerable impetus to the rise to dominance of germ theory within biomedicine. Ironically, Italian biologist Filippo Pacini had already identified the cholera bacterium and had published a scientific paper on his discovery ("Microscopical Observations and Pathological Deductions on Cholera") through the Paris Academy of Sciences. Using a microscope he had purchased with his limited savings while still a medical student, Pacini conducted histological examination of the intestinal tissues of individuals who had died of cholera in Florence and identified a comma-shaped bacillus that he named *Vibrio*. Unfortunately, as sometimes happens in science with findings that are ahead of their time, Pacini's paper was ignored for thirty years, and it is unlikely that Snow had any awareness of it. (Pacini was finally credited with his discovery, eighty-two years after his death, when the International Committee on Nomenclature adopted *Vibrio cholerae Pacini* as the official name of the microorganism that is the proximal cause of cholera.)

The Rise of Germ Theory

Despite their considerable contributions, neither Snow nor Pacini was in fact the first to propose a germ theory of disease. Almost two thousand years earlier, Marcus Varro (116–127 B.C.), the architect whom Julius Caesar had assigned to the task of building a great public library in ancient Rome (a project that went unrealized because of Caesar's assassination), had warned those looking to select hygienic locations for buildings to avoid areas near swamps, because "in swampy places minute creatures live that cannot be discerned with the eye and they enter the body through the mouth and nostrils and cause serious disease" (quoted in Amici, 2001, p. 4). How Varro, lacking the technology to identify them, came to believe in the existence of disease-causing microbes is not clear. The microscope was not invented until the late 1600s, although magnifying glasses and the use of emeralds for magnification purposes are mentioned in *Naturalis Historia,* written by Pliny the Elder, a Roman naturalist and philosopher who lived during the first century A.D. What is known is that Varro's recognition had little impact on the medical perspective of his day or subsequently and is of interest today primarily as an intriguing footnote in the history of disease understanding.

During the sixteenth century, having observed epidemics of bubonic plague, typhus, and syphilis (and having written a 1,300-verse poem in Latin hexameters focused on a fictional shepherd named Syphilus, the source of the latter disease's modern name), the Veronese physician Girolamo Fracastoro (circa 1478–1553) came to question miasma theory (as well as beliefs about divine retribution) as lacking in evidentiary support. In his major medical treatise, *On Contagion and the Cure of Contagious Diseases,* published in 1546 (and in which he dismisses his poem as a youthful endeavor), he asserted there was better support for the notion that diseases were spread by tiny living or at least lifelike seminaria (seeds) or germs (although his recommended treatment was bleeding the sufferer and administering mercury to return him or her to humoral balance). This view of disease causation has led some to nominate Fracastoro for the title "father of germ theory" (see, for example, Greenwood, 1953), although others question this titling (Magner, 2002) owing to ambiguities in Fracastoro's sixteenth-century narrative and to his speculation that seminaria might arise from poisonous emanations born of planetary conjunctions (a factor in Stephen Jay Gould's [2000] argument that the greatest "poetry" ever composed about syphilis was penned not by Fracastoro but by the scientists who methodically and meticulously developed the elegant map of the 1,041 genes that constitute the genome of the **pathogen** *Treponema pallidum,* now known to be responsible for the disease).

Less conflicted and ambiguous was the contribution of Jacob Henle (1809–1885), a prominent German pathologist after whom various structures within the human body, some of his own discovery, are named. Henle compared alternative explanations of disease in his 1840 book *Misamata and Contagion.* Although the book did not achieve instant recognition as a critical turning point in medical disease understanding, it "was retrospectively recognized as a landmark" (Magner, 2002, p. 256) with the subsequent confirmation of germ theory. This triumph was achieved when Louis Pasteur (1822–1895), demonstrated in the 1860s that specific microbes are responsible for specific fermentations and later linked microbes to disease (initially in silkworms), and when Henle's student Robert Koch (1843–1910) isolated both the microbe causing cholera and the microbe causing tuberculosis.

Aftermath of the Epidemic   Living on the cusp of the great transition from the miasmatic to the germ theory of disease causation, William Farr eventually came to embrace Snow's (and Pacini's) understanding of cholera and of infectious disease generally, as did most of his fellow biomedical physicians. His conversion to the new paradigm marked both the broader transformation going on in medicine—namely its emergence as a bioscience—and the celebration of Snow's role in that process. Indeed, in a March 2003 survey that *Hospital Doctor* magazine conducted of its readers, John Snow was voted the "greatest doctor" of all time, with Hippocrates coming in second (Oleckno, 2008). Although it has been suggested that Farr did not initially accept Snow's ideas about germ theory because, unlike Snow, he was not open to new perspectives, Eyler (2001) stresses that the reverse may have been the case: "Judged by the standards of his time Snow was the dogmatic contagionist and premature reductionist. Farr was the more cautious in weighing all evidence" (p. 230). As a result of Snow's and others' dogged commitment to an idea (and to seeking out the evidence to support it), germ theory evolved from a controversial notion into the cornerstone of biomedical disease theory. In the process, biomedicine came to privilege understanding cell biology over understanding the social origins of disease and other disorders, an emphasis that has hindered a broad ecological conception of human illness (Singer, 1986).

Separation of the Part from the Whole The scientific discoveries that propelled the acceptance of germ theory not only undercut older views of disease causation but have also contributed to the development of an understanding that differentiates biomedicine from other ethnomedical systems around the world. Davis-Floyd and St. John (1998) have called this understanding "the principle of separation," and see it as a product of "an overwhelmingly linear mode of thinking" (p. 17). This principle stipulates that each of the world's various entities is best understood when considered independently of the other entities of its natural environment. Davis-Floyd (1994) observes that "the essence of [biomedical] research and description is separation—of elements from the whole they compose, of humans from nature, of mind from body, of mother from child" (p. 1127). Similarly, George Engel (1977), an anthropologically informed physician who during his life specialized in the psychophysiological aspects of human health and illness, argued that the distinctive feature of biomedicine is its embrace of "both reductionism, the philosophic view that complex phenomena are ultimately derived from a single primary principle [in this case, that everything can be explained in terms of chemistry and physics], and mind-body dualism, the doctrine that separates the mental from the somatic" (p. 130).

Reflective of this atomistic approach to knowledge, biomedicine separates the person with an illness from his or her immediate social context and community, diseased organ systems from the whole body, and one disease from another. Further, it breaks every disease into its constituent parts and manages disease treatment through a complex and atomistic array of medical specialties. As Davis-Floyd and St. John (1998) stress, a "drive toward separation" if carried to its logical extreme, as has more or less occurred in biomedicine, can "obscure the many meanings in the non-linear" and "the interconnections and relationships between entities" (p. 17). In his widely cited article quoted earlier, George Engel (1977) maintained that biomedicine's adherence to "a model of disease [that is] no longer adequate for the scientific tasks and social responsibilities" of the discipline has led to a crisis in biomedicine. Herein lies the value of a syndemic perspective, which seeks to clarify the impact of biosocial interconnections and relationships (p. 129).

REVOLUTIONS IN BIOMEDICAL REALITIES

Although biomedicine "purports to be belief- and value free" (Gaines & Davis-Floyd, 2004, p. 100), its understanding of reality—its ontological conception of the nature of nature and of basic life processes—is rooted in a particular construction of the world, an ideology that has both driven and reflected the encompassing Western cultural worldview. Germ theory, and biomedical understanding generally, initially assumed that like cholera each infectious disease is caused by a specific, identifiable pathogen.

Although this view opened the world up to new insights (including the discovery of a wide array of pathogens), it has also carried conceptual restrictions. As Francois Jacob (1988), winner of the 1965 Nobel Prize in medicine, notes: "In analyzing a problem, the biologist is constrained to focus on a fragment of reality, on a piece of the universe which he arbitrarily isolates to define certain of its parameters. In biology [including medicine] any study begins with a 'system.' On this choice depend the experimenter's freedom to maneuver, the nature of the questions he is free to ask, and even the type of answer he can obtain" (p. 16).

When constraint is imposed on biomedical thinking, it limits not only, as Jacob suggests, the nature of the questions that are asked but also the answers that are meaningful, acceptable, even thinkable. As historian of science Thomas Kuhn noted in *The Structure of Scientific Revolutions,* a seminal book on the scientific process, this is the everyday or normal way scientific understanding operates. In any specialized subfield (including biomedicine), science tends to be guided by a **reigning paradigm,** that is, by "an entire constellation of beliefs, values and techniques, and so on, shared by the members of a given community" (Kuhn, 1970, p. xii). In common contemporary parlance, scientific thinking normally takes place "within the box," because unless doubts and uncertainties about basic assumptions have arisen to rattle confidence in that box (for example, through research findings that cannot be explained because they appear to fall "outside the box"), the box defines reality. Thus once germ theory and its "to each disease its own unique pathogenic cause" perspective gained dominance in biomedicine, a *paradigm effect* occurred, canalizing thinking and hindering attention to other ways of seeing the available evidence.

PROBLEMS WITH THE POSTULATES

Despite the compelling force of reigning paradigms, as Kuhn emphasized, science is not stagnant (by design!) and revolutions in scientific thinking are, one might argue, equally a normal part of science. Consequently, since the adoption of germ theory, scientific understanding about the causes of disease has continued, in stages, to evolve. These changes can be seen as stemming in part from problems encountered in implementing a set of postulates developed by Koch (and broadly accepted in the field as the gold standard) for determining whether a particular microbe is the cause of a specific disease. For medical science to affirm that a particular organism causes a disease, Koch (1890/1987) argued:

1. The organism must be present in every case of the disease but not in healthy individuals.

2. The organism must be capable of being isolated from the sufferer and grown in pure culture.

3. The specific disease must be reproduced when a pure culture of the organism is inoculated into a healthy, susceptible host.

4. The organism must be recoverable from the experimentally infected host.

The problems began during the period just after the achievements of Snow, Pasteur, and Koch became generally known, an epoch often thought of as the golden age of breakthroughs in medicine and infectious disease research. For Theobald Smith, a physician turned pathology researcher who was to become a preeminent pioneer in American microbiology, it was an exciting time of regular discoveries of pathogens, vectors, and disease causation. It was also a time during which diseases like hog cholera (now called classical swine fever) "swept through the countryside, causing devastating losses. During the fall months, looking across the prairies of the Middle West, one could often see smoke ascending from perhaps a half-dozen farms where pigs dead of cholera were being burned" (McBryde, quoted in U.S. Department of Agriculture and Agricultural Research Service, 2006). In 1884, as a lowly lab technician in the newly created U.S. Department of Agriculture's Bureau of Animal Industry (BAI), a center established by Congress to respond to costly waves of livestock epidemics, Smith set out to discover the cause of hog cholera, one of the most economically damaging pandemic diseases of pigs in the world.

When Smith came to this line of work, he had two years of medical training and had read, on his own, the papers of Pasteur. At the BAI he was supervised by veterinary pathologist and BAI chief Daniel Salmon (for whom *Salmonella,* the enterobacterium that causes diseases like typhoid fever, paratyphoid fever, and food poisoning, is named, even though it was actually discovered by Smith, a point of enduring tension between the two scientists; Dolmon, 1969). Having confirmed that a microbe, *Salmonella choleraesuis* (now called *Salmonella enterica*), was found consistently in pigs suffering the symptoms of hog cholera and could be isolated and grown in pure culture, having seen the disease after healthy hogs were infected with the microbe, and having recovered the bacterium from animals that had been infected in this way, Smith (although Salmon insisted on first authorship of the published findings) concluded that **Koch's postulates** had been met, and declared that the cause of hog cholera had been discovered. Notably, both Pasteur and Koch accepted this conclusion and assumed that the problem of hog cholera was well on its way to resolution (Zinsser, 1936). This proved not to be the case, as Marion Dorset, another BAI scientist, had no success with a serum made from the *Salmonella choleraesuis* bacterium during an 1897 outbreak of the disease in Iowa. Six years later, Dorset was able to show that the actual cause of hog cholera was not a bacterium at all but a virus (genetically a much simpler entity), a discovery leading to the eradication of the disease in the United States.

Why had Smith, known to be a cautious worker, gone wrong? As it turned out, swine infection with *S. enterica,* which causes its own health problems (salmonellosis and typhoid fever), was secondary to the viral infection. Smith, in other words, had unknowingly stumbled on a synergistic interaction among animal pathogens in which one (a virus) facilitated infection by another (a bacterium) producing frequent coinfection, and he had identified the wrong pathogen as the cause of hog cholera. Because of his many subsequent discoveries (such as the role of a protozoan parasite, babesia, in the development of Texas fever among cattle and the activity of ticks in its transmission), this mistake did not hurt Smith's career, but its occurrence is instructive about the potential consequences of assuming one has successfully isolated a pathogen.

Disease Carriers   Over time other problems with Koch's postulates also emerged. First, the discovery of asymptomatic **disease carriers** threw into doubt the idea that a known pathogen could not be found in healthy individuals. Mary Mallon, an early twentieth century cook for several New York families, for example, was found to be a carrier for typhoid fever (caused by *S. enterica*). Although she had no disease symptoms, she did pass on the bacterium to twenty-two members of the families she worked for and who did become sick, earning her infamy as Typhoid Mary. As a public health measure, she was forcibly quarantined in an institution on an island in the East River for much of the rest of her life. Mary Mallon was not unique; asymptomatic carriers (sometimes called *well carriers*) are now known to be a common feature in the spread of many infectious diseases, including polio, herpes simplex, and hepatitis. When Koch discovered that there were asymptomatic carriers of disease, he dropped the second half of his first postulate.

Uncultivable Microbes   It has also turned out that some microbes cannot be successfully grown in pure culture. For example, bacteria in the rickettsia family (responsible for an array of diseases, such as Rocky Mountain spotted fever) cannot live in artificial nutrient environments. Similarly, *Mycobacterium leprae,* the bacillus that causes leprosy, has never been cultivated in vitro in its classic rod-shaped form, because it appears to lack the genetic capacity to grow outside the human body. Further, although a significant number of bacteria have been isolated in the human mouth, it is estimated that only about half the species that dwell in the oral cavity can be cultured (Rolph et al., 2001).

Over time other strategies, such as molecular techniques, have been adopted to identify bacteria species that have never been cultivated. It was only with the introduction of molecular genetic strategies, for example, that the uncultivable bacterium *Tropheryma whippelii* was identified as the cause of Whipple's disease, a chronic, systemic infectious disease, most common in middle-aged men, that typically causes malabsorption in the small intestine and a wide range of other clinical manifestations including arthritis. Additionally, new culture methodologies have been invented in recent years, such as chicken tissue and embryo cultures (which can be used to grow rickettsia bacteria). Still, it is assumed by most microbiologists and pathologists that there are many pathogenic microorganisms at play in human health that have yet to be identified because of the limitations of existing technologies. Only in very recent years, as discussed in Chapter Five, have researchers discovered the viral origins of some chronic diseases previously believed not to be contagious (such as peptic ulcer disease, in which *Helicobacter pylori* plays a role, and cervical cancer, which involves several human papillomaviruses).

One consequence of encountering an uncultivable microbe is evident in the case of Lyme disease, which is caused by several species of the hard-to-culture spirochetal

Borrelia bacterium. Although Lyme disease is recognized as the most common tick-borne disease in North America and Europe, as well as one of the fastest-growing infectious diseases in the United States (with over 20,000 cases a year nationally since the turn of the twenty-first century and over 30 cases per 100,000 persons in the ten most heavily infested states), inability to culture its causative agent has led to considerable professional disagreement and intense acrimony over the guidelines to be used in diagnosis. The Centers for Disease Control and Prevention (CDC) has been forced to rely on such potentially ambiguous criteria as presentation of symptoms (which can vary considerably across infected individuals), physical findings (such as a bull's-eye rash, which does not appear in many cases), and the possibility of exposure to infected ticks (such as the black-legged tick in North America and several other tick species in Europe) based on place of residence or visitation (CDC, 2006b).

Masked Infections Problems with Koch's third postulate began with the fact that some pathogens cannot be cultured, but other difficulties have arisen as well. For various reasons (such as acquired immunity from prior exposure to a pathogen, as occurs with influenza, and genetic immunity, as seen for example in individuals who acquire a sickle cell allele from at least one parent), exposure to a pathogen does not necessarily lead to detectable infection. Of even greater importance for the issues under consideration is the fact that the presence of a second pathogen (for example, one that weakens the immune response to the presence of foreign organisms generally) can increase the likelihood that infection will develop in exposed individuals. In other words, in many instances, without the bodily effects of synergistic interaction among diseases, mere exposure to a single pathogen (including intentional inoculation) does not produce disease. At the same time, if the disease of concern is in fact the consequence of interaction among pathogens or other disease causes, it will not develop (or have the same expression) unless the new host is exposed to all those pathogens or causes.

Immune Response and the Reisolation of Pathogens In addition to the challenges to Koch's postulates already discussed, there can be difficulties with the reisolation of a pathogen from an inoculated individual because that requires the capacity to segregate and culture the pathogen. This capacity does not exist for some microorganisms (including those that infect only humans and hence, for ethical reasons, can never be tested using Koch's postulates), and it does not exist in cases of a healthy immune system because the body has eliminated the pathogenic agent (although it may exist in cases of coinfection owing to degradation of immune system capacity). Additionally, the modus operandi of some pathogens, as found for example in rheumatic heart disease (which begins with a streptococcal throat infection), involves what might be called a hit-and-run pattern, in which the organism is no longer in the host by the time the disease is evident.

Complexities of Disease Understanding Multiplying the difficulties encountered in using the postulates was the realization that a single disease might have multiple causes (a situation known as *multifactorial disease*) and that a single pathogen might produce more than one disease. These issues extend beyond infectious disease to disease with an environmental or genetic origin. For example, with regard to the first point, it is recognized that the chronic eye infection known as trachoma is a common source of blindness in developing countries. This disease has been linked to sexually transmitted infection with the pathogen *Chlamydia trachomatis*. Research by Dean, Kandel, Adhikari, and Hessel (2008), however, has found that trachoma can also be caused by *Chlamydophila psittaci* and *Chlamydophila pneumoniae*. Consequently, these researchers conclude that the existence of multiple agents causing trachoma helps to "explain the failure to detect chlamydiae among active trachoma cases, when only *C. trachomatis* is assayed," "the failure of active trachoma cases to resolve their clinical disease following effective *C. trachomatis* treatment, and the limited effectiveness of the WHO strategy to control trachoma" (p. e14). Also of note in this regard is the potential effect of interaction among copresent trachoma-causing pathogens. Similarly, coinfection with multiple strains of the microbe that causes dengue can significantly change the clinical picture and severity of that disease (a topic to be discussed in Chapter Six).

With regard to the second point, that a single cause can produce multiple diseases, consider the hepatitis B virus, which is the proximal cause of hepatitis, cirrhosis, chronic liver disease, and liver cancer (Merican et al., 2000). Moreover, the actual expression of any disease may vary widely across individuals, including affecting different organ systems in the body. Thus HTLV-1 (human T-cell lymphotropic virus type 1), a retrovirus that was once mistakenly proposed as the cause of HIV/AIDS but that actually causes adult T-cell leukemia, T-cell lymphoma, and other diseases, is expressed in three clinical patterns: cancer, autoimmune disease, and immunosuppression disease. Tuberculosis also has various expressions, depending on how the infection gains access to the body and the host's response to its presence. Although pulmonary infection through breathing in *Mycobacterium tuberculosis* is most common, it is also possible to acquire the disease by drinking infected cow's milk, leading to lesions in the intestinal track. Notably tuberculosis of the gastrointestinal tract is being seen more frequently among people with HIV/AIDS. These are examples of what have come to be called *spectral diseases*—that is, diseases with a spectrum of alternative clinical manifestations. Again, **disease interactions** may play a role in determining which of an array of possibilities finds actual disease expression in a patient or population.

Roads Less Traveled   In assessing the overall value of Koch's postulates in light of subsequent discoveries, Cochran, Ewald, and Cochran (2000) conclude that the postulates "were useful because they could generate conclusive evidence of infectious causation, particularly when (1) the causative organisms could be isolated and experimentally transmitted, and (2) symptoms occurred soon after the onset of infection in a high proportion of infected individuals. While guiding researchers down one path, however, the postulates directed them away from alternative paths: researchers attempting to document infectious causation were guided away from diseases that had little chance of fulfilling the postulates, even though they might have been infectious" (p. 406).

Modifications of Germ Theory

The result of our growing understanding about disease complexities has been a process of germ theory revision (that is, scientific evolution) at various points in time to accommodate new information. Consequently, despite its obvious power as an explanatory model, germ theory as first articulated by researchers like Snow, Pasteur, Koch, and many more is not the germ theory in vogue a hundred years later. A much more complex and nuanced comprehension about the relationship between pathogens and disease now abides, an understanding that recognizes the importance in contagious disease of **host-pathogen** interactions (and that includes an enormous increase in the appreciation of the intricacies of the immune system and the realization that symptoms may be the result of attempts by the host to rid itself of a pathogen, as occurs, for example, in cystic fibrosis); accepts three primary disease pathways (infectious agents, genetics, and body-environment interactions); includes awareness of coinfection and copresent infectious and noninfectious diseases; is cognizant of the existence of pathogens with multiple strains (with differing capacities to cause bodily damage); and is attuned to the role of biological individuality in population health. In this sense the issue of syndemics, which as indicated earlier has been a usually unanalyzed complicating factor since the earliest efforts to account for specific diseases using germ theory, presents but another stage in the normal scientific evolution of biomedical and public health thinking about disease. To the degree that it encourages a focus not just on disease interactions but on the fundamental importance of the social conditions that foster **disease clustering** and interfaces, syndemics theory also represents a **paradigm shift** in the understanding of what disease is and how it is manifested in complex biosocial feedback environments.

CONFRONTING COMORBIDITY

Over the course of time, biomedicine has encountered many patterns in nature that call into question the assumption that the principle of separation is the most fruitful approach for understanding threats to health. The most notable of these patterns is the frequent co-occurrence of more than one disease or other disorders in the same patient. The term *comorbidity* has traditionally been used in biomedicine to denote this co-occurrence (Feinstein, 1970). Some comorbid disease patterns are sufficiently regular to have acquired their own names. For example, *Austrian's syndrome,* also called *Osler's triad,* is a disease complex consisting of endocarditis, meningitis, and pneumonia caused by *Streptococcus pneumoniae* infection. It is commonly associated with excess alcohol consumption but has also been described among injection drug users. The medical literature on this condition consists primarily of individual case reports rather than focused analyses of the nature of the interactions among the three diseases.

Much of the focus in comorbidity research, in fact, has been the development of schemas (see, for example, Charlson, Pompei, Ales, & McKenzie, 1987) to assist physicians in making treatment decisions (such as whether the benefits of treating one condition in a patient with multiple health disorders will outweigh the negative effects this treatment is likely to have on the patient's other disorders). Generally speaking, such work has tended to see the diseases involved as independent entities despite their copresence in the same patient.

Health disciplines differ in the emphasis they place on assessing the nature of the relationship between co-occurring diseases and other maladies. In behavioral health, for example, a field that has evidenced a strong interest in comorbidity, a primary concern involves determining whether two apparently different problems are in fact alternate and cycling manifestations of the same condition (as may be the case in bipolar disorder). Also of interest is whether or not one disorder causes another, as happens with the abuse of alcohol or other drugs to self-medicate anxiety or depression (see Chapter Six). Additionally, it is known that there are cases in which a patient is suffering from two distinct behavioral disorders that are independent of each other but that are both the consequence of a third disorder. Finally, coexisting disorders may be traced to common risk factors, such as various injurious experiences early in life (Neale & Kendler, 1995).

Mere awareness of comorbidity as a factor in human health is not the same thing, however, as having a syndemic perspective. The differences between the terms *comorbid* and *syndemic,* as Mustanski, Garofalo, Herrick, and Donenberg (2007) aptly point out, are "not simply semantic—comorbidity research tends to focus on the nosological issues of boundaries and overlap of diagnoses, while syndemic research focuses on communities experiencing co-occurring epidemics that additively increase negative health consequences. For example, it is possible for two disorders to be comorbid, but

Why isn't there more research on syndemics? One reason can be found by looking at studies of chronic health problems. Chronic diseases like diabetes, cardiovascular disease, and cancer are recognized as significant threats to patients' quality of life. Further, it is well known that as people age, the number of chronic diseases they are likely to have goes up. However, most research on the life effects of chronic disease focuses on only one disease and its impact on patient well-being, social functioning, and quality of life. Because the co-occurrence of other diseases complicates examination of the specific effects of the chronic disease of interest, patients with comorbid conditions often are excluded from patient samples in chronic disease research. As a result the whole question of disease interaction and its significant impact on patients is often overlooked. Yet as chronic disease researchers at the Netherlands Institute of Health Services Research (Rijken, van Kerkhof, Dekker, & Schellevis, 2005) have found, patients suffering from comorbidity report the lowest levels of physical functioning. These researchers also point out that comorbid chronic diseases appear to have a synergistic effect and cause greater physical disability than would be expected from merely adding up the separate effects of individual chronic diseases.

not represent a syndemic (that is, the disorders are not epidemic in the studied population or their co-occurrence is not accompanied by additional adverse health consequences). Beyond the focus on disease clustering and interaction, the term *syndemic* also implies a focus on health disparities and the social conditions that perpetrate them" (p. 40).

Various co-occurring diseases have been described that do not (as best as is known) appear to interact in adverse ways, although in some cases the findings of different studies conflict. For example, it is known that the *Ixodes* tick that transmits the pathogen (*Borrelia burgdorferi*) identified as the source of Lyme disease can simultaneously pass on several other human pathogens, including both *Anaplasma phagocytophilum,* the bacterial cause of human granulocytic anaplasmosis, a disease that like HIV/AIDS appears to damage the immune system in a way that promotes opportunistic infection (Dumler et al., 2005), and *Babesia microti,* a protozoan parasite that causes the malaria-like disease babesiosis. Some (but not all) human studies have found that co-infection with human granulocytic anaplasmosis increases the severity of Lyme disease (Krause et al., 1996). In contrast, when mice were experimentally co-infected with *B. microti* and *B. burgdorferi,* no change was found in the course of infection of either disease as revealed by a range of measures, including pathogenic load, spleen weight, and blood chemistry (Coleman, LeVine, Thill, Kuhlow, & Benach, 2005). Rather, both diseases proceeded along their normal course of infection and caused readily identifiable, landmark symptoms specific to each disease.

In short, the mere co-presence of two or more diseases and/or other disorders is not the defining feature of a syndemic. Further, disease interaction can produce positive health effects, a condition referred to here as a *countersyndemic* (see Chapter Five). Often, however, when diseases come together in a population and in individual patients, the outcomes are neither neutral nor positive. A primary goal of this book is to advance recognition and understanding of the many instances of adverse health effects arising from connections among epidemic disease clustering, disease interaction, and **health and social disparities.**

TOWARD SYNDEMIC RECONCEPTUALIZATION

The syndemic perspective moves our conception of health beyond the narrow frames of traditional reference. An essential feature of syndemics is revealed by an unexpected life form, the lichen. Although in appearance and structure the often taken-for-granted lichen appears to be a simple plant, it in fact constitutes a symbiotic community. One member of this community is a fungus—most commonly of the Ascomycota phylum (which includes truffles and baker's yeast) but occasionally a member of the Basidiomycota phylum (which includes mushrooms and puffballs but also a human pathogenic yeast of the genus *Cryptococcus,* known in people with AIDS to produce meningitis). The other member of the lichen community is an algae—usually either (although sometimes both) green algae or blue-green algae (actually a phylum of bacteria) but also sometimes yellow-green algae or more rarely brown algae. Although plant parasitism is not unusual in nature, it is not clear that that is what is occurring with lichen. Rather, both plant "partners" appear to benefit from the relationship (a type of symbiotic connection known in biology as **mutualism**). Thus the fungi derive sugars, their only nutrient, from the algae, and the algae gain the protection of the fungi, allowing them to live in environments that they otherwise could not inhabit. Nature writer Douglas Chadwick (2003) says that because they are not a single organism but an interactive group of species, he thinks of lichens "as kind of a *doorway* between organisms [or individual species] and ecosystems. Look out one direction, and you see individual things; look the other way, you see processes, relationships—things together. This is the new level in understanding biology" (p. 119).

A parallel to the lichen case is seen in the mutualistic relationship between humans and certain lactic acid bacteria, such as *Lactobacillus plantarum*. These bacteria live, for example, on the vaginal epithelia of women. This environment provides the bacteria with a stable habitat, constant temperature, and steady supply of nutrients in the form of glycogen (which is abundant in epithelial cells). In turn, as part of the metabolism of glycogen, the bacteria produce lactic acid, resulting in a normal vaginal pH of 3.5 to 4.5, an acidity level that protects the vagina from colonization by harmful yeasts and other invasive microbes (see Chapter Six). Notably, elsewhere in the body, in the gastrointestinal tract for instance, so-called friendly bacteria (such as *Lactobacillus*) are directly involved in stimulating the immune system to produce white blood cells that are critical to fighting infection. It was recognition of this sort that led Ludwik Fleck, a Polish biologist, who like Chadwick was fascinated by lichen (and for the same reason), to write, "The [biomedical] conception of infectious disease . . . is based on the notion of the organism as a closed unit and of the hostile causative agents invading it. . . . An organism can no longer be construed as a self-contained, independent unit with fixed boundaries, as it was still considered according to the theory of materialism [that is, germ theory]" (Fleck, 1935/1979, p. 60). The bounded unit view of the organism, Fleck stressed, is a historical bias that is unbecoming to modern biology.

The significance of the kind of interspecies relationship seen in the formation of lichen is one of the recent understandings reflected in the reconceptualization of health and disease embodied in the syndemic paradigm. Motivation for the examination of syndemics is guided by Chadwick's (2003) timely warning that "[i]f we continue to focus chiefly on species—even though we embrace all shapes and sizes of them—rather than on connections, our view of nature will remain incomplete. So will our efforts at protection" (p. 125), and our approach to disease!

LOCAL KNOWLEDGE

Anthropologists and others who work with indigenous communities commonly differentiate *expert knowledge* (for example, the findings and pronouncements of scientists, anthropologists included) from *local* or *indigenous knowledge,* which is "knowledge that does not owe its origin, testing, degree of verification, truth status, or currency to distinctive professional techniques, but rather common sense, casual empiricism, or thoughtful speculation and analysis" within communities (Lindblom & Cohen, 1979, p. 12). All societies have **local knowledge** about their surrounding environment and about the nature of diseases and disease causes and effects, and this knowledge may match, overlap, or be at considerable odds with professional or authoritative knowledge on the same topic. Indeed, Latour (1979) and Wynne (1996) maintain that all knowledge, even authoritative knowledge, is local in the sense that it emerges from a local socioeconomic milieu and is shaped by local sociocultural and historical factors.

This book is primarily concerned with expert knowledge about synergistically related diseases and the sway of social environments on interactive disease processes. Yet it bears noting that local knowledge about disease interactions, or what might be called *folk syndemics,* in the sense suggested by McCombie (1987) in her discussion of *folk flu* in the American Southwest, also exists. McCombie points out that although the expert understanding is that flu is a respiratory tract infection that is caused by a virus belonging to the Orthomyxoviridae family and that results in fever, sore throat, headache, runny nose, and muscle pain, the lay or folk model of flu includes gastrointestinal symptoms. A somewhat different overlap of folk and professional disease lexicons is seen in the account by Muela, Ribera, and Tanner (1998) of *fake malaria,* a folk-labeled disease found in southeastern Tanzania that people believe imitates the symptoms of real malaria (and that would be diagnosed as such by biomedical physicians) but that is interpreted locally to be caused instead by witchcraft, not pathogens.

In the case of folk syndemics, local knowledge about disease includes cultural beliefs about disease interactions with enhanced adverse consequences. For example, Nichter (2008) reports, "In several South and Southeastern Asian countries where I have conducted research, alcohol and tobacco are thought to cause a latent illness such as TB or sexually transmitted disease to flare up or reoccur" (p. 52). From a public health standpoint, awareness of folk syndemic beliefs as a component of broader folk explanatory models of health and illness (Kleinman, 1978) may be of considerable importance in the implementation of socially acceptable and culturally meaningful interventions to address comorbid conditions.

CONNECTIONS: HUMAN AND NONHUMAN

The syndemic orientation is founded on a recognition of the fundamental importance of biosocial connections in health. It is now clear that diseases and other health conditions (such as nutritional status and stress) interact synergistically in various and consequential ways and that the social conditions of people with illnesses are critical to understanding the impact of diseases at the individual and population levels. A syndemic approach, consequently, examines both *disease concentrations* (that is, multiple, coterminous diseases and disorders affecting individuals and groups) and *disease interactions* (that is, the ways in which the presence of one disease or disorder enhances the health consequences of other diseases and disorders, paving the way, for example, for new infection or enhanced lethality). Thus one concern of the syndemic approach is the nature of the specific pathways through which diseases and other health conditions interact biologically within individual bodies and within populations and thereby multiply their overall health burden.

The syndemic perspective, however, does not stop with the consideration of biological connections (myriad, complex, and fascinating as they may be), because in the human world disease develops within and is significantly influenced by the social contexts of disease sufferers. Human social environments, including the prevailing structures of social relationships (such as social inequality and injustice) and also sociogenic environmental conditions (for example, hazards of the built environment, sales of toxic commodities, pollution, species loss, and climate change) contribute enormously to both disease clustering and interaction.

Without question, disease synergies are not limited to human populations and occur as well in the nonhuman animal world. For example, veterinary pathologists at the Indiana Animal Disease Diagnostic Laboratory at the Purdue University School of Veterinary Medicine have identified patterns of consequential synergistic interaction between a group of viruses called porcine circoviruses, first identified in Europe in 1974, and other pathogens, such as bovine viral diarrhea virus (a disease agent that may have spread to pigs from deer populations), that significantly increase the fatality rate of dually infected pigs. In recent years porcine circoviruses have spread to pig populations around the world. In places where swine are infected with other viruses in addition to the newly introduced porcine circovirus, mortality rates have jumped by 35 to 50 percent. According to Roman Pogranichniy, a Purdue virologist involved in this research, "We think that the new co-factors, including the bovine viral diarrhea virus–like pathogen and other swine viruses, work together with porcine circovirus to attack the animals' systems and become more virulent" (quoted in Steeves, 2008, p. 1). Similarly, research has shown that bacterial, fungal, and viral infections are frequent and generally worse in animals with tick-borne fever. Experimental research with sheep, for example, found not only that animals dually infected with tick-borne fever and louping-ill virus were more susceptible to louping-ill but that almost all of them died of hemorrhagic syndrome involving a systemic fungal infection with *Rhizomucor pucillus*. In contrast, none of the sheep given louping-ill virus alone developed this syndrome (Brodie, Holmes, & Urquhart, 1986). In related research Jolles and Ezenwa (2006) examined the effects of interaction of gastrointestinal worms and tuberculosis in the African buffalo and found that mortality was heightened in coinfected individuals. They noted that this pattern could be explained by the adverse effects of helminth infection on individuals suffering from TB but concluded that this simple disease dynamic model could not explain their mortality findings, and they hypothesized instead that host defenses against one infection might block simultaneous immunity to the other, an explanation that accurately reproduced their finding when tested through computer modeling. Subsequently, Jolles and Ezenwa have begun to examine disease interaction patterns at three distinct levels of biological organization: individuals, populations, and species. Their plan is to scale up their approach using a comprehensive database of parasites (a term commonly used to refer to protozoa and helminths but applicable to all disease-causing microbes) and other pathogens that infect primates, ungulates, carnivores, and humans to test whether microbe interactions determine patterns of helminth distributions across populations and species.

In light of this research the question must be asked: are disease synergies in non-human animal species syndemics, in that the structure of social relations and the issue of inequality and its health effects are not factors in the spread, clustering, and inter-action of disease entities? Of course in some animal populations, such as those of nonhuman primates, social hierarchy is an important factor in which animals get sick, as Sapolsky (2005) points out in his discussion of the ways in which characteristics of social rank among animals can have adverse adrenocortical, cardiovascular, reproduc-tive, neurobiological, and immunological consequences (and as a result, syndemic-like) effects. Among hierarchical animals, individuals may be highly stressed without being subordinated members of their group. For example, although it is easy "to imag-ine that subordination can produce an excess of physical stressors" in that subordinate animals "may have to work harder for calories, or be calorically deprived," and may be "the subjects of unprovoked displacement aggression" (Sapolsky, 2004, p. 397), among some species being at the top of a dominance hierarchy can also be stressful because of aggressive challenges from up-and-coming and would-be dominant animals or even from teams of genetically related individuals, as occurs in lion prides. Additionally, the health of animals, domestic and wild, is significantly influenced by human activity and human social structures. People regularly move animals to new environments, exposing them to new diseases. Domestic animals, like their human handlers, live in built environments that are intended to serve human needs (such as increasing milk productivity among dairy stock or producing veal by using growing stalls, hormones, and antibiotics) more than the needs of animals. Similarly, anthro-pogenic changes in physical environments can significantly affect their quality (in terms, for example, of air quality or access to food and water) from the standpoint of health (see, for example, Grandin, 1997, 1998). In other words, whatever the natural social patterns of animal species, human social structures and economies are signifi-cant factors in disease interactions that affect animal health, even in wild populations.

Nonetheless, although it is not productive to draw too fine a conceptual line sepa-rating human from nonhuman animal species—or human and nonhuman animal dis-eases, given the zoonotic origin of many human ailments and the role of animals in human therapies (Rock, Buntain, Hatfield, & Hallgrímsson, 2009)—this book under-lines the special influence of unequal social relations on health among humans in its conception of *syndemics* and applies the term *synergies* to human or animal disease interactions that lack (at least as far as is known at any point in time) an important social origin.

The tendency, perhaps accelerated in recent years, for pathogens to jump success-fully from animal to human hosts (and hence the value of paying attention simultaneously to both animal and human diseases); the requirement for the syndemic perspective to focus equally on both biological and social phenomena (and their numerous dimensions);

and the necessity of focusing on diseases of pathogenic, genetic, and environmental origin (and their interactions) all suggest the centrality of multidisciplinarity in syndemics research, an issue addressed in Chapter Two.

SUMMARY

This chapter introduced and explored the interactive, biosocial understanding of human health that underlies the syndemic perspective. It has shown how the syndemic perspective developed in response to the distinct features of earlier stages in the evolution of disease conception, especially (with the rise of germ theory and biomedicine) reductionism and mind-body dualism and the subsequent realization of the limitations of these frames of understanding.

KEY TERMS

comorbidity
disease carrier
disease clustering
disease interaction
folk syndemic
germ theory
health and social disparities
host-pathogen interactions
humors
Koch's postulates

local knowledge
masked infection
miasma
mutualism
paradigm shift
pathogen
reigning paradigm
spectral disease
vector

QUESTIONS FOR DISCUSSION

1. What are the key features of a syndemic? Why are syndemics important in public health?

2. Why are some social groups at greater risk for syndemics than others?

3. How does the emergence of the syndemics model relate to prior transitions in the conception of disease?

4. What are the key differences between the concept of *comorbidity* and the concept of a *syndemic*?

5. What are the problems that arise in describing disease interactions in nonhuman animal species as syndemics?

PART

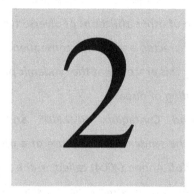

SYNDEMIC CASES

The chapters in Part Two are designed to clarify the nature of syndemics by closely examining a series of specific cases drawn from the wide range of disease interactions that have been described by health scientists.

Chapter Two, "Trucking Between the Bailiwicks: Multidisciplinarity, SAVA, and Synergies in Health," begins this examination by discussing the SAVA (substance abuse, violence, and AIDS) syndemic, the first syndemic reported in the health literature. It describes this syndemic in several different populations and concludes with a broad assessment of SAVA as a factor in public health.

Chapter Three, "Exemplars: Syndemic Case Studies," begins by examining how syndemics are made. On this foundation, it presents case studies of a number of syndemics that illustrate in detail the microlevel disease interactions within the macrolevel of disease interaction—that is, within the broad context of social and environmental determinants of disease concentration that enable synergistic disease exchange.

Chapter Four, "HIV/AIDS and Other Infections: Immune Imparity and Synde-mogenesis," continues the exploration of specific syndemics and the nature and health consequences of syndemic interactions by way of a fuller examination of HIV/AIDS, a disease involved in a remarkable number of syndemics, perhaps more so than any other known disease. Indeed, it was the multiple interactions between HIV/AIDS and a wide range of other afflictions of diverse types that prompted exami-nation of the frequency, character, and health consequences of disease interactions generally, and it was during this process that the syndemic perspective consolidated as a new, biosocial understanding of disease.

Chapter Five, "Beyond Contagion: HIV/AIDS and Noninfectious Disease Syndemogenesis," affirms the syndemogenic nature of a disease that former United Nations secretary-general Kofi Annan (2004) called, in the preface to an examination of the interaction of HIV/AIDS with noninfectious diseases of diverse types, "one of the greatest challenges facing our generation." This chapter begins by reviewing the emergent understanding of the significant role of infections generally in the develop-ment of noninfectious and chronic diseases, and follows that up with an examination of a condition known as HIVAN, which entails an exploration of the role of HIV in kid-ney disease. There is an important lesson to be learned from this discussion about the definitional boundaries of the syndemic concept. The chapter closes with a consideration of countersyndemics, a group of disease interactions that have beneficial consequences.

CHAPTER

TRUCKING BETWEEN THE BAILIWICKS

Multidisciplinarity, SAVA, and Synergies in Health

After studying this chapter, you should be able to

- Understand why, given the wide range of health and social topics incorporated into the syndemic perspective, a multidisciplinary approach is emphasized.

- Explain the etymology of the term *syndemics* as a label for adverse epidemic disease interactions in social contexts.

- Recognize the key features of the SAVA syndemic (the first syndemic described in the literature) and its specific expression among several marginalized populations.

- Understand how the published description of the SAVA syndemic helped to trigger public health efforts to move beyond narrow disease categories in order to examine the conditions that create and sustain community health.

WHY MULTIDISCIPLINARITY

Many non-Western ethnomedical traditions have taken a holistic, entwined approach in which "[m]edicine was religion. Religion was society. Society was medicine" (Fadiman, 1997, p. 60). In writing about cross-cultural misunderstandings in medical care and contrasting the holistic view with that of biomedicine, Anne Fadiman (1997) notes that "the practice of [bio]medicine has fissioned into smaller and smaller sub-specialties, with less and less truck between the bailiwicks" (p. 61). Expressive of a broad movement back toward a holistic perspective, this chapter presents the syndemics model as a multidisciplinary understanding that demands exchange and collaboration across many areas of specialization. The syndemic approach bridges public health, the social sciences, medicine, diverse environmental sciences, and biology and is framed by critical biosocial and political economic theory (for example, critical medical anthropology) concerned with explaining how biological and social factors interact to produce health and disease. To borrow Kirmayer's (2003) apt terminology, syndemics research "requires multiple languages of description" (p. 283) and analysis.

Yet achieving *multidisciplinarity*—the successful collaboration across not only disciplinary boundaries but also conceptual worlds (and languages), and perhaps even more important, the successful lifting of the blinders imposed by discipline-centered judgments (as reflected in terms like *hard science* and *soft science*)—is not ensured. For example, with reference to their respective disciplines, Cone and Martin (2003) ask: "Is collaboration between a biologist and a cultural anthropologist possible today? Would bringing insights from biological science and cultural studies together produce a synergy that scholars on both sides would find enlightening?" (p. 232). One answer to this question, one supported by the purpose of this book, is this: understanding and effectively responding to synergistic diseases requires what, following Cone and Martin, might be called *synergistic enlightenment.*

This chapter begins considering the multidisciplinary nature of syndemics research by looking at syndemic terminology, after which, it closely examines what has been called the **SAVA** (substance abuse, violence, and AIDS) syndemic, the first set of entwined epidemics analyzed syndemically in the health literature and the one often used to illustrate the nature of this multifaceted health phenomenon. An examination of SAVA reveals both the complexities of syndemics and the range of disciplines needed to understand and effectively respond to them.

THE TERM *SYNDEMIC*

The choice of the word *syndemic* to label the phenomenon of concern was carefully made. It is a *portmanteau* word, a blend that brings together two distinct concepts to convey a new meaning—like Lewis Carroll's *slithy* (formed by uniting *lithe* and *slimy*), which he coined along with similar portmanteau words for his poem "Jabberwocky," or some recent technical terms borrowed from science fiction, like Manfred Clynes's *cyborg* (created by wedding *cybernetic* and *organism*). In the case of *syndemic,* the first of the two words (and their accompanying denotations and connotations) that make up this neologism is *synergy,* derived from the Greek word *synergos,* meaning two or more agents working together to create a greater effect than the sum of each working alone, a fairly exact definition for what happens in a syndemic. The second is *demic,* a verbal suffix derived from the Greek word *demos,* or "people." It is used in *syndemic* as it has been previously used in three core public health concepts: ***epidemic,*** a disease classification that literally means "upon the people" and that is used to describe greater than expected jumps in the frequency of a disease in a given population; ***pandemic,*** an epidemic that spreads across multiple populations or even worldwide, such as AIDS; and ***endemic,*** a disease that is well established in a population and remains year after year.

Epidemiologists long have recognized that there are difficulties with terms like *epidemic, endemic,* and *pandemic,* most notably problems of imprecision. For example, there are no clear guidelines for determining what constitutes greater than expected increases in the incidence of a disease. As Gordis (1996) asks: "How do we know when we have an excess over what is expected? Indeed, how do we know how much to expect? There is no precise answer to either question" (p. 17). These terms have persisted owing to the recognition of change in disease states, such as disturbing increases in incidence and the sudden local or global appearances of new diseases, but the meanings of these terms have changed over time.

The term *epidemic* has a 2,500-year history. The Greek poet Homer provides the first recorded use—in *The Odyssey,* to describe being back in one's homeland. The term appears with a medical meaning in the Corpus Hippocraticum, a collection of writings from Hippocrates' time that describe his method; *Epidemios* is the title for seven books of the Corpus. For the writers of these documents, an epidemic was a collection of symptoms peculiar to a specific locale, such as the coughs known to occur every winter on the island of Kos. By the Middle Ages the term was being used to refer to specific, named diseases that occurred at different times and places. With the emergence of germ theory, specific epidemics were linked to specific pathogens.

As germ theory and knowledge about infectious pathogens developed, epidemics were described even more precisely in terms of particular microbial strains, as seen in the assignment of specific influenza outbreaks to particular genetic subgroups of what is known to be a diverse microbe species (see Chapter Four). Then, during the second half of the twentieth century, use of the term broadened to describe the rise in the number of cases of noninfectious diseases like cancer, drug use, or obesity (Martin & Martin-Granel, 2006).

As noted in the Preface, the new term *syndemic* was forged in the mid-1990s to label a dynamic relationship involving two or more epidemic diseases or other disorders and the socioenvironmental context that promotes their interaction, a concept not effectively communicated by older, culturally meaningful (if unclearly defined) notions like plagues; the existing and widely used concepts of epidemics, pandemics, and endemics; or newer biomedical concepts such as comorbidity. The intention was to select a manageable health term that effectively calls attention to, in Chadwick's (2003) phrase, "processes, relationships—things together" (p. 119), things that, as reflected in concepts like ecohealth, political economy of health, biosocial interaction, and psychoneuroimmunology, require collaborative strategies that cut across established disciplines of research and canalized approaches to understanding.

Like its parent concept of epidemic, the concept of syndemic is somewhat imprecise. This problem stems partly from the noted shortcomings of the original terminology but also from the challenges of differentiating two or more components of a single disease from two or more interacting diseases. Consider the relationship of type 2 diabetes, apnea (the intermittent suspension of breathing during sleep caused by the occlusion of upper airway passages), and cardiovascular disease. Recent research shows that a majority of patients with the first of these conditions also suffer from the second, which in turn is known to be a risk factor for the third. Most chronic disease specialists see apnea and cardiovascular problems as separate diseases because they have independent expression, even if one can syndemically contribute to the development of the other. Is the same true of apnea and diabetes? Research indicates that the sleep fragmentation caused by apnea alters glucose metabolism in a way that puts patients at risk for the development of diabetes (Ip et al., 2002; Tasali, Mokhlesi, & Van Cauter, 2008). In the final analysis it appears that apnea and diabetes are independent diseases—apnea is found to occur in individuals without diabetes and vice versa—but are also connected, and in interaction they constitute a syndemic with significant adverse consequences, including heightened mortality (Keller, Hader, De Zeeuw, & Rasche, 2007; Punjabi et al., 2002).

This example affirms that "disease is both pathological reality and social construction" (Hays, 2000, p. 2) and that is the actuality the syndemic term and concept encompass. The syndemic perspective recognizes the fundamental importance of the biomedical construction of disease conception, is concerned with disease-host interaction in shaping disease course and expression (and indeed makes shorthand use of common terminology in the biological sciences—for example, pathogen X causes disease Y), and even more important, calls attention to the often determinant sociocultural origins of disease (Singer, 2004b). As Tesh (1988) emphasizes, "To say that infectious diseases are monocausal confuses the agent of disease with the cause of disease. The agent of an infectious disease—a bacteria, virus, or parasite—may be necessary but it is never sufficient" (p. 61). Indeed, as Waldram, Herring, and Young (2006) stress, "the social circumstances surrounding the encounter with pathogens are of paramount importance" (p. 71).

In *War and Peace,* Leo Tolstoy (1865–1869/1998) suggests that in all areas of life, everyone tends to grasp at available causes without waiting to understand the broader canvas: "Man's mind cannot grasp the causes of events in their completeness, but the desire to find those causes is implanted in man's soul. And without considering the multiplicity and complexity of the conditions any one of which taken separately may seem to be the cause, he snatches at the first approximation to a cause that seems to him intelligible and says: 'This is the cause!'"(p. 1055). The syndemic perspective seeks to avoid precisely such narrow conceptualizing. An example of the syndemic view of disease formation is articulated by Gandy and Zumla (2003) in their explanation of the reemergence of tuberculosis as a global pandemic: "A shift of emphasis is required away from the TB bacillus as the 'cause' of the pandemic towards the social and political factors underlying the epidemiology of disease. . . . In practice, of course, there are likely to be a combination of different strategies involved in any successful attempt to control the disease, but a reliance on biomedical innovations alone cannot hope to have any lasting impact" (p. 238).

Similar arguments have been developed by Levins and Lewontin (1985), who maintain that political economy conditions are as much a cause of tuberculosis as the mycobacterial bacillus, and by Terris (1979), who points out that "the causes of cholera in India today go back hundreds of years in India's history, to the British invasion and destruction of once-flourishing textile industries; the maintenance of archaic systems of land ownership and tillage; the persistence of the caste system and the unbelievable poverty, hunger, and crowding; the consequent inability to afford the development of safe water supplies and sewage disposal systems; and, almost incidentally, the presence of cholera vibrios" (p. 204).

THE SAVA SYNDEMIC

The first syndemic to be labeled as such in the literature is a tripartite health condition called SAVA, a product of the complex interactions that occur among substance abuse, violence, and AIDS (Singer, 1996, 2006a). From the syndemic perspective AIDS, drug use, and violence in particular social contexts are so entwined with each other and each is so significantly shaped by the presence of the other two that if one tries to understand them as distinct things in the world it is hard to conceive of them accurately. The term *SAVA* emphasizes that all three health-related components are interactive. There are ways in which drug use interacts directly with AIDS, and both conditions are worsened as a result. Similarly, violence and AIDS interact in mutually accelerating ways. Drugs and violence when copresent also propel each other. In addition to being shaped by these interactions, the actual expression of a SAVA syndemic is shaped as well by local social context factors, including both the population affected and the configuration of social conditions faced by that population. As a result it is appropriate to talk about the existence of multiple SAVA syndemics, each driven by its own arrangement of populations, social conditions, and structural relationships. These points are clarified in the following discussion, which examines SAVA in four population groups that are individually defined by shared experiences and behaviors and in some cases by a shared identity: victims of domestic violence, men who have sex with men, street drug users, and commercial sex workers.

SAVA AMONG VICTIMS OF DOMESTIC VIOLENCE

Violence has been defined as "an act of physical hurt deemed legitimate by the performer and illegitimate by (some) witnesses" (Riches, 1986, p. 8). Although this understanding captures an aspect of some violence, it steers attention away from other forms, including much domestic violence, which always has perpetrators and victims but not necessarily any other witnesses.

Indeed, far from being publicly performed, domestic violence is often intentionally hidden behind closed doors and curtained windows, a secret that may not be expressed publicly. Until relatively recently, even discussion of domestic violence was kept off the stage of public discourse about social life. This has changed. Domestic violence has become a grave concern in the societies of North America and increasingly worldwide.

Research that speaks to the role of domestic violence in the SAVA syndemic includes studies both of childhood sexual and physical abuse and of **intimate partner violence.** Given the physical and emotional vulnerability of children and the (admittedly changing) societal expectations about their care, occurrences of child abuse tend to capture public attention. The headlines of newspapers routinely announce the grim statistics. Research in the United States shows that child abuse occurs in 30 to 60 percent of family violence cases in which children are present (Carter, Weithorn, & Behrman, 1999). During 2005, for example, an estimated 900,000 children in the United States were determined to be victims of abuse or neglect. It is estimated, based on cases substantiated by state and local children's protective services and included in the federal National Child Abuse and Neglect Data System, that during their first year of life 91,000 U.S. children (1 in 50) a year suffer abuse, mostly in the form of neglect (Stein, 2008). Further, at any time approximately 4 million teenagers in the United States have been victims of a serious physical assault at home, and 9 million have been witnesses to severe violence during their lifetimes (U.S. Department of Health and Human Services (HHS), Children's Bureau 2007). Each year, 3 to 10 million children in the United States witness domestic violence (Kilpatrick & Saunders, 1997). Yet awareness of child abuse and establishing legal and social definitions of what it is are relatively new developments. In DeMause's (1998) view, "the history of childhood has been a nightmare from which we have only recently begun to awaken" (p. 2).

The term *intimate partner violence* has been developed in recent years to refer to a range of abuses that occur in close personal relationships, such as those between current and former spouses, dating partners, and sexual partners. In that intimacy is culturally conceived as a positive, supportive, and indeed a cherished experience, the presence of violence and the infliction of suffering in close relationships seems particularly incongruous, resulting in a long history of denial followed more recently by increased public distress and researcher focus. The National Violence Against Women Survey (Tjaden & Thoennes, 2000), for example, conducted through telephone interviews with a nationally representative sample of 8,000 U.S. women and 8,000 U.S. men, found that about one-fourth of women and just under 8 percent of men reported that during their lifetime they had been physically assaulted or raped by a current or former spouse, a cohabitating partner, or a date.

Violence in intimate relationships has been found to take various forms, including physical brutality, sexual violence, and threats and other emotional abuse, while the frequency of such violence falls along a continuum ranging from a single, isolated incident to multi-incident battering or other abuse. The opportunity for ongoing abuse is often tied to the victim's abject fear of flight (including fear of consequences for self and others), depressive emotional state, or emotional or economic dependence on the perpetrator.

What Violence Begets and What Begets Violence

In the literature on domestic violence a common explanatory theme is that "violence begets violence" (Widom, 1989). Thus researchers have noted that low self-esteem, in conjunction with limited social support, is closely linked to *violence victimization* and the development of a life pattern of revictimization (Sobo, 1995). Prior life history is a critical feature used in explanations of domestic violence. For example, those who commit child abuse often have histories of having been abused as children themselves. Consequently, interventions often have *breaking the cycle of violence* as their objective.

Although it is likely that the psychological injuries of abuse find expression in responsive acts of violence, and in this sense domestic violence has a self-perpetuating dimension, a narrow focus on the interpersonal and phenomenological aspects of domestic violence ignores another important type of violence that many people, most notably the poor and working classes, people of color, and women and sexual minorities endure, namely *structural violence* perpetuated by the major institutions in society against denigrated and subordinated populations. As Farmer (2003) explains, structural violence refers to "a host of offenses against human dignity [including]: extreme and relative poverty, social inequalities ranging from racism to gender inequality, and the more spectacular forms of violence that are uncontested human rights abuses" (p. 1). The term *violence* in this instance, as discussed in greater detail in Chapter Six, is used to label relations of inequality that are so grave in their amplification of human pain and suffering and so damaging in their effect on well-being that they can be seen as a form of sanctioned violence (like the structuring of access to health care in terms of possession of health insurance or the exclusion of people from quality housing, or even any housing, on the basis of ethnicity and social class or the severe narrowing of life options through various mechanisms of education channeling and limited access). Although experienced individually, structural violence targets classes of people and subjects them to common forms of lived oppression. Hence the experience of structural violence has been called "social suffering" (Bourgois, Lettiere, & Quesada, 1997).

Structural violence and interpersonal violence often go hand in hand, as victims of structural violence generate physical violence from their suffering. Being taught by their day-to-day life experience that their options are few and the future unwelcoming, that their marginalized lives hold little value in the wider society, and that they are dispensable as people is the ultimate source of the trivialization of life and the explosive anger expressed through domestic violence of all sorts. It is within this type of noxious social context that the intersection of domestic violence, substance abuse, and AIDS risk is disproportionately common. Structural violence, in short, begets much interpersonal domestic violence of the varieties described in the next sections and also generates the accompanying facilitators and consequences of violence writ large and small, including drug use and AIDS risk behavior and infection.

Childhood Sexual Abuse

In recent years there has been a proliferation of research on childhood sexual abuse, with considerable attention paid to the lifetime consequences for victims, including emotional disturbances like anxiety and depression; sexual problems, including risky behaviors and sexual dysfunction; and substance-related illnesses, including eating disorders, alcohol abuse, and illicit drug abuse (Brown & Anderson, 1991). Some researchers have interpreted the eating and substance abuse patterns of victims of childhood sexual abuse as a symbolic reenactment of the earlier traumatization or, alternatively, as self-medication of posttraumatic stress, guilt, negative self-image, and depression (Teusch, 2001). The syndemic relationship between childhood sexual abuse and subsequent substance abuse is emphasized by Stewart and Israeli (2002), who note that the findings of the existing research are "consistent with a self-medication model, where traumatic familial victimization in childhood contributes to lowered self-esteem and increased depression with which victims attempt to cope through alcohol or drug abuse" (p. 105). These authors stress the development of a *vicious cycle* involving sexual and substance abuse. Notably, a pattern of adult relapse into substance abuse following treatment has been found to be associated with severity of childhood emotional abuse, sexual abuse, and overall trauma (Hyman et al., 2008).

Community studies have shown that between 7 and 33 percent of adults report childhood sexual abuse. Compared to women in the general population, women who report they were subjected to childhood sexual abuse have been consistently found to be more likely to seek treatment for both alcohol- and drug-related problems (Kovach, 1983; Rohsenow, Corbett, & Devine, 1988; Sterne, Schaefer, & Evans, 1983). Miller, Downs, and Testa (1993), for example, found that women in alcohol treatment report significantly higher rates of childhood sexual abuse than do either women in the general population or women without an alcohol-related problem receiving treatment for a mental health issue. These researchers determined that the association between childhood sexual abuse and alcohol-related problems remained even after they controlled for sociodemographic and genetic factors (for example, parental alcohol problems).

Hamburger, Leeb, and Swahn (2008) report the findings of the Youth Violence Survey, an examination of violence and its relationship to alcohol consumption in the lives of public school students enrolled in grades 7, 9, 11, and 12 in high-risk communities. In this study early child maltreatment was defined as either witnessing domestic violence or experiencing physical or sexual abuse (or both) before ten years of age. Drinking-related outcome variables included ever drinking alcohol, initiation of alcohol use during preteen years, and heavy episodic drinking. These researchers found that witnessing domestic violence, suffering physical abuse, and suffering sexual abuse were significantly associated with preteen drinking. Students who experienced one or more types of abuse were 1.5 to 3 times more likely to report initiation of drinking before the age of thirteen years. Heavy episodic drinking was associated only with childhood sexual abuse and occurred with boys but not girls. In a number of other studies, however, adult female victims of child sexual abuse have been found to have higher rates of both alcohol and other drug abuse than do either comparable women who have not been sexually abused or women in the general population (Brown & Anderson, 1991; Day, Thurlow, & Woolliscroft, 2003; Goodwin, Cheeves, & Connell, 1990; Pribor & Dinwiddie, 1992). Further, a general population study, the Los Angeles Epidemiologic Catchment Area survey, found that the 6.8 percent of women participants who reported they were victims of "forced sexual contact" before the age of sixteen were significantly more likely than other women participants to report a history of alcohol and drug dependence (Burnam et al., 1988; Scott, 1992; Stein, Golding, Siegel, Burnam, & Sorenson, 1988). Similarly, a national U.S. telephone survey (Kilpatrick et al., 1990) found that childhood sexual assault was significantly associated with current substance abuse among women.

Studies in other countries reflect similar patterns. Research with senior high school students in four provinces in central and northern China (Chen, Dunne, & Han, 2004), for example, found that both males and females who reported experiencing childhood sexual abuse were more depressed, more suicidal, and drank alcohol more frequently than other adolescents did. The victims of childhood sexual abuse were also more likely to be sexually active subsequently than were youths of equivalent age who did not suffer such abuse. Male victims were subsequently more likely to engage in violent behavior. In a Swedish study (Edgardh & Ormstad, 2000) of a representative sample of seventeen-year-olds, 3 percent of males and 11 percent of females reported childhood sexual abuse, with the mean age of onset being nine years. Thirty-three percent of the boys and 30 percent of the girls reported subsequent suicide attempts or other forms of self-inflicted harm (compared to 5 percent and 9 percent, respectively, of boys and girls who did not report sexual abuse). Use of alcohol and drugs and sexual activity before the age of fifteen were all significantly more common among abused girls (but not boys).

Childhood Physical Abuse and Neglect

In 1991, the American Academy of Pediatrics Task Force on the Future Role of the Pediatrician in the Delivery of Health Care noted that since the emergence of pediatrics as a medical specialty it has been recognized that children's health is "influenced greatly by family attitudes, environment, and socioeconomic class" (Committee on Psychosocial Aspects of Child and Family Health, 2001, p. 1227). Consequently, this specialty has accommodated a somewhat broader focus on health than have other branches of biomedicine, and the changing and emergent threats to the well-being of children that are viewed as a product of psychosocial factors are termed *new morbidities* in the pediatric literature. Childhood physical abuse and neglect, because of its long-term health effects, was quickly included under this label, and has come to be an issue of central concern within this medical discipline.

It is estimated by the HHS Children's Bureau (2007) that in the year 2005 there were about 900,000 victims of child maltreatment in the United States. Of these, the majority (63 percent) suffered neglect, followed by physical abuse (17 percent) and emotional or psychological abuse (7 percent), with the remainder suffering from sexual abuse, medical neglect, abandonment, or other less frequent types of mistreatment. The precise meanings of these terms, at least as they are used in the criminal justice system, are defined by federal and state laws. At the federal level, for example, child abuse and neglect is defined as "[a]ny recent act or failure to act on the part of a parent or caretaker, which results in death, serious physical or emotional harm, sexual abuse, or exploitation, or an act or failure to act which presents an imminent risk of serious harm" (The Child Abuse Prevention and Treatment Act, 1998).

Childhood abuse and neglect has been linked in numerous studies with a range of health problems, including a subsequent life tendency to engage in risk-taking behavior, including both substance abuse and HIV sexual risk (Hansen, Sedlar, & Warner-Rogers, 1999). Bornovalova, Gwadz, Kahler, Aklin, and Lejuez (2008), for example, carried out a study among inner-city African American adolescents of impulsivity, risk-taking propensity, and sensation seeking as possible mediators in the relationship between having a history of childhood abuse and engaging in HIV-related risk behaviors. Their research showed that suffering childhood abuse was associated with HIV risk, risk-taking propensity, and sensation seeking. Impulsivity, however, did not appear to be a mediating factor. Other research provides compelling evidence linking childhood exposure to physical abuse with youth involvement in violence, with severe childhood maltreatment being a strong predictor of teen violence (Maas, Herrenkohl, & Sousa, 2008; Wekerle & Wolfe, 1998).

Overall, the severity of the later effects of child physical abuse and neglect is tied to the severity of the maltreatment. Research on drug-involved mothers who do not maintain infant custody, for example, shows they report higher levels of personal childhood neglect and physical abuse than do those who do maintain custody (Minnes, Singer, Humphrey-Wall, & Satayathum, 2008). As this example suggests, abuse can have multigenerational consequences. Severity of consequence is also linked to the number of types of maltreatment to which children are subjected, because specific forms of childhood maltreatment do not necessarily occur in isolation. All of these points are affirmed by the findings of Bensley, Van Eenwyk, and Simmons (2000) in a population-based telephone survey for the Washington State Behavioral Risk Factor Surveillance System. They found among women that being subjected to early and chronic sexual abuse (without simultaneous nonsexual physical abuse) was associated with more than a sevenfold increase in HIV-risk behavior, whereas any sexual abuse combined with physical abuse was associated with a fivefold increase in HIV risk. Among women respondents, combined abuse was also associated with heavy drinking. Among men, any childhood sexual abuse was associated with an eightfold increase in HIV risk whereas physical abuse alone was associated with a threefold increase in HIV risk.

It is noteworthy that ethnic differences in the reporting of suspected child abuse to civil authorities reflect the broader pattern of social disparity that, it is argued in this book, fuels the SAVA syndemic. It is well known that ethnic minority children in the United States have higher rates of authenticated maltreatment than white children do (with black children having the highest rate in this group). Whereas there are just over 10 affirmed cases of maltreatment for every 1,000 white children, among black, Hispanic, and Native American/Alaska Native children there are approximately 25, 13, and 20 cases per 1,000 children, respectively (HHS, Children's Bureau, 2001). Are these differences a reflection of more abuse in minority households than in white households, or are they an artifact of increased reporting of suspected abuse involving minority children?

To help answer this question, Lane, Rubin, Monteith, and Christian (2002) conducted a retrospective chart review in an urban children's hospital, looking at the records of over 350 children below three years of age who were hospitalized for an acute primary skull or long-bone fracture between 1994 and 2000. They found that minority children of at least twelve months of age with accidental injuries were more than three times as likely as their white counterparts to be reported for suspected abuse. These researchers concluded that "[r]acial biases may have played a role in this differential reporting particularly in toddlers with accidental injuries" (p. 1608).

Although physical and sexual abuse have demonstrable adverse behavioral effects, other forms of exposure to violence can also influence drug use and sexual risk behaviors. Using audio, computer-assisted self-interviews among juvenile detainees, Voisin et al. (2007), for example, found that participants who reported witnessing community violence in the two months prior to their arrest were twice as likely to use marijuana and alcohol, get high on alcohol or other drugs during sexual intercourse, and have sex with a partner who was high as were detainees who had not witnessed violence. Similarly, in a study of risk behaviors among adolescent girls, Berenson, Wiemann, and McCombs (2001) found that girls who had witnessed violence were two to three times more likely to report using tobacco, marijuana, alcohol, or drugs before sex and having intercourse with a partner who had multiple partners as were girls who had not witnessed violence. Moreover, they found that girls who were direct victims of violence were two to four times more likely than were those who had neither witnessed nor experienced violence to have used drugs or alcohol; to have had an early sexual debut (before age thirteen); and to report intercourse with strangers, multiple partners, or partners with multiple partners, and a positive test result for a sexually transmitted disease. Girls who had both witnessed and been the victims of violence had the greatest risk for adverse health behaviors. Berenson, Wiemann, and McCombs concluded that "witnessing violence, although damaging, does not appear to be as damaging as actually being a target of violence" (p. 1241). However, both conditions, singly and even more so in combination, predict alcohol and drug use, use that is very likely, at least before the onset of addiction, due to the desire to deaden the emotion burden of involvement in violence.

Intimate Partner Violence

Although most research on intimate partner violence has been carried out in developed nations, a study of women's experiences in ten countries that are mostly developing nations (Bangladesh, Brazil, Ethiopia, Japan, Namibia, Peru, Samoa, Serbia and Montenegro, Thailand, and Tanzania), using a standardized, population-based household survey (Garcia-Moreno et al., 2006), found that the proportion of women who had ever had a male partner and who reported having ever experiencing either physical or sexual partner violence, or both, varied by country from 15 to 71 percent. The proportion of women who reported physical or sexual partner violence, or both, during the previous year ranged from 4 to 54 percent. Lifetime prevalence of intimate partner violence varied considerably by country, with two of the sites in the study showing a prevalence of less than 25 percent, seven ranging from 25 to 50 percent, and six showing from 50 to 75 percent. In all but one of the countries in the sample, women were at significantly greater risk of physical or sexual violence from an intimate partner than from other people in society. Studies like this are complicated by the varying cultural definitions of appropriate partner treatment. Violence may be severe by external standards and yet not be perceived by perpetrators as violent because of local cultural standards and understandings. As a consequence the World Health Organization (WHO) defines violence not in terms of particular cultural views but in terms of its impact on health and well-being. On this basis, WHO (2002b) reports that findings from forty-eight population-based surveys conducted around the world reveal that 10 to 69 percent of women say they have been physically assaulted by an intimate male partner at some point during their lives.

The health consequences associated with violence committed by an intimate partner include a range of physical injuries, developing various gastrointestinal disorders, experiencing chronic pain syndromes, suffering anxiety and depression, and exhibiting suicidal behavior patterns (Bonomi et al., 2006). In the United States the estimated rates of partner violence among women who use drugs are 60 to 75 percent, two to three times greater than rates found in general population samples of women (Bennett & Larson, 1994; Brewer, Fleming, Haggerty, & Calalano, 1998).

Partner violence also affects reproductive health, and among women victims can lead to gynecological disorders, unwanted pregnancy, and premature labor and delivery, as well as sexually transmitted diseases, including HIV/AIDS. The relationship between partner violence, substance abuse, and HIV risk is complex, as on the one hand it can involve substance abuse by either perpetrators or victims, or both, and on the other hand it can involve clear-cut violence victimization or reciprocal violence among partners (Amaro, Fried, Cabral, & Zuckerman, 1990; El-Bassel, Gilbert, & Wasde, 2000; Gilbert et al., 2000). Where violence victimization is a factor, it can activate a dynamic process that moves from partner battering triggered by perpetrator drug use to illicit drug use by the victim to self-medicate the damaging emotional effects of violence victimization and then to engaging in sexual and drug-related risk for HIV and related blood-borne diseases (Duke, Teng, Simmons, & Singer, 2003). Although men may be victims of intimate partner violence, the victims of this type of abuse are usually women in heterosexual relationships. Given this fact, intimate partner violence is rightly seen as part of the larger pattern of human rights abuses committed against women internationally.

Studies in various countries have found a strong relationship between intimate partner violence and child abuse (Frias-Armenta & McCloskey, 1998; Madu & Peltzer, 2000; National Research Council, 1993). Face-to-face interviews with 500 participants in rural India (Hunter, Jain, Sadowski, & Sanhueza, 2000), for example, found that the incidence of child abuse (referred to in the study as "severe disciplinary practices") was two times greater in households in which intimate partner violence occurred than it was in households where partner violence was not present. Other studies with victims of child abuse also report high rates of coming from homes in which intimate partner violence occurred as well. Even when children are not themselves direct victims of domestic violence they still exhibit significant emotional and other consequences.

In the United States, for example, it is estimated that 10 million children annually witness intimate partner violence in their homes, most commonly directed at their mother (Humphreys, 1997). Recent research has shown that children in homes in which intimate partner violence occurs are themselves at risk in various ways and may experience reduced quality of care (Bair-Merritt et al., 2008), behavioral problems, cognitive problems, and internalizing patterns, such as anxiety, withdrawal, and depression, that are consistent with being at risk for suicide (McFarlane, Groff, O'Brien, & Watson, 2003) and facing a subsequent risk of drinking and drug abuse (McNeal & Amato, 1998).

Among women, becoming the victim of intimate partner violence has been linked to experiencing childhood physical abuse or witnessing parental interpersonal violence. Bensley, Van Eenwyk, and Simmons (2003), in the Washington State Behavioral Risk Factor Surveillance System telephone survey, for example, found that women who were victims of childhood physical abuse or who had witnessed parental intimate partner violence were four to six times more likely than other women to suffer physical intimate partner violence. Women in this study who reported either of these forms of childhood trauma were three to four times more likely than others to suffer partner emotional abuse later in life. In contrast, women reporting childhood sexual abuse only were not found to be at increased risk of physical violence at the hands of their intimate partners. Similarly, Farley and Barkan (1998) interviewed 130 commercial sex workers in San Francisco concerning their lifetime experience of violence of various types and whether they had symptoms suggestive of posttraumatic stress disorder (PTSD) as defined in the criteria of the *Diagnostic and Statistical Manual of Mental Disorders.* They found that 57 percent reported sexual assault and 49 percent reported physical abuse during childhood. As adults, 82 percent reported physical abuse as part of their involvement in commercial sex, 83 percent reported being threatened with weapons, and 68 percent reported being raped. Sixty-eight percent reported PTSD symptoms. Experiencing symptoms was significantly associated with the total number of types of lifetime violence endured by a participant, as well as with childhood physical abuse, being raped as an adult, and the total number of times raped during commercial sex work.

Entwined Epidemics

As the previous discussion suggests, domestic violence in its various forms, drug and alcohol use, and HIV risk and infection are complexly entwined. Yet many aspects of these multifarious relationships remain unclear. To examine the relationships among substance abuse, violence, and HIV more closely, El-Bassel and coworkers (Gilbert et al., 2000) interviewed thirty-one women in drug treatment who reported physical or sexual violence committed by an intimate partner. Of those women who recalled recent experiences of intimate partner violence, almost all (83.8 percent) reported drug use during the incident. In 40 percent of these cases, both partners were using drugs, and in 35 percent only the perpetrator was using drugs. About one-fifth of the women (19.3 percent) indicated that they used drugs immediately after the violence had ended as a way of dealing with their emotional upset and physical pain. Additionally, about one-fifth of the women reported that they had been forced to have unprotected sex either during the most recent incident of violence or just after it ended. These researchers noted that "women in our sample attributed their experiences of abuse to their partner's drug use and to a lesser extent to their own drug use. . . . Women in this study are at very high risk of contracting HIV and HCV [hepatitis C virus], for multiple reasons. Only a minority of our sample have ever used condoms with their partners although a majority reported that they or their partners have had outside relationships" (Gilbert et al., 2000, p. 460).

Similarly, in research conducted in Hartford, Connecticut, by the Hispanic Health Council and the Institute for Community Research, my colleagues and I used street outreach to recruit a sample of 500 heroin- or cocaine-using women over the age of 18 (average age 37.8 years) and not in treatment. The sample reflected the ethnic composition of the city of Hartford, with 38.6 percent of the women being African American, 39.4 percent Hispanic, and 17.4 percent non-Hispanic white. In reviewing the findings of this study we found that each woman belonged to one of four relationship groups. About two-fifths of the women (41.9 percent) reported no incidents of physical violence between themselves and their current or most recent sex partner. Ten percent of the women reported that they were the victims of partner violence. Another 8.5 percent of the women reported that they had physically abused their current or most recent partner but were not themselves victims of partner violence. Finally, almost 40 percent reported mutual physical violence in their current or most recent relationship (Duke et al., 2006). Women who were subject to violence victimization by partners were more likely to report the more severe forms of violence, including being beaten, stabbed, or shot, than were the women involved in mutual violence with their partners: 45.5 percent versus 35.0 percent. In answering a question about whether they sold drugs in order to raise money for their partners, only 11.6 percent of the women in nonviolent relationships reported this behavior compared to 28.6 percent of the women who were victims of intimate partner violence. Only 11.8 percent of women who reported that they ever sold sex for money or drugs in order to get drugs for their partner were in nonviolent relationships, whereas 22.9 percent of those who were victims of partner violence had sold sex for this purpose. In short we found that drug-involved women in abusive relationships were significantly more likely than other drug-using women to engage in risky behaviors to raise drug money for their partner. This finding suggests that one of the ways the SAVA syndemic unfolds in this population is that some drug-involved men use particularly severe forms of violence with their partners, and these partners in turn become more likely than other drug-using women to put themselves at risk for HIV or for street violence; thus severe intimate partner violence begets HIV risk and risk for additional violence. Presumably, given the prevalence of this pattern in prior research, individuals in the sample who were subject to particularly harsh forms of violence self-medicated their emotional trauma through drug use, although we did not examine this behavior.

Following a meta-analysis of studies on the intersection of intimate partner violence and HIV/AIDS, Gielan et al. (2007) concluded, "There is a critical need for research on (a) causal pathways and cumulative effects of the syndemic issues of violence, HIV, and substance abuse and (b) interventions that target [intimate partner violence] victims at risk for HIV, as well as HIV-positive women who may be experiencing [intimate partner violence]." The examination that follows of substance abuse, violence, and AIDS among men who have sex with men (MSM) affirms that the SAVA syndemic has somewhat different dimensions in different host populations.

SAVA AMONG MSM

In North America and Europe the highest absolute number of both new HIV infections and new AIDS cases occurs among *men who have sex with men,* a term adopted in the era of AIDS to capture the diversity among men who engage in homosexual sex (including self-identified gay men, bisexual men, men who self-identify as straight but have sex with other men, and men who engage in a range of related sexual practices and identities cross culturally). For the most part, studies of HIV risk among MSM have focused on sexual risk, with comparatively little attention given to the dual risk category of MSM drug users, men who are placed in harm's way both through drug use and sexual behavior. Some studies, however, have begun to address synergisms between drug use and sexual risk among MSM.

Synergism of Drug Use and Sexual Risk Behaviors

In their comparison of sexual risk behaviors among a group of men who have sex with men and are injection drug users (IDUs) with those among a group of MSM who do not inject drugs, O'Connell et al. (2004) found that MSM who are also IDUs are younger than MSM who do not inject drugs and are more likely to be HIV-positive. Other studies also have helped to clarify aspects of the SAVA syndemic in this population. In their study of over 3,000 MSM who were fifteen to twenty-five years of age, Stueve and his study team (2002) asked their study participants about their last sexual contact with primary and secondary partners, including whether they were "high on drugs or alcohol" at the time. Almost one-fifth (18.6 percent) who reported having a primary partner said they had used drugs during their last sexual encounter, and 25 percent said they had had anal sex without a condom. Among men without primary partners, almost 30 percent reported drug use during their last sexual episode, and 12 percent reported unprotected anal intercourse. Using drugs was associated with unprotected receptive anal intercourse with both primary and nonprimary partners.

In a meta-analysis of studies that examined the relationship between sexual orientation and adolescent substance use, Marshal et al. (2008) found that lesbian, gay, and bisexual adolescents overall reported substantially higher rates of substance use compared to rates among heterosexual youths; indeed overall rates were 190 percent higher than rates for heterosexual youths, and 340 percent higher for bisexual youths compared to heterosexual youths. This body of literature has led to heightened recognition of the need for better understanding of the precise nature and pathways of the "synergism of drug use and sexual risk behaviors" and the effects of this synergism "on rates of HIV seroconversion" among MSM (Plankey et al., 2007, p. 85).

Existing research indicates that some drugs have played a particularly significant role in persistent high-risk sex among MSM. Most notable in this regard is crystal methamphetamine (Reback & Grella, 1999; Shoptaw, Reback, & Freese, 2002). Use of this drug (often called simply *crystal* on the street) was first reported in MSM communities on the West Coast of North America. The drug's appeal has been described by journalist Michael Spector (2005):

> Crystal first gained popularity in the gay community of San Francisco in the nineteen-nineties, where it became the preferred fuel for all night parties and a necessity for sexual marathons. Its reputation quickly spread. Crystal methamphetamine is highly addictive, but its appeal is not hard to understand; the drug removes inhibitions, bolsters confidence, supercharges the libido, and heightens the intensity of sex. "The difference between sex with crystal and sex without it is like the difference between Technicolor and black-and-white," one man told me . . . "Once you have sex with crystal, it's hard to imagine having it any other way" [p. 38].

Subsequently, the drug began to diffuse to the Midwest, the South, and more recently to the East Coast. In various studies use of crystal methamphetamine has been associated with sex parties, prolonged sexual events and multiple partners, and anal sex without a condom. Consequently, use of this drug is common among men diagnosed with HIV and other sexually transmitted infections (Bernstein et al., 2000). In an Internet survey of over 2,500 MSM (recruited through a banner ad posted in chat rooms and hyperlinked to the survey instrument) that investigated risk behaviors during a six-month period, Hirshfield, Remien, Walavalkar, and Chiasson (2004) found that significant independent predictors of infection with a sexually transmitted disease (primarily syphilis and gonorrhea) were use of crystal methamphetamine, unprotected anal intercourse, and having six or more sex partners during the study period. Gorman and Carroll (2000), who studied the use of methamphetamine among MSM in Puget Sound, Washington, identified a number of user subgroups: men who used this drug as part of their involvement in party circuits (affiliated, often nightlong dance events, primarily in the gay community), men who used the drug in gay baths and sex clubs, transgendered or transsexual users, and HIV-positive men who used methamphetamine to self-medicate their HIV symptoms. Ethnicity is also a factor in the patterns found in the use of this drug. Diaz (1997), for example, has described methamphetamine use among Latino MSM who favor it "as a way to deal with ambivalent feelings regarding anal intercourse," especially men who are uncomfortable taking the passive role (p. 78).

Among males with AIDS in the United States, currently 7 percent fall into the dual risk category of being both injection drug users and men who have sex with men (Centers for Disease Control and Prevention, 2008b). Unfortunately, HIV/AIDS surveillance data do not provide information on noninjection drug use and HIV infection among MSM; however, the research my colleagues and I conducted with MSM in Connecticut suggests that trading sex for drugs or money or engaging in high-risk sexual practices as a result of drug use is disproportionately common in this population (Singer & Marxuach-Rodriquez, 1996; Clair & Singer, 2009).

A Complex of Risk

Four factors have been found to increase HIV risk among men who have sex with men in the United States: use of multiple drugs, partner violence, childhood sexual abuse, and depression (Carballo-Dieguez & Dolezal, 1995; Jinich et al., 1998; Stall, Mills, Williamson, and Hart, 2003). These factors are thought to interact, producing an increase in both drug-related risk taking and high-risk sexual behaviors (Bartholow et al., 1994; Cohen & Densen-Gerber, 1982). Stall et al. (2003), who have adopted the syndemic perspective in their research among MSM, found these associations in a household telephone survey of almost 3,000 men in New York City, Chicago, Los Angeles, and San Francisco. Moreover, the percentage of MSM in their study reporting high-risk sex behaviors increased steadily from 7 percent among those with none of the four health problems to 33 percent for those suffering from all four. For men who lacked any of the cofactors, 13 percent were HIV-positive compared to 25 percent of those who reported all four cofactors. Analysis of these data in terms of *gay-related development* (that is, early, middle, or late passage through sexual orientation identity stages, such as age at first awareness of same-sex sexual attractions and disclosure of sexual orientation) found that the negative life experiences of early forced sex, gay-related harassment, and physical abuse were associated with negative health outcomes in adulthood including HIV infection, partner abuse, and depression.

Consequently, these researchers affirm the existence of a SAVA syndemic among MSM that has its roots in childhood sexual abuse that contributes to the development of depression in adulthood and the subsequent entrance into abusive adult relationships, use of multiple drugs, and high levels of HIV risk and infection. Further, being the victim of homophobic attacks contributes to serious health problems among adult gay men. All of these psychosocial factors interact and are mutually reinforcing (Friedman, Marshal, Stall, Cheong, & Wright, 2007). Relf, Huang, Campbell, and Catania (2004) measured the prevalence of *battering victimization*—which they defined as the experience of psychological or symbolic, physical, and sexual battering—in the same sample of MSM analyzed by Stall's research team. They found that rates of battering were high compared to those for heterosexual men and that HIV serostatus was associated with being the victim of physical or of psychological or symbolic violence but not of sexual violence. Further, they found that battering victimization is the key mediating variable between being subjected to childhood sexual abuse, having a gay identity, having various adverse early life experiences, and subsequent HIV risk behaviors.

Building on the work of Stall et al. with adult MSM, Mustanski, Garofalo, Herrick, and Donenberg (2007) studied an ethnically diverse, community-based sample of 310 young (sixteen- to twenty-four-year-old), self-identified MSM in Chicago. Of concern to the members of this research team were various psychosocial, behavioral, and health variables: regular binge drinking, partner violence, sexual assault, psychological distress, sexual risk taking, and HIV status. They conclude: "Our data suggest that the number of psychosocial health problems additively increase risk for HIV among urban YMSM [young men who have sex with men]. For example, each problem increased the odds of an HIV positive status by 42 percent and also increased the odds of sexual health risk behaviors. Multivariate analyses indicate that substance use and being the victim of violence show the strongest relationship to sexual health and HIV risk" (p. 44).

These studies indicate the importance of a set of factors beginning with childhood exposure to abuse and extending to later exposure to intimate partner violence, particular psychological reactions, self-medicating drug use, and high-risk sexual behavior and HIV/AIDS infection as key components of the SAVA syndemic in MSM. Further, as Mustanski et al. (2007) state, "Locating the HIV epidemic in the context of a syndemic of psychosocial risk factors underscores the existence of multiple health disparities among gay and lesbian individuals, who experience higher morbidity and barriers to care" (p. 39).

SAVA AMONG STREET DRUG USERS

Street drug users were identified as a population of critical public health concern as a result of the HIV/AIDS epidemic (Brown & Beschner, 1993). The term *street drug user* was adopted in the health and research literature during this period to refer to marginalized, inner-city drug users who have been forced by poverty, discrimination, and addiction into a far more visible and public pattern of drug acquisition and consumption than that exhibited by their wealthier suburban or rural drug-using counterparts, and who are highly at risk for HIV and a host of other diseases. The term draws attention to the context of drug use as a central social and public health issue. Taking place in abandoned buildings, dark alleyways, recessed doorways, secluded corners of urban cemeteries, rooftops and stairwells, wooded parks, deserted cars, empty lots, and similar somewhat hidden and out-of-the-way locations in busy urban settings, street drug use draws much of the media and police attention focused on illicit drug use (Singer, 2005).

Coincident with the AIDS epidemic and its rapid spread to urban drug users, a number of U.S. cities began maintaining street drug monitoring teams to assess the interface of drug activity and health risks, leading to a considerable expansion of knowledge about this population, its patterns and contexts of drug consumption, its health profile, and its intervention needs (Hopkins & Frank, 1991), and also about the role of street violence in drug use and HIV risk (Marshall, Singer, & Clatts, 1999). This important body of data collected in the new street drug monitoring studies allows detailed analyses of the patterns of violence, drug use, and HIV infection in this heretofore socially invisible and often intentionally hidden population, as discussed in the following sections.

Everyday Violence

The frequency and predictability of violence on the inner-city street is a topic regularly encountered in conversations with street drug users. A participant in one of our street drug studies in Hartford, for example, recalled the following incident: "When I was walking down the street, waiting for her [his girlfriend] to come back from her trick [commercial sex], I was going up towards Washington Street. . . . There's like this little alleyway. I take that alleyway because it's a shortcut, everybody knows that. That's where they got me. They started to attack me and one dude sliced me like that [indicating a jagged twelve-inch slash across the left side of his chest]."

The trigger for this assault was the victim's failed effort to "beat" (steal drugs from) a local drug dealer. Violence was not new to this individual. At the time of the interview, he had been using drugs heavily for twenty-two years, and as both victim and perpetrator, he had experienced drug-related violence in his life since childhood. The violence began with harsh, daily beatings administered by his father, intended to correct his alleged transgressions, and they continued throughout his adolescence as he defended his ground in the bellicose world of street-corner drug dealing, a practice taught to him by his father. During his young adulthood, violence, in the form of brutal assaults on wayward members, was a regular part of his role as an "enforcer" in a drug-selling street gang. Indeed, violence in one form or another was an enduring component in his life until he contracted AIDS through his daily drug injection (Singer, 2006c).

This individual was a participant in a study funded by the National Institute on Drug Abuse (NIDA) in which my colleagues and I examined the relationships among substance abuse, violence, and HIV risk in a sample of 224 not-in-treatment street drug users, recruited through street outreach. The study identified a wide range of types of violence exposure and involvement among participants. Seventy-four percent reported witnessing fighting in the streets of their neighborhood during the last four months (Romero-Daza, Weeks, & Singer, 1998). Violence in the streets was said to be especially common, with "once or twice a week" being the median frequency. The other most common type of recently witnessed violence was domestic violence, which, notably, was reported by 54 percent of participants. Gang violence (45 percent), robbery and muggings (42 percent), and beatings or stabbing (31 percent) were the next most common types of violence that participants reported witnessing. As these findings indicate, street drug users are experientially exposed to a considerable amount of violence on the streets and in their homes but in which they are neither victim nor perpetrator. One participant who suffered emotional consequences from witnessing violence stated: "This is haunting me still about when I seen they killed this man and everything. . . . They beat this man up and he was dead. I think all the blows and every-thing, and they took his head and hit him on the floor and that killed him. . . . And now one of my brothers is in jail 'cause he shot another man. 'Cause if he wouldn't have shot that man, he would have killed my brother for a bike the other man wanted." Witnessing violence, it became evident, is an important element in assessing the interrelationship of violence, drug use, and HIV risk.

Considering all forms of direct involvement in violence (including emotional abuse) as either victim or perpetrator, 39 percent of the sample reported being a victim over the past four months, and 30 percent reported being a perpetrator of some form of violence. Specific rates of violence victimization affirmed that exposure to violence is not a distant phenomenon in the lives of street drug users. A third of participants reported being the victims of emotional abuse during the prior four months. Additionally, 14 percent reported being the targets of physical violence, and 7 percent indicated they had suffered serious physical violence during this period. Indeed, violence is an expected aspect of everyday drug use, as noted by the following participant, who explained his strategy for defense against the constant threat of violent attack: "I was up against the corner, and I was sitting on that little bench, the little couch. A guy came up and said, 'Give me everything, your watch, everything.' He had a knife. . . . He had me trapped in the corner. And the way he had me, you know. It was like, 'give it up, and this and that.' And see, if I had seen it coming, I would grab . . . you see, I always carry a bottle. . . . I'll crack that over someone's head. They'll think twice about robbing me with a knife or not. . . . I think he was using 'ready' [cocaine]. He probably wanted to get a hit, because I had dope on me and he came in with a girl. And he was like, 'Give me the dope too!'"

Significantly, nine of the drug users in our sample responded that they had been the target of attempted murder. Participants also revealed their own role as perpetrators of violence against others during the last four months. Ten percent admitted committing acts of violence, and two respondents had attempted murder during that period.

Of the incidents of violence victimization reported by participants, 71 percent of the physical violence incidents involved the use of drugs or alcohol, and for incidents of serious physical violence that use rose to 75 percent. In cases where study participants were the perpetrator, the reported use of psychoactive substances was 75 percent when they committed emotional abuse, 80 percent when they carried out acts of physical violence against another person, and 100 percent when they committed serious physical violence or attempted deadly violence. Notably, 44 percent of our participants indicated that involvement in violence (as either victim or perpetrator) contributed to increases in their drug consumption, and 47 percent stated that it affected the kinds of drugs they used (Duke, Teng, et al., 2003). One woman participant explained:

My husband was twice my age. He used to beat me up all the time. He was a very jealous man. He wouldn't even let me look out the window. He will tear my clothes off and he will keep me locked in the house. That made me feel I needed to escape. I wanted to be like a free bird and when I finally found myself free that's when everything happened. I started with marijuana and then I moved to crack and then to heroin. Every time I had a chance to get out I would buy some rock [crack] and use it in secret. I felt trapped. I was with him for 20 years. I couldn't talk to anyone [Duke, Teng, et al., 2003, p. 30].

Among women participants (about one-quarter of the sample), 16 percent reported being victims of violence during the last four months. In cases of violence against women, the perpetrator was more likely to be a family member or someone known to the woman than was the case for male victims (100 percent versus 75 percent). Women were also more likely to increase their drug use following violence victimization and more likely to report that it was hard for them to escape exposure to violence (38 percent versus 27 percent). As one woman participant stated: "I thought that if I would leave him, my kids, you know, they're going to suffer because they didn't have a father and stuff like that, so I stayed but, after three, four years, I left. He broke my leg. He pushed me down the stairs and broke my leg. You know how you get black and blue and stuff like that? He used to hurt me like that. My body was all sore" (Singer & Weeks, n.d.).

Describing the emotional toll of being a perpetrator of violence, one participant said: "So then I started shooting up and that's when I started going crazy . . . you know like getting sick, real sick, starting to do bad things, stealing robbing . . . like taking money away from people . . . and I used to have a gun. My cousin had a gun and he used to give it to me so I can go rob people, like drug dealers, take their drugs. A lot of crazy stuff like that I come to think about now and I be like, damn, man, I could have been dead" (Singer & Weeks, n.d.).

These findings from our research in Hartford are not unique but are reflected in studies from around the country and beyond. Fuller et al. (2002) describe co-occurring patterns of adult drug injection, HIV infection, and violence victimization in a sample of street drug users in Baltimore. In another Baltimore sample, this one consisting of young adult (eighteen to twenty-nine years of age), short-term injection drug users, Doherty, Garfein, Monterroso, Brown, and Vlahov (2000) found that correlates of HIV infection were a history of sexual assault and a set of drug-use and sexual behaviors. In a study of women prisoners in a rural southern state, Fogel and Belyea (1999) found high rates of substance abuse; current patterns and past histories of violence victimization, including sexual abuse; a tendency toward multiple partners; and AIDS sexual risk. Other studies of female prisoners have produced parallel findings linking substance abuse, violence, and HIV risk (Mullings, Marquart, & Brewer, 2000).

Mullings et al. (2000) stress that childhood sexual abuse is a strong predictor of HIV drug and sexual risk, and that sexual victimization and social marginality taken together constitute a better predictor of such risk than either of these variables alone. The Vancouver Injection Drug User Study (Braitstein et al., 2003), which was designed in part to assess factors associated with sexual violence in childhood, adolescence, and adulthood, found a dose-response relationship between age at first sexual violence victimization and HIV risk behaviors. The prevalence of HIV among study participants who had ever experienced sexual violence was 25 percent, compared to 19 percent among those who never experienced sexual violence, and child sexual abuse was found to have worse consequences than later sexual violence victimization. Lindqvist's (2007) research in Sweden identified people at risk for HIV who are suffering from substance abuse, psychiatric symptoms, and violent behavior, a group he calls the "triply troubled," which is but a SAVA syndemic by another name.

A Culture of Violence?

One of the issues raised in the street drug literature is the existence of what has been called a *culture of violence,* said to be pervasive in inner-city areas populated by minority drug users (Sampson & Wilson, 1998). This "ghetto-specific" culture is said to involve the internalization of social norms of violence by inner-city dwellers and to have a life of its own beyond its expression in specific locations, so that it continues to influence behavior even when individuals move to other locations (Wolfgang & Ferracuti, 1967). Buss, Abdu, and Walker (1995) extend this understanding in their examination of the relationship of alcohol and drug use to street violence in small cities, arguing that a "culture of violence pervades the small city, as it does in large urban ghettos" (p. 75). Cultural explanations of this sort do appear to adhere to a simple and straightforward logic (that is, people must adapt to social conditions to survive, and in this adaptation they develop values and behaviors that help to perpetuate the very conditions that led to formation of the values and behaviors). However, they have been faulted on several grounds: (1) they reify culture as static and unchanging; (2) they transform culture from a tool that assists survival into a straitjacket that constricts subsequent adaptation to changing conditions; and (3) they tend to blame the victims of harsh and unjust social conditions for their own social suffering (Singer, 2007; Valdez, Kaplan, & Curtis, 2007).

As this review suggests, the SAVA syndemic is a significant aspect of the life experience of the at-risk street drug using population, and it continues to be significant for members of this population in some contexts away from the street, such as jails and prisons. Particularly severe forms of violence are found in this population both during their childhoods and in their adult lives, where everyday violence stems from conflicted relationships, conflicts over drug deals, disagreements during the sharing of drugs, incidents of police harassment, lack of reliable shelter, and drug-user-on-drug-user use of force to expropriate items of any value, however minimal. All these factors are for the most part reflections of this population's status as a marginalized, or pariah, social group; members have limited access to resources and hence must battle their similarly marginalized peers for every slight advantage. Under these conditions violence begets violence because other options are constrained and thus violence remains a possible course of action for all but the incapacitated.

SAVA AMONG COMMERCIAL SEX WORKERS

As Silliman and Bhattacharjee (2002) emphasize, "women in prostitution are particularly at risk of gender-based violence—including physical, psychological and economic violence—from pimps, buyers, police and boyfriends" (p. 210). This fact has often been hidden behind a public health focus on prostitution as a vector of disease. Note Raymond et al. (2002), "The minimal documentation of the harm and trauma of prostitution and trafficking may in large part be due to the fact that prostitution has not been recognized as a form of violence against women and the ambivalence, on the part of many researchers, NGOs and governments, to view prostitution as a violation of women's human rights" (p. 296).

Gender-Based Violence

Despite limited research until recently, it has become evident that violence is a common experience among commercial sex workers. For example, Parriott (1994) interviewed sixty-eight women in Minneapolis-St. Paul who had been involved in commercial sex for at least six months in various settings (the "street," massage parlors, and escort services), and found that 62 percent had been raped, half had been physically assaulted; and one-third had been assaulted by customers at least several times each year. About one-fourth of the women had suffered broken bones and two had been beaten into a coma. Similarly, a survey of fifty-five commercial sex workers in Portland, Oregon, found that the majority (78 percent) reported being raped by pimps and male customers forty-nine times a year on average. Additionally, 84 percent had been the victims of aggravated assault, often sufficient to require emergency room treatment; 53 percent had been sexually abused or tortured; and 27 percent had been mutilated (Hunter, 1993). In a study of 190 male-to-female transgendered individuals involved in commercial sex work in San Francisco, Clements-Nolle, Guzman, and Harris (2008) found that one-fifth reported inconsistent use of condoms during receptive anal sex in the past six months. Significant independent correlates of this behavior were histories of forced sex and crack-cocaine use.

El-Bassel's New York–based research team (El-Bassel, Witte, Wada, Gilbert, & Wallace, 2001) has focused considerable attention on these issues and has examined the key correlates of partner violence among female street-based commercial sex workers. These researchers have found that two-thirds of the women studied have experienced lifetime physical or sexual abuse, either at the hands of an intimate or commercial partner; one in eight of these women reported physical and sexual abuse by both intimate and commercial partners. Those women who during the previous year were homeless, whose main source of income was exchanging sex for drugs and money, who were injection drug users, who used sex in crack houses, and who suffered HIV/AIDS infection were most likely to report combined physical and sexual abuse.

International findings are also available. Following a study of commercial sex workers in four countries, Raymond et al. (2002) reported the existence of a complex relationship between substance abuse and violence in this population:

Some [commercial sex workers] encouraged buyers to use crack so buyers "would forget about sex altogether." Most of the women were habitual drug users (77 percent), and . . . used alcohol and drugs to deaden their feelings. [As one participant explained], "It would end up that I would just drink to get drunk to cover up what I was feeling—which was dirty and ashamed." Although many U.S. women said that they used drugs and alcohol prior to entering prostitution . . . it is simplistic to assume that they entered prostitution to support a drug habit. The cycle of substance abuse in which they are caught has its roots in the life history of abuse, neglect, and severe stress which all of the

(Continued)

respondents . . . described when asked about prior sexual abuse before entering the sex industry. [Many had] experiences of rape, incest, being witnesses to domestic violence, losing their primary home, being runaways, having a difficult home life, and economic destitution. . . . Much of their current substance abuse results from the accretion of abuse: sexual, physical, mental and economic prior to and within prostitution [p. 197].

Among street-based female commercial sex workers in India, Panchanadeswaran et al. (2008) found reports of various forms of severe intimate and commercial partner violence. Further, they found that traditional gender norms hindered the women's ability to negotiate the use of condoms with commercial sex partners. In other words, it is important to recognize that it is not just the nature of the sex trade that is at issue but also the identity of the people engaged in it: cultural subordination of women generally restricts the options available to women in the commercial sex trade.

International Cross-Border Sex Trade

A group of sex workers at special risk for the intertwined ravages of substance abuse, violence, and AIDS are those who get caught up in the international cross-border commercial sex trade (Singer, Salaheen, & He, 2004). Generally speaking, there is a strong link between migration and the geographical spread of HIV/AIDS and other infections. Studies have shown that extended or repeated overnight travel away from one's home community is associated with heightened risk for HIV infection. However, in the case of commercial sex trafficking—that is, the movement of, usually, women and girls across national boundaries for use as commercial sex workers—the link is particularly strong and its causes identifiable. Whatever their country of origin or ultimate destination, woman ensnared in the cross-border sex trade tend to come from impoverished families and the poorest (often rural) regions of their home countries, have limited formal education, and have their roots in the subordinated ethnic minority groups of their countries of origin. These factors, demarcating the weak social resources many women bring with them into the arena of commercial sex, are magnified many times in cross-border commercial sex trafficking. Women so trafficked are isolated from any means of traditional social support, often are illegal residents of the new country in which they find themselves, often have limited linguistic or cultural skills in this new country, are typically trapped in some form of debt to the traffickers, have limited knowledge of HIV prevention, and possess limited ability to negotiate preventive behaviors with clients or to access medical care through their handlers or elsewhere. Individuals' ability to protect themselves from HIV infection is measured in terms of their HIV/AIDS knowledge and learned prevention skills, social position and ability to command the labor of others on their behalf, level of emotional and material social support, possession or control over material resources such as prevention materials, freedom of movement, protection from violence, and overall health status. Looked at in terms of these measures, women in the commercial sex trade are clearly at high risk.

Explosive HIV epidemics, involving significant jumps in the prevalence of infection over a short period of time, have been recorded for a number of populations. Among female sex workers in Nepal, for example, between 1992 and 2002, there was a twenty-four-fold increase in the incidence of HIV infection. Certain conditions have been found to promote the rapid development of multiple infections. Thus, in a study of 246 young women and girls who were trafficked for commercial sex from Nepal to India (and medically examined upon repatriation to Nepal), Silverman et al. (2008) found that 30 percent tested positive for HIV infection, 20 percent for syphilis infection, and 4 percent for hepatitis B infection. Moreover, those who were HIV-positive were more likely than those who were HIV-negative to be infected with syphilis (31 percent versus 16 percent) and hepatitis B (9 percent versus 1 percent). High rates of coinfection and the rapid development of multiple infections among these women and girls, or what might be termed an explosive syndemic, occurred because of their typically young age at the time they were trafficked, inability to speak the language of their customers, limited agency to negotiate condom protection during sex, lack of social support, and being subjected to forced sex. Exemplary is Seema, a Nepalese girl who left the poverty of her home village to find work in the capital of Kathmandu when she was only twelve years old. She had dreams of becoming a movie star, but Seema was tricked into going to Mumbai and forced into prostitution (Brown, 1999). The enduring emotional effects of such inhumane treatment is seen in the high rates of anxiety, depression, and posttraumatic stress in Nepalese woman subjected to sex trafficking (Tsutsumi, Izutsu, Poudyal, Kato, & Marui, 2008). Examples like this affirm the critical importance of moving beyond biological factors in understanding syndemics.

Given their vulnerability, women involved in commercial sex in many locales have been found to have high rates of HIV infection. When the AIDS epidemic in Thailand was at its peak, for example, over 80 percent of HIV/AIDS cases in the country were attributed to commercial sex workers and clients (Viravaidya, 1993). In India, infection rates among commercial sex workers in some locales, such as Mumbai, exceeds 50 percent (DevNews Media Center, 2002). Similarly high rates of STD infection have been found in migrant sex workers in Italy (Matteelli et al., 2003).

SAVA AND PUBLIC HEALTH

Although having somewhat different components, correlates, and expressions across different places and populations, the SAVA syndemic represents a significant biopsychosocial interface in the contemporary world. Its initial description in the social science literature helped to spark efforts to build a transdisciplinary effort that seeks to elevate "public health inquiry beyond its many individual categories to examine directly the conditions that create and sustain overall community health" (Syndemics Prevention Network, 2005d). The syndemic propensities of HIV/AIDS are discussed further in Chapters Four and Five, following an examination in the next chapter of the several dimensions of syndemic complexity.

SUMMARY

This chapter and the three that follow it illuminate the nature of various syndemics and demonstrate the importance of these disease phenomena in people's lives in the contemporary world. They examine the diversity of diseases and other risks to health that are increasing their impacts on populations because of their syndemic interactions with other diseases and with unequal and unjust social conditions. As explained in this chapter, SAVA is the consequential interface of three health issues that are regularly reported in the mass media: substance abuse, violence, and HIV/AIDS. SAVA is noteworthy in the history of syndemic research because it was the first syndemic described and labeled as such in the public health literature. This chapter examined the specific mechanisms of interaction among the three conditions that constitute SAVA and the ways in which SAVA damages the health of several different populations, all of which are subject to significant social disparities.

KEY TERMS

endemic

epidemic

explosive syndemic

intimate partner violence

multidisciplinarity

pandemic

SAVA

syndemic

synergistic

enlightenment

QUESTIONS FOR DISCUSSION

1. Why does the study of syndemics promote multidisciplinary collaboration?

2. What is the origin of the term *syndemic?* What is its relationship to similar terms in epidemiology?

3. What is the SAVA syndemic? What is its historical importance in the development of research into syndemics?

4. What are some of the ways that the key elements of the SAVA syndemic interact in specific populations? What are the differences in the correlates and expressions of SAVA in these populations?

CHAPTER

EXEMPLARS

Syndemic Case Studies

After studying this chapter, you should be able to

- Define the term *microlevel of disease interaction.*

- Understand six types of microlevel interaction and how they contribute to the development of syndemics.

- Differentiate unidirectional from bidirectional disease interaction patterns in syndemics.

- Discuss how the syndemic perspective overcomes traditional barriers in disease discourse by bringing together understandings of acute and chronic diseases; infectious and noninfectious diseases; behavioral and physical health; and biological, psychological, and social factors in illness and well-being.

- Describe key features of four contemporary syndemics: the renocardiac, syndemic, the SARS–chronic disease syndemic, the asthma-influenza syndemic, and the diabulimia syndemic.

SYLLABLES IN THE BIOLOGICAL MESSAGE

The heading of this section comes from a passage in William James's *The Varieties of Religious Experience.* In this classic work on the psychology of religion, James addresses the question of whether it is regrettable that humankind has created so many different religions by arguing that "[e]ach attitude being a syllable in human nature's total message, it takes the whole of us to spell the meaning out completely." So too with the diverse processes and pathways that lead to syndemics, each is part of the total story of the syndemic phenomenon. This chapter presents concrete examples of some of the interactions that occur among diseases and other health conditions (for example, stress or malnutrition) and that lead to an increased disease burden. Of initial concern is what I call *the microlevel of disease interaction:* that is, the specific pathways and mechanisms of contact and exchange between two or more comorbid conditions clustered within a population and resulting in enhanced disease morbidity and morality.

VARIETIES OF MICROLEVEL DISEASE INTERACTION

This section introduces six ways that diseases have an impact upon each other, sometimes directly but at other times through the changes they cause to particular body systems and processes, including various layers and components of the immune system.

Enhanced Contagiousness

In the first type of disease interaction or epidemiological synergism, one disease promotes the contagiousness of another disease by helping it to gain access to vulnerable areas of the body. This type of interaction occurs, for example, between syphilis and HIV when the disruption of the multilayered epithelial barrier and genital-tract ulceration produced by the former supports sexual transmission of the latter, as discussed in Chapter Four.

Accelerated Virulence

In a second type of interaction between diseases the presence of one disease accelerates the virulence of another. Thus, as discussed more fully in Chapter Four, among patients coinfected with HIV and herpes a notable speeding up of AIDS pathogenesis occurs because of specific effects the herpes virus has on the pace of HIV viral replication. Various factors may be involved in this process, including specific herpes proteins (for example, ICP-0, ICP-4, and ICP-27) that enhance HIV replication efficacy (Schacker, 2001). In syndemics, coinfection commonly plays a role in triggering transition to a more active phase of microbe replication and resulting symptom expression.

Alterations of the Physical Body

In some syndemic interactions, such as those that occur between HIV and various opportunistic infections, alterations of the body caused by one disease promote progression of another disease. These alterations include changes in biochemistry (for example, damage or modulation of immune system components) and harm done to organ systems. Research at Japan's National Institute of Infectious Diseases, for example, has shown that some low-pathogenic respiratory bacteria that induce elastase (an enzyme that breaks down proteins) in the lungs may limit the important immune activities of neutrophils. Experiments with animal models (Ami et al., 2008) suggest that coinfection with such bacteria and SARS leads to severe respiratory disease characterized by extensive weight loss and high mortality, notably greater than that which occurs from SARS without coinfection. Bacterial alteration of the neutrophils, it appears, facilitates viral infection.

Alterations of the Emotions

As exemplified by the SAVA syndemic, social disorders have significant impacts on the emotional health of individuals and communities. Alterations of the emotions and mental health (owing to trauma or posttraumatic stress, for example), no less than physical diseases, can pave the way for other diseases to develop because our bodies biologize emotional experience (that is, transform it into bodily reactions and responses). Wright, Hanrahan, Tager, and Speizer (1997), for example, suggest that violence may be associated with the occurrence and increased severity of asthma among inner-city children. Children exposed to violence in their neighborhoods (for example, hearing gunshots or witnessing physical violence) are twice as likely as children not exposed to violence to experience wheezing and to use bronchodilator asthma medication for wheezing and almost three times as likely to be diagnosed with asthma (Wright & Steinbach, 2001). Emotional experience, in short, is a biological phenomenon of no less significance in the formation of syndemics than is disease seen as organic.

Gene Assortment

A fifth kind of disease interaction involves **gene assortment,** as seen in the movement of genes from one strain or subtype of a microorganism to another strain. HIV is characterized by a comparatively high number of mutations (because of the high error rate of its reverse transcriptase replication method), resulting in the development of multiple strains representing somewhat distinct local viral lineages. Human mobility, moreover, allows exposure to more than one strain, creating opportunities for simultaneous infection with two different strains at the cellular level (called *dual infection*), with gene mixing (that is, the movement of genes between virons of two strains) occurring during viral replication (a process called *copackaging*). In South Africa, for example, Rousseau et al. (2007) found gene mixing quite common in the subtype C strain of HIV they studied in KwaZulu-Natal province. Gene movement of this sort has had a significant impact on the evolutionary history of HIV, including enhancing HIV's overall virulence (Kijak & McCutchan, 2005). Additionally, recombination of the genomes of different HIV strains creates the opportunity for types of resistance to specific treatments that have emerged in distinct viral populations to be joined, contributing to the development of recombinant strains with multidrug resistance.

Iatrogenic Interactions

Yet another form of syndemic interaction involves the various ways in which the medical treatment provided for one disease is weakened by the actions of another disease. An instance of this pattern is seen in the case of the measles and HIV syndemic. Researchers in sub-Saharan Africa have found that HIV significantly reduces the efficacy of the measles vaccination, leading to primary and secondary vaccine failure among HIV-infected children and a high mortality rate (Helfand, Moss, Harpaz, Scott, & Cutts, 2005). Other iatrogenic syndemics have also been identified (as discussed in Chapter Eight), raising important questions about the degree of syndemic knowledge in biomedical practice (an issue also addressed in Chapter Eight).

Complexities of Interaction

Infectious agents from unrelated biological taxa can interact and cause increased disease burden. For example, a disease known as *scrub typhus* (mentioned in the Preface) is caused by bacteria transmitted by chiggers, the skin-burrowing larvae of the harvest mite, found in areas of heavy scrub vegetation. Scrub typhus has been found to interact with leptospirosis, a disease caused by a waterborne bacterium. Although these two diseases are caused by quite different microorganisms, outdoor activity in tropical settings is a shared risk factor for exposure to both and "coinfection with these two diseases is not uncommon" (Lee & Liu, 2007, p. 525). Another example of interaction by quite different pathogens is seen in the case of the virus-helminth interface described in Chapter Four. Unexpected interactions of this sort are not restricted to infectious diseases. Later in this chapter the case of diabulimia, an interaction between type 1 diabetes and an eating disorder, is discussed.

In some cases coinfection with two or more diseases can open up multiple syndemic pathways of interaction. In studies of human populations, for example, a lethal synergism has been identified between influenza viruses and pneumococcus; this is a likely cause of excess mortality from secondary bacterial pneumonia during influenza epidemics. A significant level of evidence indicates that the influenza virus alters the lungs in ways that increase pneumococcus adherence, invasion, and induction of disease. Other consequential changes, such as an alteration of the immune response that weakens the body's ability to clear pneumococcus (or alternately, an amplification of the inflammatory cascade) are also suggested by existing research.

In other cases syndemic interaction among diseases is apparent but the pathways of linkage are not yet clear. An example is the apparent interaction that occurs between type 2 diabetes mellitus and hepatitis C viral infection. Several factors are known to contribute to the onset of type 2 diabetes, particularly diet, obesity, and aging. The role of infection, however, is only beginning to be understood. It is known that risk for serious infections of various kinds increases significantly with poor diabetes control, but appreciation of more complex relationships between infection and type 2 diabetes is now emerging as well. Similarly, chronic obstructive pulmonary disease has been increasing in prevalence and has become a significant global source of human morbidity and mortality as well as rising health care costs, but the precise causes are uncertain. Intensification of the severity of chronic obstructive pulmonary disease is known to be associated with both bacterial and viral agents. Combined bacterial and viral infection has been found in about a quarter of severe cases. The exact mechanisms of interspecies interaction in such cases, however, are not well understood, leading to calls for new research (Sykes, Mallia, & Johnson, 2007).

Syndemic interactions need not involve only two diseases or other health conditions, as is clear from the case of the SAVA syndemic, where three epidemic conditions are involved. Additionally, an interaction may be **unidirectional** (one co-occurring disease or disorder affects another) or **bidirectional** (each disease finds a different expression than it would without the copresence of the other disease). The varieties of disease interaction and impact that have been described here contribute to the diversity of the syndemics that appear in the literatures of the various health sciences and of the social science of health, as discussed in the following sections in a number of exemplar syndemics.

SYNDEMIC DIVERSITY

The term *syndemics* labels diverse interacting configurations of diseases, disorders, and social conditions. Building on the case of SAVA—described in the last chapter as a tripartite syndemic that brings a behavior-linked emotional disease (substance abuse), interpersonally inflicted physical or emotional suffering (violence victimization), and an infectious disease (HIV/AIDS) together in the context of a particular set of social conditions (for example, inner-city poverty, discrimination, and blocked social advancement)—the remainder of this chapter presents case studies of four additional syndemics that emerge through a diverse array of connections among a contrasting assortment of diseases, disorders, and disparities. This discussion of syndemic variet-ies considers the specific diseases involved in each syndemic, several key dimensions of these diseases and their interactions (including *acuity* versus *chronicity, behavioral* versus *physical health, unidirectional* versus *bidirectional causality,* the *biopsychosocial mechanisms of syndemic interaction*), and the social and environmental factors that influence syndemic production. These four syndemics are

- The renocardiac syndemic

- The SARS–chronic disease syndemic

- The asthma-influenza syndemic

- The diabulimia syndemic

RENOCARDIAC SYNDEMIC

Chronic kidney disease is known as a quiet epidemic. This designation is a consequence of the fact that the onset of kidney disease is slow and symptoms are not evident until damage is considerable. As a result, although it is estimated that almost 20 million people in the United States have kidney disease, many do not know it. The course of this disease has five identifiable states. The fifth stage, also called the *end stage* (an administrative term signifying eligibility for Medicare payment for dialysis and trans-plantation), is kidney failure, a lethal condition (unless there is intervention) that is becoming increasingly common (by 2 percent a year) and is already requiring 400,000 people in the United States to receive dialysis treatment or a transplanted kidney to survive. This number has doubled in each of the last two decades and is expected to surpass 650,000 by 2010 (United States Renal Data System, 2000). Notably, kidney disease is not distributed equally across ethnicities or social classes. In the United States the incidence of end-stage kidney disease is significantly higher among blacks, Native Americans, and Asians than it is among whites. Hispanics have a higher incidence rate for kidney disease than do non-Hispanic whites (Tell, Hylander, Craven, & Burkart, 1996). The poor overall are also at greater risk than other economic groups for the development of kidney disease. Thus, by merging U.S. Bureau of the Census data with a database of patients who have initiated kidney dialysis treatment in the states of Georgia, North Carolina, and South Carolina between January 1998 and December 2002, Volkova et al. (2008) found that neighborhood poverty was strongly associated with higher rates of end-stage renal disease for both blacks and whites. There were ethnic disparities here too, however, with blacks being at greater risk across all levels of poverty. As Volkova et al. (2008) note, this finding suggests that the renal health of blacks may suffer more from living in poverty than does the renal health of whites. This suggestion has been interpreted as reflecting the fact that poor blacks face a double burden: poverty and color discrimination.

Health writers have regularly commented that the general population lacks a sound understanding of the kidneys, their complex role in sustaining life, and the diseases that put them at risk. As Peter McCullough, preventive medicine chief at William Beaumont Hospital in Michigan, observes, "The average patient knows their cholesterol. The average patient has no idea of their kidney function" (quoted in Neergaard, 2007). Research has shown that each of the body's two kidneys contains approximately 1 million filtering units called nephrons; each nephron is composed of a miniature filter and a tubelike structure lined with cells that process the filtrate and reabsorb water and useful body chemicals. Matter that is not retained is eliminated from the body. In kidney disease the nephrons are damaged and lose their capacity to filter the waste and surplus products of metabolism out of the bloodstream. Normally, the kidneys filter approximately fifty gallons of blood every day and produce about half a gallon of urine. Although the kidneys perform this vital filtration function, their broader role is to preserve the volume and chemical composition of the extracellular fluid that bathes and protects the body's tissues. In other words the "principle function of the kidney is not excretion, but regulation" (Cameron, 2002, p. 3). Additionally, the kidneys have a major role in regulating the blood levels of various minerals, including calcium, sodium, and potassium, and they produce several hormones, such as erythropoietin, which signals the bone marrow to produce red blood cells. As this multitude of vital functions suggests, kidney health is critical to overall health.

A feature of kidney disease of special interest from the syndemic perspective is that it appears to cause an acceleration of heart diseases, including myocardial infarction, heart failure, arrhythmias, and cardiac death. Moreover, this syndemic interaction, here named the *renocardiac syndemic,* causes people to die of cardiovascular problems long before their kidney disease reaches end stage (Schrier, 2007). At the same time, the pathway of interaction is not unidirectional: heart disease can set off kidney disease as well. Ronco, House, and Haapio (2008) comment that the "term 'cardiorenal syndrome' has generally been reserved for declining renal function in the setting of advanced congestive heart failure. Considering the complex and bi-directional relationship between the heart and the kidneys, we postulate refining the definition to recognize the symbiotic nature of these organs."

Several large research projects have offered some insight into the nature of these chronic disease interactions. In one of these projects McCullough et al. (2002) enrolled over 800 consecutive patients being evaluated for possible acute myocardial infarction following hospital admission with chest pains. They found that patients with advanced kidney disease (identified from renal function) or already on dialysis had higher rates of hypertension and evidence of coronary disease than the rest of the patients did. The most frequent in-hospital complication in the subsample with advanced kidney disease was the development of heart failure, which occurred in 36.5 percent of those with a low creatinine clearance rate. Creatinine is a compound formed by the metabolism of creatine, a biochemical that supplies energy for muscle contraction. Healthy kidneys excrete creatinine into the urine as metabolic waste. Measurement of blood creatinine levels is commonly used to evaluate kidney function. At thirty days after intake, this subgroup of patients had the highest rates of cumulative myocardial infarction, development of heart failure, and death (40 percent).

In another study McCullough et al. (2002) tracked over 35,000 people, with an average age of fifty-three years, who volunteered for a kidney function screening. These researchers used three markers of kidney function: the rate at which kidneys filter blood; levels of the protein albumin in the urine, a known sign of kidney dysfunction; and anemia, which is a sign that the kidneys are not properly signaling the bone marrow to produce red blood cells. They found that the odds of having cardiovascular disease rose as each of these kidney markers worsened. Most striking to these researchers was the death rate among participants, a relatively young group. In all, 191 participants died during the study, with those who had both kidney dysfunction and known heart disease having three times the death rate of those with only heart disease. Similarly, the Health, Aging, and Body Composition study (Deo et al., 2008) found that weakened kidney function is a strong predictor of cardiovascular death in individuals who do not have a prior history of cardiovascular disease.

In a meta-analysis of research on the relationship between kidney failure and cardiovascular risk, Vanholder et al. (2005) used a PubMed search to identify eighty-five relevant publications, eighty-two of which supported a link between these two conditions. In six studies in which chronic kidney dysfunction and cardiovascular disease were particularly well defined, the results confirmed the impact of kidney dysfunction on heart problems. Consequently, Vanholder et al. (2005) concluded that there is "a significant relationship between the markers of renal dysfunction and overall mortality and/or cardiovascular morbidity or mortality. One of the most relevant findings of this analysis is that the increase in cardiovascular risk occurs very early during the evolution of chronic renal failure" (p. 1053). Moreover, the studies reviewed by Vanholder and coworkers suggest (but do not confirm) several potential mechanisms by which kidney dysfunction could affect the heart. One candidate involves the accumulation in the body of nitrogenous waste products (a condition known as uremia) because of the failure of the kidneys to eliminate them. These noxious solutes may have damaging effects on the cardiovascular system, as several studies have identified a link between uremia and heart disease.

As noted, cardiovascular disease also has an impact on renal disease. That cardiovascular disease contributes to kidney problems is not a surprising finding, in that it involves narrowing of the arteries in all parts of the body, including the kidneys. But there also appear to be other ways in which the kidneys might be affected by developing heart problems. To investigate whether cardiovascular disease is a risk factor for either the development of kidney disease or the progression of existing kidney disease, Elsayed et al. (2007) combined the data for almost 14,000 participants in two longitudinal, community-based studies, the Atherosclerosis Risk in Communities Study and the Cardiovascular Health Study. Various heart-related health conditions, including silent myocardial infarction and angina, were used to define cardiovascular disease, and kidney function was defined in terms of rising creatinine levels and declining kidney function. Findings showed that having cardiovascular disease at the study baseline was associated with increased serum creatinine levels and declines in kidney function over time, suggesting that cardiovascular disease plays a role in kidney disease.

An additional suspected linkage in the development of kidney and heart disease lies in the bone marrow. Both the heart and the kidneys are known to send electrical signals to the red bone marrow found at the center of the larger bones to produce a type of stem cell that helps keep body organs in good working order. Stem cells from the bone marrow help the body form new heart muscle and blood vessels to replace damaged or worn tissue. Additionally, animal studies have found that these cells can reverse kidney damage. This research has been carried out with a group of genetically engineered mice that are missing genes needed to create the kidneys' blood filtration system, causing the mice to develop kidney failure. In mice given a bone marrow transplant, however, transplanted stem cells moved into the damaged areas of the kidney and began making repairs (Orlic et al., 2001). In both kidney and heart disease the triggering signals that activate body repair activities are diminished, producing a decline in the body's built-in ability to repair itself. The morbidity and mortality consequences of this decline can be severe.

In sum, research into cardiovascular disease and renal disease affirms multiple forms of deleterious interaction between these diseases, and barring intervention, the renocardiac syndemic significantly accelerates bodily decline and demise with significant public health impact.

SARS–CHRONIC DISEASE SYNDEMIC

The World Health Organization (2003) has dubbed SARS (severe acute respiratory syndrome) "the first severe and readily transmissible new disease to emerge in the 21st century." The first cases of this twenty-first-century disease occurred in Guangdong Province in the south of China during the time that our Hartford-based research team, in collaboration with local Chinese public health workers and social scientists, was involved in a study of syringe sharing among Chinese injection drug users in the Province (Duke, Singer, Li, & Pelia, 2003). The first official report of an outbreak of what appeared to be an atypical expression of pneumonia was based on 300 cases in Guangdong, in 5 of which cases the patient had died; it was sent by Chinese health officials to the World Health Organization (WHO) on February 11, 2002. Noteworthy in the report was the fact that almost a third of the cases were among health care workers. It was not until April of the following year that WHO was finally granted permission by the Chinese government to send an epidemiological team to Guangdong to assess the outbreak and to help identify the new disease.

Meanwhile, in February 2003, a Chinese physician, Dr. Liu Jianlun, from Zhongshan University in Guangdong, one of the health care providers treating the early cases of the new disease, made what he intended to be a short trip to Hong Kong. He stayed on the ninth floor of the Metropole Hotel in the Kowloon district, one of the most densely populated areas on the planet. Also staying in the hotel in a ninth-floor room at this time were Sui-chu Kwan and her husband, visiting from their adopted home of Toronto, Canada. Through some chance encounter between Dr. Jianlun and Sui-chu Kwan, perhaps merely riding together on the same elevator, the latter was infected with SARS and carried the disease back with her to Toronto.

Upon his arrival in Hong Kong Dr. Jianlun had felt well enough to go shopping and sightseeing with his brother-in-law, but by the next day he sought urgent care and was admitted to an intensive care unit, where he died of respiratory failure on March 4, 2003, having been exposed to the disease through his patients in Guangdong. His brother-in-law also died. Three days after Dr. Jianlun's death, Chi Kwai Tse, the forty-three-year old son of Sui-chu Kwan, showed up at the emergency room at Toronto's Scarborough Grace Hospital complaining of a cough and a fever. Because he was having a hard time catching his breath and appeared very anxious, he was admitted to the hospital and assigned a bed in the emergency room's observation ward, separated from other patients by only a sliding cloth curtain. Tse told the nurses that his seventy-eight-year-old mother, Sui-chu Kwan, a diabetic, had died at home two days earlier from what had been diagnosed as a chest infection of unknown origin, following her return from Hong Kong.

At first, doctors believed that Tse had tuberculosis, a disease that is not uncommon in the low-income, ethnically diverse Toronto neighborhood where he lived. But this diagnosis was soon in doubt because of the rapid decline in Tse's condition. Six days after being admitted to the hospital he too was dead. Then his wife died as well. Two of his siblings also got sick but recovered. Others who had had contact with Tse were also exhibiting respiratory symptoms, including Joseph Pollack, a patient with a heart condition who had been in an emergency room bed near Tse. After exposure to Tse, Pollack began coughing and registering a fever, and soon joined the list of local fatalities in what was quickly shaping up to be a frightening epidemic with an unknown cause. Within a few days a number of hospital staff began showing up as patients, all of them exhibiting fever and respiratory symptoms. Between February and September 2003, Health Canada reported on 438 probable or suspect cases of the new disease, primarily among people living in the Greater Toronto Area, and 43 of these patients died (Borgundvaag et al., 2004).

A major cosmopolitan city, Canada's largest urban area, and its economic capital, Toronto is known for its world-class leisure attractions and telecommunications, aerospace, transportation, publishing, software, and sports industries. It is generally not thought of as a center of contagious epidemics. As a result, the sudden appearance of the deadly disease of SARS produced an economic shock wave in The Big Smoke (one of Toronto's affectionate nicknames). Toronto businesses were hit hard, especially the tourism sector. Cancellations at area hotels led to an estimated $40 million in lost revenues during the month of April 2003 alone; audiences at the city's many playhouses and theaters dwindled; restaurants lost as much as 30 percent of their clientele; hundreds of tour bus rides were halted as were a series of major conferences and conventions, including one on health care. The Canadian Tourism Research Institute estimated that altogether the economic impact of SARS on Toronto's gross domestic product was $1.5 billion, or about 15 percent of the city's economy (Conference Board of Canada, 2003). Put simply, syndemics can be costly not only to human life and well-being but to fiscal health as well.

Outbreaks of the new infection also began appearing in hospitals in Hong Kong, Viet Nam, Singapore, the Philippines, and elsewhere in Asia, ultimately producing 8,422 cases and 916 deaths (with a case fatality rate of 11 percent) across twenty-nine countries and regions on five continents during the first wave of the epidemic.

In Hong Kong recognition of the new contagion began on March 10, 2003, when eighteen health care workers in a medical ward of the Prince of Wales Hospital, a public hospital located in Sha Tin in the New Territories district, reported that they were sick. Phone calls from workers at Prince of Wales Hospital to absent staff revealed that over fifty hospital employees had developed a fever and other symptoms. Twenty-three of these health care workers were admitted as patients on March 11 (cases were admitted at Queen Mary Hospital, Kwong Wah Hospital, and Pamela Youde Nethersole Eastern Hospital as well). These patients were screened for common viruses, including influenza viruses, respiratory syncytial virus, adenovirus, parainfluenza viruses, mycoplasma, and *Chlamydia pneumoniae*. None of these pathogens appeared to be the source of the new ailment. Ultimately, the index case was identified as a twenty-six-year-old ethnic Chinese man who had been admitted to the hospital on March 4. The patient had reported that he had begun having symptoms, including fever, chills, diarrhea, and cough, prior to his admission to the hospital. He had been housed in a general medical ward with no specific isolation precautions. Two days after this man was admitted to the hospital, other patients in the hospital also began reporting these symptoms, suggesting he had been the source of their infection. With antibiotic and other treatments the health of the index patient eventually improved and within a month he was symptom free. The infection continued to spread to new cases, however. By March 25, 156 patients had been admitted to the hospital, over 80 percent of whom had had direct or indirect contact with the index case. Of note, of these patients 19 had comorbid conditions, including diabetes; heart problems; and liver, kidney, and lung diseases. By the eleventh day of the outbreak, 5 of the 156 patients had died, all of whom had suffered from comorbid conditions.

Eventually, the novel disease spread outside the hospitals and over 1,500 cases were identified (Riley et al., 2003). Contaminated sewage was found to be responsible for an outbreak of over 300 cases in the Amboy Garden apartment complex. The immediate social impact was significant. Schools were closed in Hong Kong, and more than 1,000 people who had had contact with an identified patient were placed in quarantine (Lee et al., 2003). In a subsequent study of 1,755 cases of SARS in Hong Kong, involving 302 deaths, Leung et al. (2004) found that the time between a patient's first developing symptoms and being admitted to the hospital ranged from two to eight days and that among those who died of the new disease, the mean time from symptom onset to death was about twenty-four days. Predictors of worse outcomes included increased age, being male, and suffering from a comorbid condition.

In Vietnam, another country struck by the outbreak, SARS began to show up on February 26, 2003, with the admission to Bach Mai Hospital, a private hospital in Hanoi, of a traveler from Hong Kong, Johnny Chen, a Chinese American who had stayed on the same floor of the Metropole Hotel as Dr. Jianlun. Sixty-one patients were eventually hospitalized with SARS, in two Vietnamese hospitals, and six of them died. All SARS patients in the country were socially or behaviorally linked through one of the involved hospitals (as patients, staff, or visitors) to the first case (Ha et al., 2004). Ultimately, through strict infection control and diligent contact tracing, Vietnam became the first country to successfully contain its SARS outbreak.

In Singapore the Ministry of Health was notified on March 6, 2003, that three people who had traveled to Hong Kong in February had been admitted to local hospitals for pneumonia. These patients also had stayed at the same hotel as Dr. Jianlun. Soon other patients with similar symptoms were being hospitalized as well. The disease spread outside the hospital to taxi drivers, coworkers of the initial patients, and others. By April 30, 201 probable cases and 722 suspect cases had been reported in Singapore (Leo et al., 2003).

Through diffusion of this sort in and out of hospitals and also as a result of rapid international travel, SARS quickly became a global disease. Before long a coronavirus, termed *SARS Co-V,* a member of a family of large, single-stranded RNA viruses, was identified as the source of the new infection. SARS Co-V is spread primarily through coughing and sneezing that expels moist droplets containing the virus. Isolation of the virus in fecal and urinary samples suggests other routes of transmission as well. Within the body this virus targets the epithelial cells of the lower respiratory tract, resulting in diffuse lung damage, especially to important structures involved in gas exchange with the blood. Several other cell types may be infected, including the mucosal cells of the intestines, tubular epithelial cells of the kidneys, neurons of the brain, and several types of immune cells (Gu & Korteweg, 2007).

Epidemiological investigation has suggested an animal origin for SARS-CoV. The importance of zoonotic diseases (that is, those of animal origin) in human health is reflected in the fact that the major human emerging infectious diseases in recent years, including AIDS, Ebola fever, and avian influenza, have had their origin in interspecies transmission from animals. Since the appearance of the first cases of SARS in Hong Kong in 2003, intensive efforts have been invested in identifying an animal source of SARS-CoV (Vijaykrishna et al., 2007).

Research in China linked SARS-CoV to palm civet cats (a relative of the mongoose), raccoon dogs, and ferret badgers sold in local food markets in Guangdong. At the open-air Qingping market, for example, a variety of mammals, birds, and amphibians are on sale to roaming shoppers. Subsequently, horseshoe bats of the genus *Rhinolophus* were identified as a natural reservoir of SARS-like coronaviruses. Vijaykrishna et al. (2007) concluded that "bats are likely the natural hosts for all presently known coronavirus lineages and that all coronaviruses recognized in other species were derived from viruses residing in bats" (p. 4012).

As mentioned earlier, in some locales comorbidity with diabetes was found to be associated with death and with poorer outcomes (with a relative risk of 3.1), such as intensive care unit admission and clinical need for mechanical ventilation. Individuals with cardiopulmonary disease were also at heightened risk if infected (Chan et al., 2003). A review by Chen et al. (2005) of the clinical features and outcomes for 67 SARS patients in Taiwan, for example, found that an age greater than sixty-five years and preexisting diabetes mellitus were independent predictors of acute respiratory distress symptoms. Whereas the overall mortality rate in this group of SARS patients was 31.3 percent (21 out of 67), the mortality rate for patients who developed acute symptoms was 63.6 percent (21 out of 33). Similarly, in Taipei a study of the clinical characteristics of patients who died of SARS found that among 36 probable cases and 17 suspected cases, 8 patients died. Of the fatal cases, all except 3 had comorbid chronic conditions, such as diabetes mellitus, hypertension, coronary artery disease, or chronic obstructive pulmonary disease (Wong et al., 2003). In Hong Kong an analysis of over 1,700 SARS patients (Leung et al., 2004) determined that the case fatality rate for patients with comorbid chronic conditions was 46 percent, compared with 10 percent for patients who lacked such conditions. In short, diabetes, cardiopulmonary disease, and several other chronic conditions have been established as independent predictors of mortality as well as level of morbidity in SARS patients (Yang et al., 2006). In all the studies described earlier the comorbid conditions involved were characterized by either decreased cardiopulmonary capacity or a compromised immune system, suggesting two ways in which SARS and chronic diseases interact. As Gu and Korteweg (2007) comment with reference to the role of immune function in the course of a SARS infection, "A compromised immune response may lead to aggravation of SARS-CoV-induced lung injury, which otherwise might not have been so widespread and devastating" (p. 1145). Additionally, these researchers note that prolonged infection with SARS or treatment of the disease with high doses of corticosteroids (or both) appears to result in opportunistic infection by various other pathogenic agents, such as methicillin-resistant *Staphylococcus aureus.* The SARS epidemic of 2003, in sum, did not exact its toll alone; its most severe and deadliest effects, those that pushed SARS into the headlines and caused apprehension worldwide, were the result of interactions with several chronic diseases.

In the SARS epidemic a phenomenon appeared that has also been seen with some other diseases, including rubella, laryngeal tuberculosis, and Ebola—namely that a few individuals appear to have spread the disease to many others. In the case of SARS, exposure to certain infected individuals was far more likely to be associated with contracting the disease than was exposure to other infected people. Individuals who appear to be more efficient in transmitting the disease have been termed *superspreaders.* Dr. Liu Jianlun was clearly a superspreader in Hong Kong, for example. Superspreading might result from a particular combination of host, environment, and virus interactions. The most probable explanation is that it involves far greater than average viral shedding (that is, coughing or sneezing out water droplets with high viral loads). This may result from the patient's being at an advanced stage in the disease course, when the immune system's ability to contain the pathogen is diminished. Additionally, there is some evidence that the presence of comorbidities results in high viral loads and heightened shedding. In other words, syndemic factors may play a role not only in how well an individual fares once he or she contracts SARS but also in how infective he or she is and how likely to contribute to the spread of SARS.

ASTHMA-INFLUENZA SYNDEMIC

Allergic diseases constitute the sixth leading cause of chronic illness in the United States, directly affecting the lives of 17 percent of the population. Asthma is a prominent allergic disease, characterized by episodic inflammation and narrowing of the small airway passageways in the lungs. This restriction causes the airways to be sensitive, and as a result they have strong allergic reactions (which are immune system responses) to various triggers, including pollens, cockroach excrement, molds, perfumes, and other chemicals regularly released into indoor and outdoor environments. (In just the last fifty years humans have originated approximately 60,000 new varieties of such triggers; Unklesday, 1992.) In an allergic reaction the immune system has identified a particular irritant as a significant threat to which it mounts a major defensive reaction. Once the tissues lining the air passages have been overstimulated by an allergenic substance, reexposure or even cold air, exercise or exertion, or stress can trigger an asthmatic attack. Asthmatic attacks are episodic, occur especially at night or early in the morning, and are characterized by symptoms like wheezing, coughing, chest tightness, and shortness of breath. The condition can range from mild to severe; so too can individual asthmatic episodes, which at their worst can be fatal.

According to the Centers for Disease Control and Prevention, in 1980 asthma affected only about 3 percent of the U.S. population (Moorman et al., 2007), but the rate of affected individuals has been steadily climbing in recent years, especially in low-income, urban, ethnic minority neighborhoods. In 2001–2003, asthma directly affected the lives of about 7 percent of the U.S. population (Moorman et al. 2007). Asthma among children has been increasing at an even faster pace, with the percentage of children with asthma jumping from 3.6 percent in 1980 to about 9 percent in 2005 (Akinbami et al., 2005).

Today, asthma is the most common chronic medical condition among children in the United States. Nearly one of every ten U.S. children has asthma; however, the disease is not equally distributed across ethnic groups. Asthma prevalence among American Indians, Alaska Natives, and African Americans is 25 percent higher than it is among white people (Akinbami, Rhodes, & Lara, 2005). Among Puerto Ricans the rate of asthma is 125 percent higher than it is among non-Hispanic white people and 80 percent higher than among non-Hispanic black people. Puerto Ricans also have far higher rates of asthma than other Hispanic subgroups do. For example, among people diagnosed with asthma, people of Puerto Rican descent are more likely to have had an asthma attack during the preceding twelve-month period (62.3 percent) than are persons of Mexican descent (51.4 percent). Similarly, the poor are more likely to have asthma than are people from wealthier social strata (Moorman et al., 2007).

Research in Connecticut (a state with a comparatively large Puerto Rican population) among school-aged children, for example, found that socioeconomic status (SES) has a significant impact on asthma rates. Schools with students classified as having a high SES have the lowest prevalence rates (Schwab, Cullen, & Schwartz, 2000). Similarly, Miller (2000), using multivariate models, found that asthma prevalence and asthma-related hospitalization and emergency room visits in Connecticut declined with increased income levels for the children of all ethnic groups except African Americans. Additionally, lower SES has consistently been found to be associated in Connecticut with increased asthma severity and mortality. This is particularly true in Hartford, the impoverished capital city of Connecticut. In 2003, inner-city asthma hospitalization rates (51.5 per 10,000 people) were significantly higher in Hartford than they were for the state of Connecticut as a whole (22.4 per 10,000 people) or for the United States as a whole (37 per 10,000 people) (American Lung Association, 2003). Overall hospitalization rates for Hispanic and African American youths in Connecticut in 1999 were five times higher than they were for white children (Schwab et al., 2000).

The prevalence of asthma is increasing not only in the United States but worldwide. A number of developed countries now have levels of asthma that are even greater than U.S. levels, including Australia, in which 13 percent of the population suffers from this disease, and New Zealand, which at 20 percent has the highest known incidence rate. Asthma is much less common in developing countries, as would be expected given the likely role of industrial pollutants in triggering this condition.

Given its growing prevalence, asthma presents an interesting arena for conceptualizing syndemics because coinfection with various viruses (for example, respiratory syncytial virus and influenza A virus) is high among people with asthma. Further, infants and young children with asthma who also suffer from infection with viruses have a higher probability of asthma exacerbation and of asthma attacks of greater severity than do children with asthma who are not coinfected (Zhao, Takamura, Yamaoka, Odajima, & Iikura, 2002), suggesting the likelihood of a synergistic interaction.

What has been called the *asthma-influenza connection* (Petaschnick, 2004) is of particular interest from a syndemic perspective because it involves adverse interaction between a chronic disease and an acute disease. This interaction has drawn medical attention because people with asthma have been found to have a high risk of developing complications when suffering from an influenza infection. Although often confused with the common cold by those it infects, influenza (a name derived from the Italian word for influence) is a significant infection characterized by an array of symptoms, primarily fatigue, fever, chills, muscle and head pains, sore throat, and coughing. Although the incidence of influenza varies widely from year to year, in an average year in the United States over 200,000 hospitalizations are linked to this disease (Thompson et al., 2003). People tend to confuse bouts of influenza and colds because, like cold viruses, the pathogens that cause influenza infect the upper respiratory tract—the nose, throat, and major air passages leading into the lungs. In these areas the influenza virus targets and kills cells making up the ciliated epithelia that line the surface tissue. These cells have tail-like projections 5 to 10 micrometers long that beat in coordinated waves, sweeping mucus (which traps small particles such as bacteria), dirt, and other foreign matter out of the lungs and thus serving an important immune function. Smokers, for example, are more prone to infection because tobacco smoke destroys these ciliated cells (although they regenerate once smoking ceases). Because influenza also kills these cells, it "can pave the way for other microbes to enter areas of the upper respiratory system damaged by the virus and spread into the lungs or occasionally other parts of the body" (Barnes, 2005, p. 338). This continues until the immune system overcomes the virus and new ciliated cells develop.

Research has revealed that the genome of the virus that causes influenza, more popularly known as the *flu* since early in the twentieth century, is composed of eight single strands of RNA. When the cells of an organism (human, water fowl, pig, or other species) are coinfected by two different influenza strains, genetic mixing occurs, leading to the rise of a novel strain. Biomedicine has responded to this pattern. Each year WHO uses early case reports to predict the strains most likely to be dominant and useful for developing an appropriate vaccine. The U.S. Food and Drug Administration (FDA) maintains the Vaccines and Related Biological Products Advisory Committee (VRBPAC), and the specialists on this committee then make recommendations for the content of each year's U.S. vaccine, actually a cocktail of targeted vaccines for three influenza strains. Sometimes the predictions of the strains that will be most prevalent are incorrect, and influenza then takes a higher than usual toll. For the years from 1979 to 2001, for example, Dushoff, Plotkin, Viboud, Earn, and Simonsen (2005) calculated that the average annual number of deaths due to influenza in the United States was approximately 41,000. In the 2007–2008 season, however, many people were infected late in the flu season, even those who had been vaccinated, by a strain not covered by the available inoculation (Dao et al., 2008). As a result the number of deaths attributed to influenza was above the average for seventeen consecutive weeks (Centers for Disease Control and Prevention, 2008a). That means, according to Theodore Eickhoff (2008), a voting member of the VRBPAC, that the "pressure to develop a four-component vaccine will likely be substantial in the future." Moreover, thinking of the impact of major influenza pandemics of the past (see Chapter Seven), Eickhoff (2008) notes that the significant jump in influenza cases "did not take long to back up local health care systems, reminding us once again that our health care system has virtually no excess capacity, and it does not take much of an increase in demand to overwhelm the system. [An influenza] pandemic of moderate severity, such as we experienced in 1957–1958 and again in 1968, would likely collapse our present health care system. One shudders to think what a 1917–1918 severity pandemic might do."

Or what a syndemic, which can introduce challenges far above those created by influenza alone, might do.

Contributing to the annual health impact of influenza are interactions with other diseases. Influenza is particularly dangerous when it leads to pneumonia, which can be fatal in vulnerable populations, such as the very young, the malnourished, and those under considerable stress. Moreover, as Randolph Lipchick, professor of medicine in the Division of Pulmonary and Critical Care Medicine at the Medical College of Wisconsin, observes: "Individuals with asthma are at high risk of developing complications after contracting the influenza virus. . . . When these individuals get an upper respiratory infection like influenza, they frequently have a flare-up of their asthma. Respiratory infections are more serious in patients with asthma, and can often lead to pneumonia and acute respiratory distress. . . . It isn't just adults with asthma who are adversely affected by the influenza virus, but children as well" (quoted in Petaschnick, 2004). Indeed, according to the National Foundation for Infectious Diseases (2004), "During the 2003–2004 influenza season, 153 influenza associated deaths in children younger than 18 years were reported to the CDC. Of those 2 to 17 years of age who died who had a known underlying risk, 43 percent had asthma" (p. 4).

Studies with animal models suggest the nature of the synergistic interaction that may occur between asthma and influenza. Research by Riese, Finn, and Shapiro (2004) with mice, for example, found that influenza infection affects a component of the immune system known as the helper T cell, which comes in two varieties: Th1 and Th2. Each produces its own type of cytokine, a hormonal messenger that controls the activity of immune cells, especially those involved in immune inflammation reactions. As Playfair (2004) explains, each of the thirty or so varieties of cytokine has a specific function, such as stimulating immune cells "to enlarge, to divide, to release antibody, to switch from making IgM to IgG, etc." (p. 126). Th1 cytokine triggers a proinflammatory response that helps the body fight infection by both activating body defenses at the site of infection and by slowing the flow of blood that would otherwise carry a virus from the site to other parts of the body. Excessive inflammation, however, is dangerous and results in tissue damage. This is where Th2 plays a role because it tends to trigger an anti-inflammatory response. Excessive production of Th2, however, weakens the protective functions of inflammation. In a healthy body there is a natural balance between Th1 and Th2, allowing sufficient inflammation to effectively fight a particular infection without going overboard and damaging body tissues. There is some evidence to suggest that a bodily imbalance in favor of Th2 can lead to the development of allergic hypersensitivities. Further, in mice, influenza infection has been found to enhance subsequent allergen-triggered asthma symptoms. The mechanisms involved in this process are dendritic cells (immune cells, found on the inner linings of the nose, lungs, stomach, and intestines, that display fragments of foreign antigens on their surfaces to be read and responded to defensively by other immune system cells) and interferon gamma, an immune-modulating cytokine (Dahl, Dabbagh, Liggitt, Kim, & Lewis, 2004). Even after the immune system successfully clears influenza from the body, these durable immune components remain in the lungs, attenuate pulmonary inflammation, and trigger asthmatic reactions. It is likely that other respiratory viruses produce a similar response in asthmatics. With rising rates of asthma (a pattern likely to continue given global warming and other global pollution) and the always pending threat of new influenza strains, the asthma-influenza syndemic is likely to be of increasing importance in human health in future years.

DIABULIMIA SYNDEMIC

Diabulimia is a syndemic involving type 1 diabetes and the food disorder known as bulimia, one of several food disorders that interact syndemically with diabetes. Behaviorally, this syndemic is manifested in the underuse of insulin as an intentional weight-loss strategy. It has developed among (primarily) young individuals who have both bulimia (or another restrictive food disorder) and type 1 diabetes and who have recognized certain possibilities in the function of insulin, a hormone that plays a central role in the body's metabolism of sugar, starches, and other food components into energy for daily activities (Hoffman, 2001). Among other effects, insulin stimulates body muscle and fat cells to take in glucose from the circulating blood system. Disruptions of this vital process result in the development of a glucose starvation state involving high blood glucose levels (and urination of glucose), poor protein synthesis, inadequate glucose storage in liver and muscle tissues (which the body relies on as a source of needed energy during the night and other fasting periods), blood vessel damage, and a condition known as diabetic acidosis (or ketoacidosis) in which the body burns stored fat instead of glucose. Rapid burning of body fat leads to the development of ketones (a waste product of using fat for energy) in the blood and mounting body acidity. The health consequences, such as neuropathy, blindness, kidney disease, and renal failure, may be severe, and without medical intervention, life threatening.

It is estimated that more than 20 million U.S. adults and children have diabetes, about 7 percent of the total population. The World Health Organization (2004a) estimates that globally at least 170 million individuals suffer from diabetes. Moreover the number of diabetes cases has been going up around the world, and it is expected that there may be almost 350 million cases by 2030. Diabetes-related complications are major causes of morbidity and mortality for these individuals.

There are two primary forms of diabetes (a third form is associated with pregnancy). Most people (90 to 95 percent) with this disease have what is known as type 2 diabetes, a condition that usually involves inadequate insulin production and ineffective use of available insulin, a state known as insulin resistance. Type 1 diabetes is an autoimmune (that is, an aberrant immune response) disease in which the body's immune system destroys the insulin-producing beta cells normally clustered on the islets of Langerhans on the surface of the pancreas. The result is hyperglycemia (that is, an overload of blood sugar). The trigger for this autoimmune response is not known, although some suspect there is viral involvement (for example, viruses from the Coxsackie virus family, which stimulates the onset of German measles, may be involved). There may be a genetic propensity for type 1 diabetes as well, and genes in the human leukocyte antigen region on the short arm of human chromosome 6 have been proposed as a likely candidate (Donner et al., 1997). Other causes, such as various infections and dietary patterns, have also been suggested.

Whatever its exact cause(s), type 1 diabetes can be controlled through the injection of manufactured insulin (created in a laboratory using a genetically altered strain of the *Escherichia coli* bacterium). This usually requires a person with diabetes to administer regular doses of insulin through self-injection. Studies of medical adherence in people with diabetes show that various unintentional factors, including depression, certain personality attributes (for example, poor internal locus of control or low adaptability capacity), poor memory, inadequate health literacy, and challenging and conflicted family environments (Alan et al., 1990; Hauser et al., 1990; Kravitz et al., 1993; Lin et al., 2004) reduce the quality of diabetes self-care. In contrast, in cases of bulimia or anorexia nervosa, individuals may select to limit insulin intake to achieve weight loss (as well as avoid the weight gain that can be associated with insulin use). Sufferers of these often brutal eating disorders, which involve abnormal body perception and intense sensitivity to being perceived as fat, engage in various techniques (depending on the particular disorder) such as obsessive dieting, intensive exercise, compulsive use of laxatives, and regular vomiting as strategies for experiencing a sense of control in their lives (Singer & Singer, 2008). As Stuart Brink, a senior pediatric endocrinologist at the New England Diabetes and Endocrinology Center in Massachusetts, observes, "You don't have to vomit. You don't have to purge. You don't have to use laxatives. . . . You just have to let your sugar stay high" (quoted in Mendelsohn, 2008). Exemplary is the case of Kate, a nineteen-year-old sophomore, as described by Cooper (2008):

> Kate first developed eating disorder symptoms late in high school, by which time she had been managing her diabetes in a relatively independent manner for about seven years. During her junior year, Kate got a stomach virus and couldn't keep food down. When she recovered, she was pleased to see a thinner image in the mirror. Although she'd been taught the serious risks associated with withholding insulin, she began to skip shots with the intention of losing weight. And later, during her senior year of high school, a troubled Kate began to binge-eat. "It was a tough year," she said, "and I didn't know how to deal with anything, so I began to eat obscene amounts of food, and then I would beat myself up for eating so much when I was supposed to be on a diet. . . . It's so intense, . . ."I can't stop. It's a nightmare" [p. 1A].

Significantly, the control needs of young people with eating disorders may be in conflict with the actions of worried parents who may feel they must be actively involved in ensuring that their children maintain vigilant glycemic monitoring (through regular blood sugar testing) and management (through dietary adherence, regular exercise, and timely insulin injection) to avoid the life-threatening complications of diabetes. Parent-child conflict in such situations may propel insulin restriction behavior. Conversely, perceived intrusive parental control may contribute to the emergence of eating disorder patterns among young diabetics. As Goebel-Fabbri, Fikkan, Connell, Vangsness, and Anderson (2002) emphasize, "Once an eating disorder and recurrent insulin omission becomes entrenched, a pattern develops which is hard to break—one of chronic hyperglycemia, depressed mood, fear of bodyweight gain, and frustration with diabetes management" (p. 155).

These researchers conducted an eleven-year follow-up study with 234 women with type 1 diabetes that suggests the significant health consequences of diabulimia. At baseline 30 percent of these women reported insulin restriction. At the time of the follow-up, 26 women of the total sample had died, with those who had reported insulin restriction at baseline having a threefold increased level of risk for mortality. In addition those who had reported insulin restriction and had died had done so at a younger age than women who did not report restricting insulin intake (forty-five versus fifty-eight years). Those who had reported insulin restriction and were still living had higher reported rates of kidney disease and foot problems at follow-up. Note Goebel-Fabbri et al. (2008), "Our data demonstrate that insulin restriction is associated with increased rates of diabetes complications and increased mortality risk" (p. 418). In another study, Bryden et al. (1999) examined the interface of eating disorders and insulin misuse in a sample of 76 male and female adolescents with type 1 diabetes over an eight-year period. On average, female participants were overweight during adolescence, and both sexes were overweight as young adults. As they grew older, concern about weight and body shape increased significantly for both sexes, expressed as increased levels of dietary restraint (although none of the participants met existing criteria for either anorexia nervosa or bulimia at intake or follow-up). At follow-up, 30 percent of the female participants, but no male participants, reported underuse of prescribed insulin to control weight.

An important component of diabulimia is societal and corporate emphasis on thinness. Women and girls in particular are regularly exposed to the message that in order to be happy, successful, and popular, they must be thin. Corporate participation in the promotion of a cultural ideal of thinness is seen in movies and television programming targeted to young adult females; magazines and novels aimed at female readers; and patterns of model selection, messages, and products in commercial advertising. As aptly described by Kathryn Putnam Yarborough (1999) of the Center for Eating Disorders at St. Joseph Medical Center: "It is hard to not be affected by the media bombarding us constantly with the message, 'Thin is in!' On TV commercials we are told to 'lose weight fast' or 'exercise for thirty minutes' to have a beautiful body. Magazines displaying thin, attractive women try to convince us that we are not okay until we 'slim our thighs.' The overriding message is that we need to change something about ourselves in order to be loved or successful. In particular, if we have thin, fit bodies, 'our lives will be perfect.'"

Fashion models, for example, whose body weight tends to be far lower than the average body weight of females of comparable height in the general population, are rewarded, glamorized, and held up as a cultural ideal. Notably, research with fashion models has found that they report significantly more symptoms of eating disorders than do controls of the same age and of comparable social and cultural backgrounds (Preti, Usai, Miotto, Petretto, & Masala, 2008). Being preoccupied with having a thin body and experiencing social pressures such as media modeling, concern with weight and shape, peer concern with thinness and dieting behaviors, and weight teasing by peers are known risk factors for the onset of eating disorders (Thompson & Hammond, 2003; Taylor et al., 2003). In an examination of the effects of exposure to reality TV cosmetic surgery programming, for example, 147 women participants were assigned to one of two groups; one group watched *The Swan* and the other watched a home improvement program (*Clean Sweep*). Participants were surveyed at the end of the video viewing and at the two-week follow-up; results showed that compared to the women who watched the home improvement program, women who watched the cosmetic surgery program exhibited a higher level of internalization of a thin body ideal at baseline and expressed lower self-esteem at follow-up. The researchers (Mazzeo, Trace, Mitchell, & Gow, 2007) concluded that media emphasis on thinness and body image may be contributing to disordered-eating attitudes and behaviors among young women, especially those who have internalized a thin body ideal. As this study suggests, corporate profit seeking is a critical component of the biopsychosocial interaction that underlies the diabulimia syndemic.

In recent years it has also been discovered that abusive drinking (or other drug use) and eating disorders are sometimes linked, a condition sometimes referred to colloquially as *drunkorexia*. This condition has been documented by Food for Thought: Substance Abuse and Eating Disorders, a study carried out by the National Center on Addiction and Substance Abuse (CASA) (2003) at Columbia University. The study found that in the United States, as many as half of the individuals suffering from an eating disorder also abuse alcohol or other drugs (compared to about 9 percent in the general U.S. population). At the same time, 35 percent of individuals diagnosed with a substance abuse disorder also suffer from an eating disorder. According to Joseph Califano, former U.S. Secretary of Health, Education and Welfare, and the president of CASA, "For many young women, eating disorders like anorexia and bulimia are joined at the hip with smoking, binge drinking and illicit drug use. . . . This lethal link between substance abuse and eating disorders sends a signal to parents, teachers and health professionals— where you see the smoke of eating disorders, look for the fire of substance abuse and vice versa" (National Center on Addiction and Substance Abuse, 2003). To limit their caloric intake, many people with eating disorders avoid alcohol. Some, however, use alcohol and other drugs to self-medicate anxiety. And yet others use alcohol, as well as stimulants like cocaine and methamphetamine, to suppress their appetites. Many of these patterns are also being recorded in other societies. For example, high rates of alcohol abuse have been described by Suzuki, Takeda, and Matsushita (1995) among Japanese high school students suffering from anorexia.

SUMMARY

This chapter has described four exemplar cases to illustrate several dimensions of **syndemic complexity.** The first case, the renocardiac syndrome, involves bidirectional interaction between two chronic diseases that have been called *sedentary diseases* because of their frequency among populations and groups with less active life patterns. These diseases occur at notably higher rates among ethnic minority populations, an association that has been explained in terms of lower socioeconomic status; poorer diets; and living in higher density, more dangerous, and more stressful social environments (Franks, Muennig, Lubetkin, & Jia, 2006). The second case, the SARS–chronic disease syndemic, involves adverse interactions between an acute disease and several chronic conditions, such as diabetes, that are disproportionately common among the poor. In this instance the chronic conditions were found to contribute to enhanced severity and lethality in an infectious disease. The third syndemic, asthma-influenza, reverses the direction of enhancement found for SARS and chronic diseases; in the asthma-influenza syndemic the infectious disease plays a role in triggering and intensifying chronic disease episodes. Again, the chronic disease of concern was found to be significantly more frequent among the poor and among ethnic minority populations. The final case, the diabulimia syndemic, an entwining of diseases of body and mind, reveals another aspect of the role of political and economic factors in the emergence of syndemics. Here the group of concern is females who are subject to social manipulation, including those of relatively high SES and with wealthier families. Add to this profile of syndemic complexity the case of SAVA (discussed in the prior chapter), and it is evident that syndemics cut across (and hence blur the boundaries that divide) traditional dimensions of disease classification (for example, chronic versus acute conditions, behavioral versus physical disorders, and infectious versus noninfectious diseases). Indeed, as discussed in Chapter Five, in some cases the distinctions traditionally assumed between noninfectious chronic diseases and acute infectious ones have in recent years faded altogether.

KEY TERMS

accelerated virulence
asthma-influsenza syndemic
bidirectional disease interaction
diabulimia syndemic
drunkorexia
enhanced contagiousness

gene assortment
iatrogenic interaction
renocardiac syndemic
SARS–chronic disease syndemic
syndemic complexity
unidirectional disease interaction

QUESTIONS FOR DISCUSSION

1. Differentiate microlevel and macrolevel disease interactions.
2. Describe the various ways in which diseases interact at the microlevel.
3. Identify the key features of the renocardiac syndemic.
4. Why did having a prior chronic disease affect SARS patients?
5. What is the nature of the disease interaction in the asthma-influenza syndemic?
6. How do emotional and biological health interact in the diabulimia syndemic?

CHAPTER

HIV/AIDS AND OTHER INFECTIONS

Immune Imparity and Syndemogenesis

After studying this chapter, you should be able to

- Explain the key role of interactions between HIV/AIDS and other diseases in producing the devastating global toll of HIV/AIDS.

- Understand the specific ways in which HIV/AIDS acts together with various transmittable diseases categorized as *opportunistic* because they are most apt to cause infection in the presence of specific health conditions.

- Recognize how HIV/AIDS interacts with other infections, including major scourges like sexually transmitted diseases, tuberculosis, and malaria, that are not limited to opportunistic contagion.

- Describe the specific channels and mechanisms through which HIV contributes to the impact of other infectious diseases and how, in turn, these other diseases amplify the adverse outcomes of HIV/AIDS infection.

- Appreciate the fundamental role of social conditions in increasing the likelihood that HIV/AIDS will interact with other infectious diseases.

ASSESSING THE HIV/AIDS SYNDEMICS

Over 25 million people in the world have died of AIDS, making this disease one of the most deadly pandemics in recorded history. Each day almost 7,000 people become infected with HIV and over 5,700 die as a result of HIV/AIDS. The number of people living with HIV/AIDS worldwide was estimated to be approximately 33 million in 2007 (UNAIDS & World Health Organization, 2007). In the United States, approximately 1 million cases of AIDS have been reported, disproportionately among ethnic minority populations. The disease is nearly seven times more frequent among African Americans and three times more frequent among Hispanics than it is among non-Hispanic whites (Fenton & Valdiserri, 2006).

The full impact of HIV/AIDS, and the reason it is a leading cause of mortality worldwide (and the primary cause of death in some places, like sub-Saharan Africa), stems from its syndemic interaction with various other diseases. HIV has been found to work together with a wide array of pathogens that cause hepatitis, tuberculosis, malaria, leishmaniasis, herpes and other sexually transmitted diseases (STDs), and many other diseases. At the same time, HIV/AIDS disease interacts adversely with various noninfectious diseases and disorders, not only interpersonal violence and drug abuse (as described in Chapter Two) but also kidney disease, food insufficiency, behavioral health problems, and cardiovascular diseases, among others.

This chapter's discussion of the nature of HIV and its frequent role in the emergence of syndemics, a process called **syndemogenesis,** begins with an examination of interactions between HIV/AIDS and other infectious diseases. In part because of the damage it wreaks on the immune system, HIV/AIDS is a critical element in the rise of new syndemic interactions that involve both unidirectional and bidirectional influences (that is, HIV/AIDS has an effect on other diseases and other diseases in turn have an effect on HIV/AIDS). Indeed, HIV/AIDS first came to light because of its role in the sudden appearance in young men of a cancer (or cancer-like infection) known as Kaposi's sarcoma (KS), which was first described over 100 years before the HIV/AIDS epidemic but previous to it was seen primarily in the elderly or in people being treated with immune suppression drugs following an organ transplant. A treatable but not yet curable disease, which shows up as dark, raised blotches on the skin, oral cavity, GI tract, lungs, and lymph nodes, KS is caused by an infection with sarcoma (KS)–associated herpesvirus (Olsen, Chang, Moore, Biggar, & Melbye, 1998). Before long, HIV/AIDS was linked not only with KS but with a host of other opportunistic infections of diverse origins as well.

This chapter discusses several AIDS-associated opportunistic infections and then considers a range of infections, including malaria and tuberculosis, that are known to interact adversely with HIV/AIDS and that may be opportunistic at times but are not found only among individuals with compromised immune systems. These diseases have caused epidemics independent of HIV/AIDS (although often in syndemic interaction with other diseases). (Chapter Five addresses the syndemic interaction of HIV/AIDS with noninfectious diseases, for which the channels of influence may be different.)

OPPORTUNISTIC INFECTIONS AND HIV/AIDS

The role of HIV/AIDS in opening the door to numerous other infections and other disorders is, in the third decade of the epidemic, a well-known story. By definition, as established by the Centers for Disease Control and Prevention (CDC), diagnosis of AIDS requires laboratory confirmation of HIV infection in a person who also has a CD4 T-cell count of less than 200 cells/μl or who has an opportunistic comorbidity. The list of often life-threatening conditions that make up the inventory of AIDS and opportunistic disease syndemics is frighteningly long and biologically varied, including various bacterial and mycobacterial infections (for example, *Mycobacterium avium* complex, bacillary angiomatosis, and tuberculosis), fungal infections (for example, candidiasis, aspergillosis, cryptococcal meningitis, and histoplasmosis), protozoal infections (for example, microsporidiosis, *Pneumocystis carinii* pneumonia, and toxoplasmosis), viral infections (for example, hepatitis, herpes, and progressive multifocal leukoencephalopathy), and malignancies (for example, non-Hodgkin's lymphoma, cervical cancer, and anal cancer).

In Puerto Rico, for example, where AIDS is comparatively prevalent, Gomez, Fernandez, Otero, Miranda, and Hunter (2000) report finding the following rates of **opportunistic infections** among over 900 HIV/AIDS patients recruited for a prospective longitudinal study of the natural history of the local AIDS epidemic: *Pneumocystis carinii* pneumonia, 38.5 percent; candidiasis, 28.4 percent; toxoplasmosis, 20.3 percent: wasting syndrome (discussed later in this chapter), 16.5 percent: and tuberculosis, 11.9 percent. (These percentages total more than 100 because some patients had more than one opportunistic infection.) Other samples have displayed different tapestries of opportunistic diseases, but whatever the array of conditions and their relative prevalence, the entwining of these diseases with HIV/AIDS is complex. Pugliese, Andronico, et al. (2002), for example, have conducted research showing that human papillomavirus (HPV) correlates with greater immunosuppression in HIV-positive women. In other words, in this syndemic interaction HIV-associated damage to the immune system facilitates HPV infection, which can trigger the development of cervical cancer. Among women in the United States, drug use and sexual relations with a drug user are the most common routes of HIV infection, adding yet another health condition to the intricate development of an HIV-related cancer.

SEXUALLY TRANSMITTED DISEASE SYNDEMICS

Although spread in several ways, HIV/AIDS is primarily a sexually transmitted disease, and this is the major means of its diffusion worldwide. Within its range, which is essentially global at this point, it encounters and interacts with many other sexually transmitted infectious diseases. Some of these interactions have been mentioned in previous chapters, such as the role of other sexually transmitted diseases (STDs) in causing lesions that enhance the ability of HIV to infect human bodies. Other kinds of interaction between HIV/AIDS and STDs are also of concern in syndemics research.

Pugliese, Torre, et al. (2002), for example, investigated the effect of coinfection with HIV and human herpesvirus type 8 (HHV-8) among women. They found that compared to HIV-positive women who tested negative for HHV-8 infection, those who were coinfected with both viruses exhibited accelerated deterioration of their immunological and hematological statuses (Pugliese, Torre, et al., 2002). This suggests a consequential interaction with important implications for individuals at risk for sexually transmitted diseases.

STD/HIV Prevalence

Existing research has shown that rates of other sexually transmitted diseases in people living with HIV infection vary from 15 to 25 percent, depending on the population (Kalichman, Rompa, & Cage, 2000). To investigate the extent of STD clustering, Miller, Liao, Wagner, & Korves (2008) administered a structured questionnaire to over 200 women involved in drug use in Brooklyn, New York. In addition to HIV, the women were screened for herpes simplex virus-2, syphilis, gonorrhea, chlamydia, and trichomoniasis. Seventeen percent of the women in the sample tested positive for HIV infection, and almost 80 percent of this subgroup was infected with herpes simplex virus-2; in addition, 37 percent had trichomoniasis, 11 percent tested positive for chlamydia, and 2 percent had a gonorrheal infection. Few of the women were aware that they suffered from sexually transmitted diseases other than HIV. Excluding HIV, the average number of STDs per study participant was 1.3, with HIV-infected women being significantly more likely to test positive for multiple STDs. Further, HIV-infected women were more likely to be involved in commercial sex transactions, and those who reported crack cocaine use were more likely to suffer from multiple sexually transmitted diseases. Similarly, a study of primarily poor HIV-positive women in Rio de Janeiro, Brazil, found that although some STDs (for example, chlamydia and gonorrhea) were not common, others were quite prevalent, with 50 percent of participants having a coinfection with human papillomavirus (Grinsztejn et al., 2006). These studies affirm common patterns of sexually transmitted disease clustering at both individual and group levels.

In recent years, there have been notable increases in HIV rates among men who have sex with men in the United States, Europe, and in other developed countries. Evidence suggests that an important contributing factor in this rise in HIV infection (following earlier declines) is the cohort of recently infected individuals with acute HIV infection, a phase in the natural history of HIV/AIDS characterized by very high HIV loads but negative HIV test results (at least with standard HIV detection technologies in use in most community settings). Because coinfection with HIV and the pathogens that cause other sexually transmitted diseases heightens the risk of HIV transmission over a longer period of time than acute HIV infection (which is relatively brief acting alone), syndemic interaction also may be of considerable importance in current rising rates of HIV among men who have sex with men (Buchacz et al., 2008).

Syndemic Patterns of Herpes

One group of pathogens with members commonly transmitted through sexual contact consists of the herpes viruses, a group that has attracted increasing attention since the 1960s. From a syndemics standpoint, herpes viruses are noteworthy because they tend "not to act alone, and instead require some other agent of disease, genetic weakness, or physiological upset for the development of herpes vesicles, small blisterlike sores" (Barnes, 2005, p. 31). The interaction of the herpes viruses with HIV has been the subject of extensive research. Over thirty studies have demonstrated that herpes simplex virus type 2 (HSV-2) is associated with two to four times greater risk for HIV infection, especially in the Americas, Africa, and Asia. Indeed, as Corey, Wald, Celum, and Quinn (2004) point out, "Of all the sexually transmitted diseases (STDs), there appears to be true epidemiologic synergy between these 2 viruses, in that HIV-1 incidence is increased in parallel with HSV-2 prevalence among HIV-1-negative and -positive persons, and HIV-1 prevalence increases HSV-2 incidence" (p. 435). When co-occurring, the natural course of both diseases is altered.

That herpes is a more significant factor in the transmission of HIV than are other STDs is seen in a revealing study by Gray et al. (2001) of the probability of HIV-1 transmission per sexual event (coitus) among monogamous, heterosexual, HIV-1-discordant couples (with the HIV-positive partner not receiving highly active antiretroviral therapy [HAART]) in Rakai, Uganda. Although symptoms of or laboratory-confirmed infection with gonorrhea, chlamydia, and trichomoniasis did not increase the per event risk of HIV transmission, the HIV-negative partner was five times more likely to become infected with HIV during a single sexual contact if he or she was already infected with herpes. This enhanced susceptibility was greater if the HIV-negative partner had evident herpes symptoms but was still significant in asymptomatic infected partners.

Various studies suggest that the interaction between herpes and HIV is conditioned by the recentness of the HSV-2 infection. In a study in rural Tanzania of over 750 adults, del Mar Pujades Rodriguez et al. (2002) found that increased risk for HIV infection was greater in people who had been infected with HVS-2 within the last two years than it was in those with older HIV infections. Similar findings were obtained among male and female STD clinic patients and commercial sex workers in Pune, India (Reynolds et al., 2003), and men who have sex with men in the United States (Renzi et al., 2003). The significant role of herpes in HIV prevalence is also suggested by the research by Weiss et al. (2001) in four urban African populations. They found that the frequency of HSV-2 was a primary predictor of whether a population had a high or low prevalence of HIV infection.

The bidirectionality of this syndemic is seen in the fact that the presence of HIV appears to promote herpes epidemics. Studies in both Zimbabwe and Uganda have found higher rates of HSV-2 acquisition among HIV-positive individuals than among the HIV-negative (Kamali et al., 1999; McFarland et al., 1999). An alternative interpretation of the findings of these studies, however, is that individuals who have contracted HIV engage in more frequent sexual risk than other people do and that this increases their likelihood of also acquiring herpes.

STD/HIV Infection Risk and Cultural Context

Risk for STD infection is highly contextualized and varies by population and social and geographical setting. In research that my colleagues and I conducted on **sexually transmitted disease syndemics** in several cohorts of sexually active emergent adults (eighteen to twenty-four years of age) living in inner-city Hartford, Connecticut (Singer et al., 2006), for example, we found high rates (11 to 22 percent) of individuals reporting they had been told by a doctor or nurse that they had a sexually transmitted disease, with females being more likely than males to report having ever had an STD. Infection rates appeared to reflect a tendency to suspend condom use early in a relationship on the grounds that participants believed they had moved past a casual level of interaction into a more serious romantic phase, one that contradicted continued condom use in that it communicated lack of trust to a partner. At the same time, however, participants feared getting too deeply involved with a single individual as this increased the potential for feeling hurt and suffering embarrassment if it were found that this partner had cheated on them (something most participants believed would happen) or if this partner eventually rejected them. In response, participants adopted an emotional protective strategy of maintaining various kinds of relationships "on the side," in addition to their main partner. Moreover, primary relationships were often relatively short lived because of the multiple challenges to sustaining them in a resource-poor, stressful, and unsupportive social environment, one in which arrest for various offenses was common, residential stability uncertain, and regular employment hard to acquire. As a result, participants engaged in a series of overlapping romantic and sexual relationships that often did not include consistent condom use. Risk for HIV and other STD infections in these cohorts was, in short, the consequence of a cultural logic of emotional self-protection (for example, by having multiple relationships, allowing the seriousness of any one relationship to be denied) in a context of challenging social conditions that in themselves put participants at risk for diverse emotional and physical assaults.

Our investigation of sexual behavior and health risk among inner-city youths and young adults in Hartford was part of a two-site, CDC–supported study that employed both qualitative and quantitative approaches to data collection. Identification of sexual behaviors began with a series of focus groups, during which we learned about various types of casual and romantic relationships and a range of sexual practices. In-depth, individual sexual life history interviews informed us about many participants' early age of sexual debut; clarified how participants' relationships began, progressed, and ended; and revealed participants' tendency to engage in multiple, overlapping relationships as a way of limiting their investment in any single bond and the emotional upset of rejection or relationship failure. Having a subgroup of participants maintain coital diaries and conducting a survey taught us about the contexts and frequency of various sexual behaviors and the number of partners typical of our participants. All of these methods contributed to our appreciation of how poverty and discrimination influenced sexual decision making and behavior in this population.

HEPATITIS AND HIV/AIDS SYNDEMIC

The viral diseases of hepatitis and HIV/AIDS have been called the *twin epidemics* (Highleyman, 2003), in part because of their similarities and in part because of the consequences of coinfection. Of special concern with regard to coinfection is the liver disease hepatitis C, which is stimulated by the hepatitis C virus (HCV).

HIV/HCV Cotransmission

Both HIV and HCV are rapidly replicating RNA viruses, and both are transmitted through blood-to-blood contact and exchange. A common route of cotransmission is multiple-person syringe use (often referred to in the literature as *syringe sharing*) among injection drug users (Singer et al., 2000). Segurado, Braga, Etzel, and Cardoso (2004), for example, carried out a cross-sectional study to determine the prevalence of HCV infection in a cohort of people living with HIV/AIDS in Santos, Brazil. They found that the cohort's overall rate of HCV seroprevalence was 36 percent. However, the rate was significantly higher (85 percent) among injection drug users compared to noninjection drug users (21 percent). Further analyses of study data revealed that HCV infection among injection drug users was independently associated with syringe sharing. In contrast, no association was found with a person's lifetime number of sexual partners, having a history of STD infection, or having had sex with commercial sex workers. Among noninjection drug users in the sample, HCV infection was independently associated with having a sexual partner who was an injection drug user. Similarly, in Madrid, Spain, a study of patients admitted to a large HIV/AIDS treatment facility between 1996 and 2000 found that over 80 percent overall were current or former injection drug users. Of these, 12 percent had been admitted because of chronic viral liver disease. Looked at over time this group had increased from 9 percent (1996) to 16 percent (2000). Over the same period of time the percentage of deaths due to liver disease in this population increased from 9 percent to 45 percent (Martín-Carbonero et al. 2001).

These similarities between HIV and HCV notwithstanding, there are important differences between these two viruses as well. Unlike HIV, HCV does not integrate into human cells, is not easily transmitted sexually (unless a person is immunocompromised), and among injection drug users, rates of HCV infection are far higher than rates of HIV infection, reaching 90 percent in some populations.

Health Consequences of Coinfection

Interaction between HIV and HCV in coinfected individuals has significant health consequences. Worldwide, one-third of HIV-infected individuals suffer from chronic hepatitis C virus infection. In Western countries, liver disease is the second leading cause of death among people with HIV/AIDS, and hepatitis C virus infection accounts for the majority of cases of liver disease in this population. An array of studies show that HIV infection leads to hepatitis infections that are more aggressive than those in individuals not infected with HIV (although effects in the reverse direction—HCV on HIV—are less clear). Specifically, HIV infection in a person with hepatitis C is associated with higher levels of the hepatitis C virus in the bloodstream, more rapid progression to liver disease, and increased rates of both cirrhosis and liver cancer. These negative outcomes appear to be the consequence of the inability of the immune system to contain HCV when under assault from HIV. Even in cases where it appears that the body has been able to clear HCV, as the immune system deteriorates, HCV replication renews (Kim et al., 2006). Additionally, it has been found that HCV and HIV coinfection can complicate treatment. Some anti-HIV drugs have proven to be hepatotoxic (poisonous to the liver) in people suffering from liver damage due to chronic hepatitis. Moreover, the different drugs used to treat HIV and hepatitis can interact, producing undesirable side effects.

TUBERCULOSIS AND HIV/AIDS SYNDEMIC

Science historian J. N. Hays (2000) has written that "AIDS is . . . the logical partner of tuberculosis" (p. 302). By this he meant, in part, that this epidemiological partnership involves the teaming up of a new and in some ways still emergent disease with a classic disease of the past (whose historical impact is revealed in one of its many nicknames: the "captain of all the men of death"). What was old has become new again and that which is novel has acquired an ancient partner. As a result, as succinctly described by Barnes (2005), "The fear of tuberculosis has returned" (p. 157).

The historical depth of tuberculosis (TB) is revealed by the earliest scientific evidence of the disease. Analyzing the metacarpal of an extinct long-horned bison radiocarbon dated to 17,870 (plus or minus 230) years before the present, Rothchild et al. (2001) found evidence of pathological changes suggestive of TB infection. A bovine form of TB continues to exist, and was likely the source of human infection, dating to the domestication of cattle.

Unknown at the time Hays made the observation quoted here was the fact that the pathogens involved in AIDS and TB—one a virus, the other a bacterium—are partners in another sense as well: they share a common infectious strategy. Both subvert the surveillance functions of dendritic cells to avoid immune system detection, though in different ways. HIV is able to bind with a receptor component of dendritic cells and is transported by those cells to lymphoid tissues, where the virus can infect and reproduce in T cells. *Mycobacterium tuberculosis,* the primary pathogenic cause of tuberculosis, also affects dendritic cells (and by way of the same cell component), primarily to down-regulate the cells' signaling role in mounting immune responses to the detection of pathogens (van Kooyk, Appelmelk, & Geijtenbeek, 2003). Also like HIV, *M. tuberculosis* has an immune cell as its primary target, only in this case it is the *macrophage* (a name derived from the Greek words for "big eater" and reflecting the generalized role of these cells in engulfing and digesting both pathogens and the debris of cell breakdown, a process known as phagocytosis).

The understanding of the human relationship with tuberculosis has been significantly informed through the recent development of a new scientific discipline, *paleomicrobiology,* a field devoted to the study of ancient pathogens through the direct detection, recovery, and analysis of their DNA from fossil material (or in some instances even from preserved soft tissues or from soils in which bone and tissue were once buried). Zink et al. (2003) used the methodologies of paleomicrobiology to analyze the bone and soft tissue samples derived from eighty-five ancient Egyptian mummies from several tomb complexes in Thebes West for the DNA of ancient *Mycobacterium tuberculosis.* Twenty-five samples indicating presence of the bacterium were obtained from individuals from several of these tomb complexes (dating from 2050 B.C. to 500 B.C.). Similarly, Konomi, Lebwohl, Mowbray, Tattersall, and Zhang (2002) analyzed tissue samples from the genital areas of twelve mummies from the Andes Mountain region of South America (dating from 140 A.D. to 1200 A.D. and now in the possession of the American Museum of Natural History collection in New York). *M. tuberculosis* DNA was detected in two of these samples.

Identification of this airborne microbe dates to the golden age of germ theory. It was first isolated and described in 1882 by Robert Koch, an achievement that earned him the Nobel Prize in Physiology or Medicine over twenty years later. Its genome was sequenced in 1998. Other mycobacterial species, including *M. bovis, M. africanum, M. canetti,* and *M. microti,* have subsequently been identified, but these have not for the most part been found to cause tuberculosis except among the young and adults with compromised immune systems. *M. bovis,* however, is the source of about 3 percent of pulmonary TB cases and 9 percent of all nonpulmonary cases in humans worldwide.

Today tuberculosis is responsible for one in every four preventable deaths worldwide. Nearly 2 billion people, over one-third of the world's population, are infected with *M. tuberculosis,* with new infections occurring at the rapid pace of one per second (World Health Organization, 2008d). Most of these individuals, however, are asymptomatic, and only 5 to 10 percent of people who are infected with *M. tuberculosis* (and who are not coinfected with HIV) will actually become sick at some time during their lives. Left untreated, half of those who do become sick would die of the disease.

Syndemic Patterns of Tuberculosis

TB is like HIV/AIDS in another respect as well: it tends to be involved in syndemics featuring complex biosocial interactions. Thus TB is most common in "populations rendered susceptible by instability of residence, mixing of populations, forced migration, breakdown of government and social institutions that provide order and protection, major life-threatening events, poor sanitation, high rates of certain other diseases, such as measles, [and] exposure to chemicals and particles which irritate the deep lung" (Wallace & Wallace, 1998, p. 84). A further connection between these two diseases, one Hays had in mind in his characterization of tuberculosis and AIDS as partners, is the role the latter disease is playing in resolving an old curiosity about tuberculosis: why do such a small percentage of those who are infected ever develop symptoms? This feature of TB is poignantly described by Paul Draus (2004), a health research scientist, in the case of his grandfather. In 1962, while working in his garage in Chicago, Draus's grandfather, then fifty-four years old, slipped and banged his chest against his car. When the pain did not resolve he visited his doctor, who upon examination told him he had a tumor. He was admitted to the hospital for surgery uncertain if he would ever leave. When he awoke from the operation, he was initially put in a postoperative recovery room but a little later was suddenly and without explanation moved to an isolation room. Hospital staff entered and left his room wearing masks, but no one explained why he was being secluded, and he was, Draus reports, "confused, alienated, and afraid" (p. 1). Finally, his son's fiancée, a nursing student, arrived for a visit and discovered the reason for his special treatment. What was in his chest was not a tumor but an old TB infection, dating to his youth, that had reactivated and was once again infectious. Draus's grandfather had been diagnosed with TB during his earlier outbreak but, like many others who contracted the disease in the era before antibiotics, had been sent to a sanatorium and had recovered. He thought he had fully recovered, in the sense that the pathogen had been destroyed. But what in fact had happened, as is commonly the case in otherwise healthy adults, his immune system had responded to the detection of the tuberculosis bacteria by encasing them in scar tissue; there they had remained in a dormant stage for decades. His aging body, damaged over the years by heavy smoking and alcohol consumption, ultimately suffered a weakening of his immune defenses and the microbe began reproducing once again. A different path to the same end was trod by Eleanor Roosevelt, who died of a reactivated case of bone marrow tuberculosis—acquired years earlier during her activist visits to tenements and settlement houses—triggered by the impact of her arthritis medicine on her immune system.

In the contemporary world, HIV is having the same effect on individuals harboring *M. tuberculosis* as the ravages of age and toxic chemicals had on Draus's grandfather and arthritis medicines had on Eleanor Roosevelt. Specifically, HIV completes a task that *M. tuberculosis* often is unable to achieve on its own in an otherwise healthy host, blocking immune response sufficiently to allow the infectious agent's free replication. Even though, as Geijtenbeek et al. (2003) observe, "The ability of *M. tuberculosis* to exist as a latent infection of the host suggests that mycobacteria are able to suppress cellular immune responses" (p. 7), they, unlike HIV, are not by themselves able to devastate the immune system.

Bidirectionality of Effect

As a result, people infected with HIV who are also exposed to *M. tuberculosis* are 800 times more likely than people exposed to *M. tuberculosis* but not infected with HIV to develop active TB (Lockman et al., 2003; Narain, Raviglione, & Kochi, 1992). In South Africa, for example, between 50 and 80 percent of TB patients are HIV positive (National Department of Health [South Africa], 2006), and HIV has played a central role in causing the soaring rates of TB infection in that country and in developing countries. Asia has the highest number of cases of tuberculosis (60 percent of the global total) and has experienced a striking rise in HIV seroprevalence (22 percent of the global total), resulting in growing rates and consequences of coinfection (Vermund & Yamamoto, 2007). It is estimated that between 9 and 14 million Americans are infected with TB bacteria. As of 2005, the CDC estimated that 9 percent of all U.S. TB cases and nearly 16 percent of cases among individuals between the ages of twenty-five and forty-four were among people coinfected with HIV. Among coinfected individuals, 63 percent are black (CDC, 2007; Glynn & Rhodes, 2005).

The HIV/AIDS and TB interaction is bidirectional and takes several forms. On the one hand, HIV infection, in addition to increasing the risk of reactivation of latent tuberculosis, also plays a role in the progression of a TB infection, specifically in the acceleration of tuberculosis infection within the body—including those strains of TB bacteria that are drug resistant—and in the interpersonal transmission of the disease. Individuals coinfected with HIV and TB are thirty to fifty times more likely than people with only latent TB infections to progress to active (that is, symptomatic and infectious) TB. Also, unlike distinctly opportunistic infections associated with HIV, tuberculosis may arise throughout the course of HIV infection. Pulmonary TB, the disease known as *consumption* during the nineteenth century, can occur very early during HIV infection, whereas TB infection in other parts of the body, known as extrapulmonary or atypical TB, follows the appearance of the more profound immunodeficiency caused by long-term HIV infection. On the other hand, it appears that TB infection in an HIV-uninfected individual results in activated T cells that are more susceptible to HIV infection upon exposure. Further, TB accelerates the course of HIV infection by stimulating viral replication and accelerating the decline in the body's census of CD4 T cells. TB modulation of the host immune system includes dysregulation of host cytokines, chemokines, and chemokine receptors on the surface of leukocytes, an activity that diminishes the ability of the immune system to slow HIV pathogenesis. A T cell activated in response to *M. tuberculosis* infection and infected by HIV produces more human immunodeficiency virus than a quiescent cell, increasing HIV expression (Toosi et al., 2004; Villacian, Tan, Teo, & Paton, 2005). Moreover, malnutrition often accompanies HIV and TB, and because it negatively affects both of these infections, the interaction of these three significant threats to health has been described as a source of "triple trouble" for human well-being (van Lettow et al., 2003).

The Urgency of Drug Resistance

This complex array of synergistic interactions affirms Hays's idea that AIDS is the "logical partner" of tuberculosis. Together they overwhelm immune defenses, giving them the well-deserved nickname of the "deadly duo." As Swaminath and Narendr (2008) stress, "The global impact of the converging dual epidemics of tuberculosis (TB) and human immunodeficiency virus (HIV) is one of the major public health challenges of our time" (p. 527). The sense of urgency common in discussions of this syndemic is fueled at least in part by the growing spread of drug-resistant, multidrug-resistant, and extensively drug-resistant (XDR) forms of TB. In 2006, for example, in Tugela Ferry, a hamlet just north of Durban in KwaZulu-Natal province in eastern South Africa, an outbreak was reported among HIV-infected individuals (Gandhi et al., 2006) of extensively drug-resistant TB (that is, three of the six medicines used as the last line of defense against TB proved ineffective against this new TB strain).

Fifty-three cases were identified, almost all of which (52 cases) died following a median survival time after diagnosis of just sixteen days. Following the initial report, over 250 additional cases were identified, with mortality dropping to 85 percent. Many cases of multidrug-resistant TB were also reported in Tugela Ferry, 90 percent of these patients were coinfected with HIV, and they had a morality rate approaching 70 percent. Since the initial outbreak, additional cases have been found at thirty-nine hospitals in South Africa's other eight provinces. As Erstad (2006) stresses: "As part of a syndemic, XDR TB will have disastrous and fatal effects on people and health care in South Africa and even poses a threat to world health. At the time of the emergence of XDR TB in South Africa there was no therapy available in the country. The extreme strain has spread to all provinces in the country, being prevalent in almost 10% [of] all tested [multidrug-resistant] TB cases" (p. 47).

Reflecting a growing frustration that this syndemic is being overlooked, Nesri Padayatchi, an epidemiologist and expert on drug-resistant TB with Caprisa, a Durban-based AIDS research consortium, has proclaimed, "It's an emergency, and we're not reacting as if it were an emergency" (quoted in Wines, 2007).

Beyond interaction with HIV, tuberculosis is part of another syndemic of growing importance, TB and diabetes. A growing concern of public health officials is that the increasing prevalence of diabetes may threaten global efforts to control TB. In a metastudy assessing research conducted using different designs and in diverse regions of the world, Jeon and Murray (2008) found that suffering from diabetes increases the risk of developing active TB by three times in TB-infected individuals compared to people who infected but do not have diabetes. At greatest risk are younger people and populations with high rates of TB. Given the rising global rates of diabetes, which are expected to double by the year 2030, and the increasing presence of drug-resistant TB, this syndemic has the potential to have a significant impact on human health. This potential is suggested by Jeon and Murray's calculation that in Mexico, diabetes accounts for 67 percent of the active TB cases found among people suffering from diabetes (representing 11 percent of the active TB cases in the Mexican population). In developing countries where the incidence of TB is even greater and the mean age of the population is lower, as in India, diabetes may account for over 80 percent of the incident pulmonary TB among people with diabetes (representing approximately 15 percent of the incidence of TB in the total population) (Stevenson, Forouhi, Roglic, Williams, & Lauer, 2007). Several mechanisms of interaction among people with poorly controlled diabetes have been suggested by various studies, including an impact on the Th1 and Th2 cell balance that results in a drop in Th1 immunity; a reduced capacity for oxidative killing by neutrophils; and reduced leukocyte bactericidal activity. In short, existing studies strongly support the view that diabetes directly impairs the innate and adaptive immune responses that counter the proliferation of *M. tuberculosis* and keep TB inactive. The impact of TB on diabetes is less clear, and it is possible that TB and diabetes form a unidirectional syndemic. Together, in interaction, these two potentially lethal diseases have been described as "a brewing double trouble" for human health (Kant, 2003, p. 83).

MALARIA AND HIV/AIDS SYNDEMIC

The connection between malaria and HIV/AIDS, the former a vector-borne disease and the latter transmitted through various body fluid exchanges, represents the coming together of two major pathogenic killers in the contemporary world.

One of the earliest scourges known to human societies, malaria has left deep and enduring footprints across human history. Reference to this debilitating and deadly disease is found in ancient Chinese, Indian, Egyptian, Greek, and Roman documents. The misery it inflicts on the human body was attributed in the pre-germ-theory era to toxic fumes rising from decomposing matter in swamps, marshes, or other torpid bodies of water, as noted in Chapter One. Followers of Hippocrates' methods thus explained that the source of this affliction was the drinking of long-stagnant water. Two thousand years later, one of Shakespeare's characters, the slave Caliban, curses Prospero, his master, saying, "All the infections that the sun sucks up / From bogs, fens, flats, on Prosper fall and make him / By inch-meal a disease!" (*The Tempest,* II, ii), affirming the long persistence of traditional beliefs about diseases from this source. In all, Shakespeare mentioned ague in eight of his plays, including *The Tempest* (Reiter, 2000). Even after the development of germ theory, the source of malaria was initially misidentified by Edwin Klebs, the German pathologist who first isolated the diphtheria bacillus, and Corrado Tommasi-Crudeli, an Italian bacteriologist, as a microbe living in damp soil, an organism they named Bacillus malariae. It was not until 1888 that the French physician Charles-Louis-Alphonse Laveran accurately identified one of the pathogens that cause malaria—for which he won the Nobel Prize in 1907—and that malaria's true complexities as a vector-borne disease transmitted by mosquitoes began to be known to science.

Impact of the Malaria Epidemic

It is widely recognized that the "global impact of malaria is staggering" (Jones & Williams, 2004, p. 156), and that efforts to stamp out the disease, such as the United Nations' Global Malaria Eradication Programme, launched in 1955, have ended in failure. The disease is especially prevalent in the *malaria belt,* a broad tropical swath across the middle of the planet. It is estimated that there are 300 to 500 million cases of malaria each year in Africa alone, resulting in 1.5 to 2.7 million deaths, most of them (90 percent) among children under five years of age. Two thousand children die each day from this disease in Africa, making it the leading cause of death of African children. Malaria is the reason almost a fourth of all Zambian babies do not live to experience their fifth birthday. Those who survive infection suffer recurrent attacks as the pathogen moves through its developmental phases, including the process of schizogony (also known as merogony), a type of asexual reproduction peculiar to pathogenic protozoa (Finkel, 2007). Children who have endured an initial bout of malaria may suffer lifelong health challenges, including significant neurological problems.

Actual disease patterns vary depending on the local endemicity of the pathogen. In some parts of Africa the disease has achieved holoendemic status: virtually everyone is infected. In places where people experience repeated exposures over time, a degree of immunity develops. It limits severe disease expression but rarely fully eliminates reinfection and hence does not stop subsequent subacute expression of the disease.

There are over 3,500 mosquito species on planet earth, and all of them require blood to carry out their reproductive process, but only a small number feed on humans. Of those that do, several are transmitters of pathogens that produce disease in humans (including yellow fever and dengue), but only an *Anopheles* mosquito can transmit the sporozoites (the developmental stage prior to the infection of a new host) of any of the four species of protozoa of the genus *Plasmodium* connected to human malaria: *P. falciparum, P. vivax, P. ovale,* and *P. malaria,* with *P. falciparum* being the most widespread as well as the most lethal. Others of the 200 or so species in the genus *Plasmodium* infect a wide range of other hosts, including lizards, birds, water buffalo, bats, and monkeys.

The consequences of contracting malaria are well known and include extreme anemia, fatigue, fever, headache, and chills over a number of days. Additionally, the disease increases pregnant women's risk of miscarriage, stillbirth, or delivering low birth weight infants. The pattern is well described by van Eeuwijk (2000) for three villages in Minahasa, a peninsular region in Indonesia, where "malaria remains the main source of sickness . . . [and] causes 62 percent of all illness cases in the villages . . . [taking] a heavy toll on human lives, particularly babies and children under five. Four to five times a year every villager suffers from regular malaria attacks" (p. 89).

The health and social costs of malaria have been so great and have burdened human populations for so long that an array of adaptations—genetic (for example, red blood cell deformities that prevent pathogen reproduction), settlement, subsistence, dietary (for example, consumption of oxidant-rich plants), and ethnomedical—have evolved that assist people in coping with the effects of this punishing disease (Brown, 1998; Greene & Danubio, 1997; Livingston, 1958).

New Patterns of Dispersion

In recent years, malaria has been dispersing to new areas or reconquering old territories from which it had been largely eradicated (for example, by the use of DDT, now banned owing to its significant environmental effects). In part the spread of malaria reflects direct human action, such as the building of dams and canals, and the political and economic factors that shape such development initiatives.

Construction of the Indira Gandhi canal in Rajasthan, India, for example, was primarily responsible for a significant outbreak of malaria there (Mankodi, 1996). Stagnant water in the main canal coupled with long-standing rainwater near villages was found to create huge breeding sites for mosquito vectors (Tyagi, Yadav, Sachdev, & Dam, 2001). World Bank–imposed structural adjustment policies that led to high food prices, greater health care costs, decreased wages, increased unemployment, and loss of both prevention and treatment initiatives magnified the impact of the outbreak (Manfredi, 1999). Further, malaria is associated with the tropics and owing to global warming— also in no small part a human-caused transformation of the environment—malaria could become a planetwide threat. Notes Berger (2000): "Milder temperatures have contributed to the spread of mosquito-borne diseases in Africa. Richards Bay, South Africa, for example, which was once malaria-free, had 22,000 cases in 1999. Malaria has also reached highland regions of Kenya and Tanzania where it was previously unknown. In the Andes of Colombia, disease-carrying mosquitoes that once lived at altitudes no higher than 3,200 feet have now appeared at the 7,200-foot level" (pp. 36–37). (Global warming is discussed further in Chapter Eight.)

Despite the importance of climate change in the spread of malaria, other factors, including syndemic interaction with HIV, may be of even greater significance in some local contexts (such as Kisumu, Kenya, as described in Chapter Nine).

Syndemic Patterning: The Silent Alliance

Various studies affirm the involvement of malaria in adverse syndemic interactions, including interaction with HIV/AIDS, an interface that Van geertruyden and D'Alessandro (2007) refer to as a "silent alliance." The character of this alliance is succinctly summarized by Abu-Raddad (2007), who comments that "scientific findings suggest a vicious cycle of interaction between [these] two diseases. HIV infection facilitates malaria acquisition. In turn, the immune reaction against malaria makes dually infected persons twice as infectious for HIV. Therefore, HIV fuels malaria and malaria fuels HIV."

Research in Kenya (Gallagher et al., 2005) with HIV-infected women, for example, found that compared to matched HIV-negative women they were two times more likely to have peripheral blood malaria or placental malaria (two alternative expressions of the disease) and more than two times more likely to have lymphatic filariasis. In addition, women with HIV and malaria exhibited a somewhat increased risk for mother-to-child HIV transmission. Although the Gallagher study also found that mother-to-child transmission of HIV was significantly higher in women who were coinfected with one or more helminth species than it was in women without this parasitic infection (helminth infections are discussed later in this chapter). Similarly, research in South Africa (Grimwade et al., 2003, 2004) found increased malarial severity in HIV-infected adults but not children. Further, it is of note that families living in the same dwelling with an HIV-infected family member had higher rates of malaria among HIV-negative children than did families that did not have an HIV-infected member.

A review of the pathophysiological mechanisms of disease interaction carried out by Renia and Potter (2006) identified cell-based immune responses to HIV and malaria as the biological explanation of the adverse consequences of dual infection. The development of a degree of immunity to malaria is based on the release of proinflammatory cytokines and their antibodies and on the production of counter-regulatory cytokines that interfere with the first stage of plasmodium development after the infectious agent enters the human blood system. Failure to develop these responses because of HIV infection has significant consequences. Thus in a prospective cohort study in South Africa, Cohen et al. (2005) found that the severe malaria symptoms occurred more often in HIV-infected patients with a low CD4 T-cell count. Individuals who had not built up prior malaria immunity and were also HIV-infected were significantly more likely to suffer severe malaria than were nonimmune individuals who were HIV-negative. Among individuals who came from a region of the country with high malaria endemicity, HIV serostatus did not increase the likelihood of suffering severe malaria.

Other research in sub-Saharan Africa supports and extends these findings. In a Ugandan study, Whitworth et al. (2000; see also French et al., 2001) found that suffering bouts of malaria symptoms was significantly more common among HIV-positive than HIV-negative participants. The risk of clinical malaria and the parasite load tended to increase with HIV-caused drops in CD4 T-cell levels. In cases where malaria infection precedes HIV infection, the body's initial immune response to the virus may (temporarily) inhibit parasitic development (Whitworth et al., 2000). Research by Grimwade et al. (2003, 2004) suggests that the immunological responses to infection described previously also differ between adults and children. This body of research affirms a significant level of biological interaction between HIV and malaria with grave consequences for dually infected individuals, especially those without prior malaria exposure.

Overall it is evident that Abu-Raddad (2007) aptly labels the HIV and malaria syndemic a "vicious cycle of interaction," one likely to worsen with the ever wider dispersion of malaria to previously malaria-free zones as a result of global warming.

Beyond the HIV and Malaria Coinfection

Today researchers are recognizing that important interactions occur in cases of coinfection with malaria and filarial worms. Both of these threats to human health are commonly are found in the same populations and in some parts of the world both can be transmitted by the same mosquito vector, *Anopheles gambiae*. Helminth coinfection appears to affect how well the immune system responds to malaria in animal research; coinfected mice, for example, develop more severe disease, assessed both in terms of level of anemia and loss of body mass, than do mice infected with malaria alone (Graham, Lamb, Read, & Allen, 2005). Human research in Georgetown, Guyana, in South America, where filarial worms and malaria are well established, found that of almost 800 people tested for filariasis during a one-year period, 13 percent were positive for worm infection; of these, 3 percent were coinfected with malaria (Chadee, Rawlins, & Tiwari, 2003). Similarly, of over 500 people tested for malaria, 4 percent were positive for the disease; of these, 3 percent were coinfected with filarial worms. Comparable results are reported for a study in Orissa, India (Ravindran Sahoo, & Dash, 1998). Although concomitant infection in these examples is low, interaction between these two pathogenic species inside a common vector or host could have important implications for the health of coinfected individuals and for the health of communities as global warming enables mosquitoes to carry these two pathogens to new areas. One barrier to this outcome, noted by Muturi et al. (2006) as a result of their research in Kenya, is that coinfected mosquitoes may have a lower level of survival than singly infected mosquitoes. Testing of mosquito populations in two locations that overlapped found that under 2 percent had concomitant infections. Nonetheless, in a hospital study of pregnant and postpartum Nigerian women, Egwunyenga, Ajayi, Nmorsi, and Duhlinska-Popova (2001) found that mothers infected with malaria but free of intestinal helminths delivered babies of a higher birth weight on average than did mothers coinfected with malaria and worms. This difference was enhanced in first-time mothers. Other studies show increased severity of malaria episodes in coinfected individuals, but this finding is not consistent across existing research (Hotez, 2006).

VL AND HIV/AIDS SYNDEMIC

Leishmaniasis is a disease triggered by a number of protozoal species within the large *Leishmania* genus. The name acknowledges William Leishman, a physician in the British Army in India, who in 1901 developed one of the earliest stains for one of the protozoa that cause this sometimes mild but potentially deforming disease.

Leishmaniasis has been called one of the important **neglected tropical diseases** (Hotez et al., 2006)—a group of approximately fifteen parasitic infections caused by worms (lymphatic elephantiasis, onchocerciasis, ascariasis, hookworm, whipworm, dracunculiasis, schistosomiasis, oriental liver fluke, and cysticercosis), bacteria (trachoma, leprosy, and Buruli ulcer), and protozoa (human African trypanosomiasis, Chagas' disease, and leishmaniasis). Food-borne trematodiasis and several other parasitic infections are also sometimes added to this list. These infectious diseases, which contribute to as many as 500,000 deaths annually, are among the most common pathogenic threats to health globally, especially in developing tropical countries, and yet they have not attracted significant global health and pharmacological attention. At special risk are the poor in both rural areas and urban slums. As the Global Network for Neglected Tropical Diseases emphasizes, "The greatest impact of these diseases is the way they promote poverty, stigmatize, disable and inhibit individuals from being able to care for themselves or their families." Because they tend overwhelmingly to be diseases of the poor, "there are few or no commercial markets for drugs and vaccines against the neglected tropical diseases, and the pharmacopoeia for these diseases has remained essentially unchanged since the middle of the 20th century" (Hotez et al., 2006).

Despite its neglect, leishmaniasis has been a bane of human populations since ancient times. In the New World, pre-Colombian Incan pottery from Ecuador and Peru displays images of facial lesions and deformities that closely resemble the effects of this disease and suggest that it afflicted Incan civilization. In the Old World, in India, the Sanskrit term *kala azar* ("black fever") has been applied to this disease for centuries. The disease was first described in the biomedical literature in 1756 by Alexander Russell (Gelpi, 1987). Following examination of a Turkish patient with what was then called Aleppo boil, Russell wrote that the disease "leaves an ugly scar, which remains through life, and for many months has a livid colour" (World Health Organization, 2008c). In South America, *chicleros,* traditional collectors of chicle, the milky sap obtained from the bark of sapodilla trees that was used in the making of chewing gum before the introduction of synthetics, were frequently exposed to sand flies carrying leishmaniasis, giving rise to the term *chiclero ulcer.*

Transmission of Leishmaniasis in the Era of HIV/AIDS

Leishmaniasis is a vector-borne condition spread by several different families of sand flies (small biting insects, two to three millimeters in length, that resemble mosquitoes both in their appearance and in their reproductive need for blood to nourish their eggs). It is estimated that the global prevalence of this disease is 12 million cases, with an annual incidence rate of 1.5 to 2 million cases. Leishmaniasis is today becoming an urban disease as a consequence of human migration to cities and the adaptation of sand flies to urban environments (World Health Organization, 2002a).

The most common symptoms are skin sores, as seen in recent years on soldiers returning from the U.S. war in Iraq. In the infection's most severe form, called visceral leishmaniasis (VL), lesions caused by the disease can result in disabling disfigurement involving partial or even total destruction of the mucous membranes of the nose, mouth, and throat cavities and surrounding tissues. Other significant symptoms, which may not show up for several months or even years after the onset of infection, include damage to the spleen and liver. VL is especially prevalent in India, Bangladesh, Nepal, Sudan, and Brazil, with a total of half a million new cases and 5,000 VL-related deaths a year in these countries. Sand flies that harbor a strain known as *Leishmania infantum* are spreading northward in Europe in response to changes wrought by global warming, and in coming years contemporary disease models predict "a dramatic increase" in visceral leishmaniasis in northern Europe (Kuhn, 1999, p. 2).

The epidemiology of visceral VL is undergoing important changes as a result of increasing levels of coinfection with HIV. HIV and VL coinfection has been reported in over thirty countries in Africa, Asia, Europe, and South America. World Health Organization surveillance indicates that over 70 percent of HIV cases in southern Europe are coinfected with VL (Molina, Gradoni, & Alvar, 2003). In particular, Spain, Italy, and southern France are seeing a growing incidence of coinfection among youths, including those engaged in injection drug use (which may be serving as a vector-free route of VL transmission). People with HIV who are coinfected have a reduced immune capacity to contain the initial infection and keep it from progressing to VL. Specifically, control of leishmanial infection requires a competent Th1 inflammatory response which, as HIV infection progresses, is increasingly diminished, allowing latent leishmanial infection to become active, propagate, and spread within the body. In coinfected individuals, leishmaniasis has been found to "be particularly severe and unresponsive to treatment" (Oliver, Bararo, Medrano, & Moreno, 2003, p. S85). VL, in turn, has been found to enhance HIV infection through several complex biochemical pathways.

Biology of Interaction

The biological basis for syndemic interaction between leishmaniasis and HIV arises from the fact that both HIV and several leishmanial protozoa, such as *L. donovani,* invade and multiply within immune cells produced in either the bone marrow or lymphatic system, such as the macrophage. This process involves various processes and several phases of the protozoan life cycle. When a female sand fly infected with leishmanial protozoa bites a person to extract blood, it injects the parasite in its promastigote form (that is, bearing a flagella or tail to facilitate mobility) into the host. When a macrophage subsequently encounters the promastigote, it quickly engulfs but does not destroy it. Rather, inside the macrophage the parasite loses its outer structure (including lipophosphoglycan, a molecule found on its outer surface, which transfers to the surface of the macrophage) and tail, but retains its internal components, called the phosphatidyl inositol core, or core-PI. This transfer of lipophosphoglycan appears to assist the survival of the core-PI inside the macrophage by preventing the launching of the phage's normal lethal microbicidal activities in defense of the body (Turco, 1999). Notably, lipophosphoglycan also has been found to be a powerful activator of HIV replication and leishmaniasis is believe to stimulate HIV replication through several additional mechanisms as well (Wolday, Berhe, Akuffo, & Britton, 1999). As Oliver et al. (2003) state: "In addition to its capacity to activate HIV-1 replication, the [lipophosphoglycan] molecule can also stimulate the release of several inflammatory molecules, such as prostaglandin E [which] plays a role in the development of HIV-1-related pathogenesis, particularly in those coinfected with leishmania" (p. S81).

As Harms and Feldmeier (2002) observe, "Leishmania/HIV coinfection is . . . an example of a deadly gridlock with detrimental interactions in both directions" (p. 484). The consequence is a significantly higher mortality rate and lower mean survival time in coinfected individuals compared to the rates for those with parasitic infection alone (World Health Organization, 1999). VL and HIV, in particular, represent a growing syndemic, one with potential to spread to many parts of the world as a result of global warming and the resultant climate-facilitated diffusion of sand flies to new environments. Syndemics of this sort are called *ecosyndemics* (Baer & Singer, 2008), because the disease clustering and interaction involved is being driven by anthropogenic environmental changes (see Chapter Eight).

HELMINTHS AND HIV/AIDS SYNDEMIC

Parasitic infection with various **helminthss,** or parasitic worm species, is yet another neglected tropical threat to the health of the poor in developing countries. There is also evidence suggesting that some of these organisms interact with HIV infection, both increasing susceptibility to HIV and exacerbating HIV progression in coinfected individuals.

A number of channels have been identified through which this syndemic disease promotion occurs. One such channel stems from the immune cell environment as HIV infection progresses; eventually a point is reached when the infectable cells in the blood stream (others may be dormant in the body) that the virus can use for further replication are in short supply. In individuals who are also suffering from helminth infection, however, the number of activated immune cells exposed to HIV infection goes up. A second channel involves an increase in Th2 cells in helminth-infected individuals (which, some have suggested, is a form of worm-induced immune system dysregulation that facilitates parasitic infection). This may create a biochemical environment that favors HIV replication because Th2 lymphocytes may be more susceptible than Th1 lymphocytes to HIV infection. Some researchers, however, have questioned this idea, owing to the health status of many helminth-infected individuals (see, for example, Brown, Mawa, Kaleebu, & Elliot, 2006). Other mechanisms arising from the enhanced immune activation typically provoked by helminths have been suggested as well (Bundy, Sher, & Michael, 2000). Helminth-induced chronic immune activation may prove to be the critical factor in HIV and helminth interaction. Support for the importance of HIV and helminth interaction is seen both in the fact that research in Ethiopia has found that the HIV viral load is higher in coinfected individuals than it is in those suffering HIV infection alone, and in the fact that effective treatment of worm infestation produces drops in the HIV viral load (Bentwich, Maartens, Torten, Lal, & Lal, 2000).

Elephantiasis

Although in certain regional environments helminth infection is widespread and expected, especially among children, one parasitic infection that is especially dreaded is elephantiasis, a disease that acquired its name from the effects it has on sufferers, namely the enlargement of the lower legs (and also arms, genitals, and breasts) because of thickening of the skin and underlying tissues. This disease is found in over eighty countries in Africa, the Indian subcontinent, South Asia, the Western Pacific, the Caribbean, and South America. Across its range of distribution, elephantiasis puts more than a billion people at risk of infection. Moreover, rates of infection are increasing in many affected regions of the world. The rapid growth of urban populations in impoverished and medically and socially underserved shantytowns and similar slum areas of megacities in developing countries has contributed to the creation of multiple potential breeding sites for the mosquito vectors that transmit the parasite from one person to the next.

The World Health Organization (2000) reports that over 120 million people are infected and must endure the development of the seriously incapacitating, disfiguring, and stigmatizing symptoms of this disease. Although not everyone who is infected develops the dreaded visual expressions of elephantiasis, they nonetheless may suffer significant internal damage to the lymphatic system and kidneys as the disease develops. Moreover, because sufferers can be physically incapacitated, the disease has significant economic implications, contributing to lost income, household failure, and further impoverishment (Coreil, Mayard, Louis-Charles, & Addiss, 1998).

The Primacy of Secondary Infection

The worms that cause elephantiasis are known as lymphatic filaria. Upon entering the body (following the bite of an infected mosquito), the threadlike, filarial worms (either

Wuchereria bancrofti or *Brugia malayi*) begin circulating in the blood and lodging themselves in parts of the lymphatic system, an essential component of the immune system and responsible for maintaining the delicate fluid balance between body tissues and blood. Immune response is critical in that both chronic and acute manifestations of filariasis are more common in refugees or other newcomer populations (for example, soldiers) than in local populations that have been continually exposed to infection (beginning in utero). Manifestations seen in newcomer populations but not in lifelong residents of endemic areas include hives, rashes, asthma symptoms, and other allergic reactions to an unfamiliar stimulant.

Only in recent years has it become clear that many of the symptoms of elephantiasis (especially disfiguring, inflammation-mediated filarial disease) are not directly caused by the helminths but are the result of secondary bacterial skin infections. Elephantiasis itself appears to be a product of a syndemic interaction between the parasitic worm and a species of bacteria known as *Wolbachia,* which, it is beginning to be realized, may be the most common infectious bacterium on Earth. The worms responsible for elephantiasis are infested by these quasi-symbiotic bacteria (indeed, the death of the bacteria usually results in the death or sterility of the worm), as are other types of roundworms and numerous insect species as well. To a significant degree, the **pathogenicity** of the helminths is a consequence of the intense response of the human immune system to *Wolbachia* exposure, which suggests why newcomers to an endemic area have atypical reactions to filarial infestation (Hoerauf et al., 2003). Thus Taylor (2003) reports that the development of acute and severe inflammatory responses in people infected with either *Brugia malayi* or *Onchocerca volvulus* (a worm transmitted by blackflies that causes onchocerciasis, a major source of blindness) following antifilarial chemotherapy is associated with the release of *Wolbachia* into the blood system.

Recent research in Tanzania examined possible syndemic interactions between HIV and filarial worms (especially *W. bancrofti*) in coinfected adults. These individuals exhibit somewhat higher HIV loads and lower levels of the CD4 immune cells targeted by HIV than do individuals not infected with filariasis, but these differences did not reach statistical significance (Nielsen et al., 2007). Research in Kenya (Gallagher et al., 2005), however, with a small sample of eighty-three HIV-positive women, found these women to be more than twice as likely to have lymphatic filariasis infection than were individuals in a matched HIV-negative sample. Although women with HIV and malaria had somewhat heightened risk for mother-to-child HIV transmission, mother-to-child transmission of HIV was found to be significantly greater in women who were coinfected with one or more worm species than in women without helminth infections.

Schistosomiasis

Other worm infections, such as schistosomiasis (also called bilharzia, after Theodor Bilharz, the German physician who first described schistosomes), also produce adverse health consequences in coinfected individuals (Secor & Sundstrom, 2007). These blood-consuming worms derive their name from the fact that they travel through human bodies in pairs, male and female, with the latter living in a slit in the body of the former (the name *schistosome* is ultimately derived from Greek words meaning "split body"). Another peculiarity of this parasite is that it lacks an anus and thus eliminates waste through regurgitation. Through several tricks of the pathogenic trade (for example, possessing molecules that disable components of the immune system, intercept immune system messages, and possibly disguise the organism as being a natural part of the body), schistosomes are able to limit detection and reaction by the human immune systems (Skelly, 2008).

It is estimated that at least 200 million people are infected with schistosomiasis (about one-tenth of these severely so), primarily in tropical and subtropical environments. Once inside the human blood system, individual schistosomes can survive for decades. Their eggs can elicit damaging immune system responses that can lead to internal bleeding and possibly cancer of the colon. Research has shown that schistosomiasis sufferers who are coinfected with HIV are more susceptible to subsequent reinfection by the parasite than are individuals who are HIV-negative, suggesting that immune system cells attacked by HIV participate in resisting schistosome infection (Karanja et al., 2002). Moreover, in laboratory and animal model studies, schistosomes have been found to accelerate HIV disease progression by facilitating the infection of cells by HIV, although it is not certain (because of ethical issues in carrying out confirmatory research) that these findings translate into actual patterns in the human body (Secor, Karanja, & Colley, 2004).

Additionally, schistosomiasis has been found to facilitate HIV infection. For example, a study of over 500 sexually active women in rural Zimbabwe—almost half (46 percent) of whom had genital lesions caused by *Schistosoma haematobium* infestation—found a significant association between HIV infection and genital schistosomiasis. Whereas 41 percent of the women with laboratory-confirmed genital schistosomiasis were HIV-positive, this was true of only 26 percent of the HIV-negative women. This finding indicates significantly heightened susceptibility to HIV when worm-induced genital lesions occur (Kjetland et al., 2006). Additionally, all seven women who became HIV-positive during the study period had signs of *S. haematobium* infection at baseline.

Hyperinfective Syndrome

Another helminth of concern is *Strongyloides stercoralis,* a parasitic roundworm that in infected individuals lives in the mucosa of the small intestines and causes what is usually an asymptomatic or mild respiratory and gastrointestinal condition called strongyloidiasis (Igra-Siegman, Kapila, Sen, Kaminski, & Louria, 1981). This disease, which first came to biomedical attention through the work of several French physicians treating soldiers returning from French colonies in Southeast Asia, is found as well in parts of Africa and Central and South America. Owing to its unusual life cycle, which allows it to pass through all its developmental phases and to reproduce within the human body (a cycle not characteristic of most parasitic worms), this helminth can cause helminth and intestinal bacteria syndemic infections. As the organism migrates between the intestines and the lungs during its development, it can serve as a transportation device, hauling attached intestinal bacteria that can set off significant bacterial infections in the respiratory system. Further, if not kept in check by the immune system, strongyloidiasis can develop rapidly into what is known as disseminated strongyloidiasis, or **hyperinfective syndrome,** a severe disease with a mortality rate of over 80 percent in some contexts (Marcos, Terashima, Dupont, & Gotuzzo, 2008).

Herein lies the potential for helminth interaction with HIV. Research with HIV patients by Feitosa, Bandeira, Sampaio, Badaró, and Brites (2001) in Bahia, Brazil; Pinlaor, Mootsikapun, Pinlaor, Pipitgool, and Tuangnadee (2005) in Khon Kaen Province, Thailand; and Gomez et al. (1995) in rural Tanzania found heightened presence of *Strongyloides* in HIV-positive individuals. Parallel work by Viney et al. (2004, p. 2175) did not, however, replicate these findings nor suggest that HIV infection facilitates the development of hyperinfection, and hence further research is needed to resolve the role, if any, of HIV in promoting disseminated strongyloidiasis. One source of information on this issue is case reports of lethal coinfection of HIV and strongyloidiasis (for example, Harcourt-Webster, Scaravilli, & Darwish, 1991; Lessnau, Can, & Talvera, 1993). These suggest that interaction may occur at advanced stages of HIV progression.

HTLV and Helminth Interactions

In contrast with the uncertainty of HIV and *Strongyloides* connections, it is well established that another RNA virus, human T-cell lymphotropic virus type 1 (HTLV-1) (discussed in Chapter One), promotes hyperinfectious strongyloidiasis (Marcos et al., 2008). In the United States HTLV-1 has about half the prevalence of HIV infection and is found disproportionately among injection drug users (IDUs), especially in the southeast. Rates of HTLV infection among IDUs ranging from 0 to 50 percent have been found in studies in several cities, especially among African American drug users (Cantor, Weiss, Goedert, & Battjes, 1991). Worldwide, HTLV-1 infects an estimated 20 million people and has become a global epidemic (Edlich, Arnette, & Williams, 2000). This virus, which infects primarily T cells, is able to modify the body's immune response in a way that decreases the body's existing helminth defense mechanisms (by inducing lymphocyte proliferation and secretion of high levels of Th1 cytokines) (Carvalho & Porto, 2004; Porto et al., 2001).

HTLV-1, like HIV, interacts as well with *Schistosoma* species of helminths. For example, in a clinical study comparing HTLV-1 infected patients and HTVL-1 seronegative controls, Porto et al. (2004) found that the prevalence of the schistosomiasis-causing species *S. mansoni* is higher in HTLV-1 infected subjects than in HTLV-1-seronegative controls. These researchers found that HTLV-1 "modified the clinical outcome of schistosomiasis and altered the immune response to parasitic antigens. Additionally, HTLV-1 coinfection reduced the efficacy of antischistosomal drugs" (Porto et al., 2004, p. 427). At the same time, it bears mentioning that evidence exists that some helminth parasites, especially hookworm and the snail-borne flatworms that cause schistosomiasis, interact with and exacerbate serious infectious diseases other than HIV or HTLV-1 infections, such as pulmonary tuberculosis. Additionally, several studies have examined interactions between HTLV-1 and HCV, the virus that causes hepatitis C. In one such study, a nine-city comparative assessment of U.S. drug users, Hisada, Chatterjee, Zhang, Battjes, & Goedert (2003) showed that coinfection is associated with a higher viral load of HCV. In another, HTLV-1 and HCV coinfected individuals in Miyazaki, Japan, were found to be at greater risk for the development of liver disease, liver cancer, and death than individuals were who were not coinfected (Boschi-Pinto et al., 2000). Moreover, HTLV-1 and HIV are themselves interacting diseases in coinfected individuals (Page et al., 1990).

Overall it is clear that helminth and HIV/AIDS syndemics are frequent in some sociogeographical environments; that the effects of coinfection tend to be bidirectional; that the specific biochemical, signaling, or other mechanisms of interaction are starting to be identified; and that significant treatment implications arise as a result of the clustering and interaction of HIV and worms.

SUMMARY

This chapter continued the exploration of specific syndemics begun in Chapter Two. The nature and complexities of syndemic interaction generally have been examined through the special case of HIV/AIDS, a disease that is more syndemically interconnected with other diseases and health challenges than is any other known infectious disease. The tendency of HIV/AIDS to interact with so many other health conditions can be explained in terms of its role in damaging the human immune system. HIV/AIDS is known to throw open the castle gate, allowing the entry of a range of infectious diseases, those labeled opportunistic and those that infect large numbers of individuals even without the multiplying effects of coinfection with HIV. At the same time, the presence of other diseases has been shown to foster the progression of HIV/AIDS toward greater levels of sickness, possibly including the death of the patient.

KEY TERMS

drug resistance
helminth
helminths and HIV/AIDS syndemic
hepatitis and HIV/AIDS syndemic
hyperinfective syndrome
malaria and HIV/AIDS syndemic
neglected tropical diseases

opportunistic infections
pathogenicity
sexually transmitted disease syndemics
syndemogenesis
tuberculosis and AIDS syndemic
tuberculosis and diabetes syndemic
VL and HIV syndemic

QUESTIONS FOR DISCUSSION

1. Why is HIV/AIDS described as syndemogenic?

2. Explain why some of the diseases with which HIV/AIDS interacts are described as "opportunistic."

3. Describe the bidirectional interactions that occur between hepatitis and HIV/AIDS in coinfected individuals.

4. How significant is tuberculosis as a global health problem? In what ways is tuberculosis like HIV/AIDS? How does HIV/AIDS affect the disease course of tuberculosis? How does tuberculosis affect the disease course of HIV/AIDS?

5. Why is the malaria and HIV/AIDS syndemic having a major impact on public health in Africa? Where else is this syndemic likely to have an important effect on public health?

6. What is leishmaniasis? Describe how the epidemiology of visceral leishmaniasis (VL) is undergoing changes as a result of increasing levels of coinfection with HIV.

7. What are the various channels of HIV/AIDS interaction with parasitic worm diseases? Discuss the role of chronic immune activation in this interaction.

8. Describe the role of helminths and secondary bacterial skin infections in the syndemic development of the lymph system disease elephantiasis.

CHAPTER

BEYOND CONTAGION

HIV/AIDS and Noninfectious Disease Syndemogenesis

After studying this chapter, you should be able to

- Describe the role of infectious diseases in chronic health problems.

- Understand how HIV/AIDS interacts with noninfectious diseases like malnutrition, cardiovascular problems, and mental health conditions.

- Identify the key differences between syndemics and countersyndemics.

AN AGING EPIDEMIC

In 2008, the *New York Times* featured an article by Jane Gross titled "AIDS Patients Face Downside of Living Longer." The article's message was contextualized by several painful prior decades of the AIDS epidemic, a period during which AIDS in developed nations slowly transitioned from an acute disease that robbed the lives of the young and vigorous to a chronic disease that could be kept at bay for years through a demanding but increasingly manageable regimen of pharmaceutical treatments (and lifestyle changes). Reporting on an emergent discovery about long-term AIDS survivors, Gross (2008) commented: "The graying of the AIDS epidemic has increased interest in the connection between AIDS and cardiovascular disease, certain cancers, diabetes, osteoporosis and depression" (p. 1). Indeed, even more trenchant than the growing concern being expressed in the AIDS treatment world and among AIDS patients about the early onset of a range of chronic diseases among middle-aged people with many years of exposure to potent AIDS medications, as reported by Gross, is the uneasy realization that in addition to its multiple adverse interactions with other infectious diseases, HIV also appears to work together in harmful ways with various chronic diseases not known to be spread by pathogens. This is alarming news because many noncommunicable diseases are expected to increase dramatically worldwide during the twenty-first century. The global prevalence of diabetes mellitus, for example, may almost double from the 124 million sufferers estimated in 1997 to 220 million by the year 2010 (Amos et al., 1997). The prospect for yet another way in which HIV can make life for humans a challenge, especially for those who have escaped its destructive capacity despite infection, magnifies this pathogen's already iniquitous reputation.

INFECTIOUS AND CHRONIC DISEASE CONNECTIONS

In the United States there are 90 million people living with chronic diseases, and together these diseases account for 70 percent of all deaths. A majority of U.S. adults and children who have health insurance are taking prescription medications for chronic health problems, and one-fifth are using three or more medications (Medco Health Solutions, 2008). The World Health Organization (2002b) projects that by the year 2020, the chronic health problems faced by developed countries will be a factor in a similar proportion of deaths worldwide. It further estimates that about 70 percent of deaths from ischemic heart disease, 75 percent of deaths from stroke, and 70 percent of diabetes-related deaths will occur in the developing world. In this light, it is significant that among the numerous new discoveries about infectious diseases that have occurred in the often grim shadow of the AIDS pandemic and the renewed focus on contagion it provoked, is the key role of infections as "determinants, not just complications, of chronic diseases" (O'Connor, Taylor, & Hughes, 2006, p. 16).

Although the idea that there may be an infectious cause of noninfectious disease is several centuries old, empirical evidence for this view awaited the new arsenal that now equips biological research (for example, the advent of the polymerase chain reaction technique for synthesizing DNA, mass spectrometry, electron microscopy, enhanced antigen and antibody detection techniques, and growth-promoting factors that improve the cultivation of microbes). In the absence of these powerful technologies, infectious diseases and chronic diseases were constructed in the medical and public health imaginations as different worlds wholly separated by an unbreachable wall. (Many members of the general public thought the same way, although some groups have maintained other beliefs about certain diseases, for example, that cancer is contagious.) Then the roles of *Helicobacter pylori* in the development of both peptic ulcer disease and gastric adenocarcinoma and the role of the human papillomavirus in the onset of cervical cancer were discovered, and the wall began to crumble.

H. pylori, for example, a spiral-shaped pathogen that lives in the mucus layer of the stomach, duodenum, and less frequently, the esophagus, is a common source of infection in the world, especially in developing countries, where infection rates of up to 10 percent of children and 80 percent of adults have been detected through laboratory assessment, even though sufferers may be asymptomatic. In the United States about 20 percent of people under forty years of age and half of those over sixty years are believed to be infected. Generally, inadequate sanitation facilities and practices, lower socioeconomic class, and crowed living conditions have been linked to a higher prevalence of *H. pylori* infection. In South Korea, for example, Malaty, Kim, Kim, and Graham (1996) found that 22 percent of children were infected, in inverse relationship to socioeconomic class: 12 percent of children among upper-class families, 25 percent among middle-class families, and 41 percent among lower-class families. Similarly, *H. pylori* infection in the United States is approximately twice as frequent among African Americans and Latinos as among non-Hispanic whites and is also inversely related to socioeconomic class in these ethnic populations (Graham et al., 1991). As a result, intrafamilial and institutional clustering of *H. pylori* infection is common (Brown, 2000).

Those individuals who do experience symptoms of *H. pylori* infection have nausea, vomiting, and stomach pain. First isolated in humans in 1982, *H. pylori* has been linked in various publications with **zoonotic transmission** from cats (although transmission from humans to cats, an example of *reverse zoonosis,* is also possible) and from sheep and may also be spread by houseflies (Handt et al., 1994). Human-to-human transmission (though oral-to-oral or anal-to-oral routes), however, appears to be the most common route of disease spread. The channels through which *H. pylori* triggers peptic ulcers and gastric adenocarcinoma are under study in various laboratories around the world. Robinson et al. (2008), for example, have found that compared to individuals without ulcers, individuals who have peptic ulcer disease have a 2.4-fold reduction in T-helper cell levels. These findings suggest that *H. pylori* induces a regulatory T-cell response and that ulcers develop when this regulatory response is inadequate.

As a result of the discoveries about the disease roles of *H. pylori* and human papillomavirus, in October of 2002, the Institute of Medicine of the National Academies held a groundbreaking workshop, "Forum on Microbial Threats" (Knobler, O'Connor, Lemon, & Najafi, 2002), intended to implement a state of the art review of the linkages that have been identified in recent years between infectious agents and chronic diseases. The workshop, a dialogue among representatives from a variety of sectors of the health research, care, and policy worlds, explored a range of factors that drive infectious etiologies of chronic diseases to prominence, and sought to identify more effective disease prevention and health promotion strategies and more focused research agendas in light of developing knowledge. In particular, various cancers, **autoimmune or immune-mediated diseases,** and neurodevelopmental disorders were discussed as potential candidates for having an infectious origin. Some participants expressed the belief that some chronic conditions outside these three disease categories will be discovered to have their origin in infection as well. Consequently, one product of the workshop was the expectation that the already growing list of chronic diseases proven to have an infectious origin (see Table 5.1) will grow further as unexpected links between infectious and noninfectious diseases are identified in the coming years.

Australian pathologist John Robin Warren first saw the small curved bacteria known as helicobacters in 1979, during a biopsy of the mucous membrane of a gastritis patient's stomach. In this sighting, Warren rediscovered a bacterium first described, initially in animals and then in humans, at the end of the nineteenth century. Although originally identified in patients with gastric cancer and peptic ulcers, the role of bacteria in these diseases was overlooked. The cause of cancer was unknown, and for many years spicy food or life stress was presumed to produce stomach ulcers. Working with fellow Australian physician Barry Marshall in Perth, Australia, Warren began trying to culture the bacteria he had seen. After a series of unsuccessful attempts the two physicians finally began growing bacterial colonies in the laboratory in the early 1980s—thanks to an experimental error. They mistakenly left their samples incubating for five days over a long holiday weekend (previously their lab technicians had discarded samples if no bacteria appeared after two days of culturing) only to discover on their return that their efforts had finally been rewarded. They began publishing a series of papers in the *Lancet*, a British medical journal, and elsewhere, asserting that most stomach ulcers and gastritis were caused by bacterial infection (Marshall & Warren, 1984). Their reports suggesting a bacterial cause for chronic gastritis, duodenal ulcer, and gastric ulcer were at first met with skepticism from many of their peers. To prove that *H. pylori* causes gastritis and to fulfill the second of Koch's postulates (see Chapter One), Marshall drank a beaker of the microorganism and within a few days began suffering from nausea and vomiting (Marshall, Armstrong, McGechie, & Glancy, 1985). Examination revealed signs of gastritis and the presence of *H. pylori*. In 2005, Warren and Marshall received the Nobel Prize for their pioneering research.

In addition to addressing specific acute and chronic disease relationships, workshop speakers focused on three types of relationship between infectious and chronic diseases:

- The role of infectious agents in producing chronic disease or long-term disability through increasing severe tissue damage and organ decomposition (as seen, for example, in the impact of the hepatitis B virus and hepatitis C virus on chronic liver disease)

- The ways in which the initial stages of an infection can cause later or lifelong deficits or disabilities (as seen, for example, with poliovirus and late-onset neurological deterioration)

- Infectious predisposition to chronic sequelae (as seen, for example, in maternal infection during pregnancy that even without direct infection of the child increases that child's risk for chronic neurological and pulmonary deficits)

From a syndemic perspective, recognition of these linkages is a momentous advance. At the same time, not everyone infected with *B. burgdorferi* develops Lyme disease and not everyone exposed to *H. pylori* suffers from peptic ulcer disease, and the same patterns hold for other infectious agents now tied to chronic health conditions. The wider social context and its impacts on individuals and communities, including their physical and emotional health, remain critical elements in disease course and outcome. Moreover, although a number of unexpected ties have been uncovered and there is little doubt that additional linkages between infectious agents and diseases labeled as chronic are likely to be identified, thus far there has been no avalanche of new discoveries.

TABLE 5.1. Known Infectious Determinants of Chronic Diseases

Infectious Agent	Chronic Disease or Condition
Human papillomavirus	Cervical cancer
Hepatitis B virus	Liver cancer, cirrhosis
Chlamydia pneumoniae	Atherosclerosis
Vaccinia virus	Postinfectious encephalomyelitis or acute disseminated encephalomyelitis (ADEM)
JC virus	Progressive multifocal leukoencephalopathy (PML)
Various viruses	Multiple sclerosis
Enteroviruses	Type 1 diabetes mellitus
Toxoplasma gondii	Schizophrenia, congenital toxoplasmosis
Herpes simplex virus type 2	Schizophrenia
Jaagsiekte sheep retrovirus	Ovine pulmonary adenocarcinoma
Propionibacterium acnes	Chronic inflammatory acne

(Continued)

TABLE 5.1. Known Infectious Determinants of Chronic Diseases (*Continued*)

Infectious Agent	Chronic Disease or Condition
Cryptosporidiosis and intestinal helminth infections	Disabilities including growth shortfalls, fitness, and cognitive impairment
Helminth infections	Epilepsy
Plasmodium falciparum	Epilepsy, cognitive development, childhood anemia
Treponema pallidum	Congenital syphilis
Maternal rubella virus	Congenital rubella
Perinatal HIV	Developmental disabilities
Perinatal herpes viruses	Neurodevelopmental disabilities
Haemophilus influenzae type b	Nervous system impairment, meningitis
Japanese encephalitis virus	Neuropsychiatric sequelae
Measles virus	Developmental disabilities
Poliovirus	Paralysis
Chlamydia trachomatis	Trachoma
Human T-cell lymphotropic virus type 1	Adult T-cell leukemia or lymphoma, autoimmune disorders, infections associated with immunosuppression
Human herpes virus type 8	Kaposi's sarcoma
Borna disease virus	Neurodevelopmental disorders

Source: Knobler et al., 2002, table S-1.

KIDNEY DISEASE AND HIV

The role of kidney disease in the renocardiac syndemic was examined in Chapter Three. Another potential kidney-related syndemic involves HIV infection. Studies have shown that kidney function is abnormal in up to 30 percent of HIV-infected patients and that kidney disease in HIV patients is associated with higher morbidity and mortality than found among HIV patients without renal pathology (Gupta et al., 2005). Between 1995 and 2000, the number of HIV-infected individuals in the United States with end-stage renal disease doubled. Additionally, there is a growing body of evidence suggesting that HIV-infected African Americans are at notably increased risk of developing kidney disease, including end-stage renal disease (Lucas et al., 2007).

To investigate the relationship between kidney disease and HIV, Choi et al. (2007) tracked the development of end-stage renal disease in a national U.S. sample of over 2 million U.S. veterans over a period of about three and a half years. At the beginning of the study over 15,000 patients in the sample had been diagnosed with HIV and over 400,000 had a diagnosis of chronic kidney disease. About 1,000 participants suffered from both diseases. In addition, 7.3 percent of white patients with HIV also had kidney disease, and 6.9 percent of black participants had both conditions. Among individuals who did not have HIV, however, 19.7 percent were white and 10.5 percent were black. Similarly, among individuals who suffered from diabetes and also had kidney disease, 28.5 percent were white and 19.5 percent were black. By the end of the study, among the HIV-infected patients, 208 were being treated for kidney disease; most of these cases (86 percent) were among black participants, and the incidence of kidney disease among black participants with HIV at this time was approximately ten times the incidence among white participants with HIV.

Among patients in the study who had both HIV and renal conditions, the most common cause of the kidney disease was human immunodeficiency virus–associated nephropathy (HIVAN), a disease characterized by direct viral infection of and damage to kidney cells by HIV. It was first reported among black patients in New York in 1984 and is still primarily found among young black men. There is growing evidence that HIV infects cells in the kidney, primarily the renal glomerular and tubular epithelial cells, which are part of the basic filtration structure of the kidney, and that these cells may provide nonimmune system sites for HIV replication. Several HIV genes, especially those known as nef and vpr, have been found to play important and synergistic roles in the pathogenesis of HIVAN (Wyatt, Rosenstiel, & Klotman, 2008). Even though syndemic-like in several ways, it is not certain that HIVAN is best described as a kidney disease and HIV syndemic, for the same reason that direct immune system destruction by HIV is not termed a syndemic. Although HIVAN is a severe condition whatever label is used, on a positive note, Ahuja, Grady, and Khan (2002) report that the "survival of HIV-infected dialysis patients in the United States has remarkably improved" as a result of AIDS treatment (p. 1892), although this has not been found by all researchers (for example, Rodriguez, Mendelson, O'Hare, Hsu, & Schoenfeld, 2003). Researchers tend to agree, however, that the survival of

HIV-positive patients remains low when compared to that of age- and gender-matched HIV-negative patients, and barriers to treatment adherence are suspected to be part of the explanation.

As this example suggests, it is important to differentiate syndemics from two or more different but linked expressions of the same disease, such as diarrhea and vomiting in cholera, or asthma, chronic bronchitis, and emphysema, which according to the so-called Dutch hypothesis (Kraft, 2006), should be considered not as separate diseases but as different expressions of airway obstruction disease. For this reason, identification of the nature and channels of disease interaction is key to the syndemic approach. Since the idea of syndemics was proposed, the term *syndemic* has been adopted to label various kinds of interaction within and beyond the arena of health. The term can be more useful, however, if it is restricted to a specific set of meanings as delineated in this volume.

As it happens, there may well be a syndemic dimension to HIVAN after all, given its frequent association with illicit injection drug use (Fine & Atta, 2007; Shahinian et al., 2000), and there may be utility in carefully assessing this condition in light of syndemic interactions and processes. Certainly HIVAN is a health disparity in greater need of explication.

FOOD INSUFFICIENCY AND HIV

Although the HIV/AIDS epidemic has been global in its toll, sub-Saharan Africa has endured the worst of it. As reported by the World Health Organization (2003), in this region HIV/AIDS "has had a devastating impact on health, nutrition, food security and overall socioeconomic development" (p. 3). In sub-Saharan Africa the epidemic rages among various populations in which malnutrition also has reached epidemic proportions. This copresence is of note here because undernourishment exacerbates HIV/AIDS infection by lowering individual and community capacity to respond effectively to the disease (van Lettow, Fawzi, & Semba, 2003). Attention to this dangerous interface reflects a growing recognition that narrow or single-track approaches (for example, focusing just on the distribution of AIDS medicines) are insufficient to either comprehending or building public health measures that reflect the complexity of factors influencing contemporary human health, in Africa or elsewhere.

Nutrition and the Immune System

Biological interaction between malnutrition and HIV/AIDS is centered in the body's complex and multilayered host immune system. In fact, malnutrition and HIV are the two most common causes of acquired immune dysfunction globally, and the patterning of immune system suppression caused by malnutrition is similar in many ways to the immune effects of HIV infection. When these two conditions are concurrent, "their effect on the immune system is synergistic" and severe (Anabwani & Navario, 2005, p. 98).

Research has established that to maintain body weight and physical activity levels, **macronutrient** (protein-energy) needs increase during infection (for example, by 10 percent for asymptomatic HIV/AIDS patients and 20 to 30 percent for symptomatic patients); that because of its need to replace immune cells expended on fighting pathogenic invasion, the immune system is a major consumer of **micronutrients;** and that inadequate nutrition plays an important role in immune dysfunction and AIDS progression among HIV-infected patients (Bogden et al., 2000). Inadequate diet influences an array of immune system functions, causing a reduction in the development of antibodies, a reduced concentration of immunoglobulin, a decreased presence of lymphocytes, a reduced production of interferon, and a lowered level of natural killer T cells and T-cell subsets (for example, helper cells) and interleukin-2 receptors (part of the immune system's signaling system and instrumental in triggering immune response to infection) (Chandra, 1997; Scrimshaw & SanGiovanni, 1997). As Goldberg (2000) emphasizes, "Nutritional deficiencies have been linked to decreases of all cellular and serum immune functions" (p. 1645). Indeed, "[a]ll types of immune cells and their products (that is, interleukins, interferons, and complements) depend on metabolic pathways that use various nutrients as critical cofactors for their actions and activities" (Anabwani & Navario, 2005, p. 98). Interleukins are important in mounting initial immune responses to HIV, and the success of these responses helps determine the length of the initial, symptom-free stage; interferons inhibit viral replication within other cells, especially by RNA-based pathogens like HIV; and complements assist biochemical reactions that clear pathogens from the body.

Fighting Disease and Protein-Energy Inadequacy

Three primary connections have been found between the development of a compromised immune system and inadequacies in the quantity and quality of food intake.

Protein-energy. First, the capacity of the immune system to fight infection is affected by inadequate protein-energy (and possibly fat) intake, with protein-energy insufficiency being one of the primary causes of immunodeficiency in the developing world (Field, Johnson & Schley, 2002; Jolly & Fernandes, 2000). This connection is understandable given the high energy and amino acid demands of immune cells for the successful completion of normal processes, such as cell division. There are multiple potential immunostatus consequences of macronutrient insufficiency. As Chandra (1997) observes, "Protein-energy malnutrition is associated with a significant impairment of cell-mediated immunity, phagocyte function, the complement system, secretory immunoglobulin A antibody concentrations, and cytokine production" (p. 460). One specific impact of protein-energy insufficiency that has grave importance for the well-being of the immune system is the atrophying of the lymphoid organs, including substantial reductions in the size of both the thymus and the spleen. Lymphocytes produced by the thymus, which in the past were thought to be immunoincompetent, have been shown in more recent years to be helper cells that enable lymphocytes derived from bone marrow to mature into antibody-forming cells.

Nutrients that block oxidative stress. Second, specific nutrients, like vitamins C and E, selenium, and N-acetylcysteine (derived from the amino acid L-cysteine), as well as dietary compounds like bioflavonoids and proanthocyanidins, help to block the development of **oxidative stress,** a condition that damages the body's cells, including immune cells, and accelerates their destruction (Troy, Derossi, Prochiantz, Greene, & Shelanski, 1996). A growing body of research suggests that oxidative stress may contribute to pathogenesis by pushing cells into a highly activated state, enhancing viral replication, weakening cell repair activity, decreasing immune cell proliferation, and contributing to loss of immune function (Romero-Alvira & Roche, 1998; Rosenberg & Fauci, 1990). The potential for oxidative stress is rooted in normal oxygen metabolism, which is necessary for survival but can put cells at risk because of the consequent formation of a type of toxic oxygen cell known as an *oxidant.* Oxidants, such as some free radicals and peroxides, lack a full complement of electrons. Under normal conditions the body's natural antioxidant networks maintain a delicate oxygen balance, limiting oxidant formation and resulting cell damage through enzyme-driven cell repair and oxidant removal molecules like glutathione, an intracellular antioxidant that promotes T-cell proliferation and activation. Notably, evidence has accumulated in recent years suggesting that HIV-infected individuals are under chronic oxidative stress and as a result their need to ingest and metabolize foods containing antioxidant nutrients that can be used to maintain antioxidant processes is elevated above the level a noninfected individual typically needs. N-acetylcysteine, for example, increases cellular levels of glutathione, and vitamin C contributes to internal recycling of glutathione and thus increases glutathione availability. Dietary insufficiency (as well as environmental exposures to tobacco smoke and other pollutants, excess alcohol consumption, and infectious agents) can tip the metabolic balance, leading to the overproduction of oxidants, oxidative stress, cell damage, and cell demise (Fiers, Beyaert, Declercq, & Vandenabeele, 1999).

In HIV/AIDS patients, oxidative stress appears to contribute in several ways to HIV disease pathogenesis, including greater viral replication, decreased immune cell proliferation, loss of immune function, cell death, chronic weight loss, and increased sensitivity to the toxicities of HIV drugs (Pace & Leaf, 1995). Existing research indicates that development of a compromised antioxidant status begins early in the course of HIV infection and appears to contribute to disease progression in a number of ways, many of which are not as yet fully understood (Bogden et al., 2000).

Micronutrients. Third, various immune system components and processes depend on the consumption of specific micronutrients, and it is likely that almost all dietary nutrients have quite specific roles to play in maintaining an optimal immune response (Ferencík & Ebringer, 2002). Inadequate intake of micronutrients—a condition sometime referred to as the *hidden hunger*—including vitamins, minerals, trace elements, essential amino acids, and linoleic acid, is known to damage immune system response in three identifiable ways (Calder & Kew, 2002; Wintergerst, Maggini, & Hornig, 2007).

One way stems from the fact that micronutrients, including vitamins A, C, and E and also a trace element like zinc, help to strength the skin and mucosa. Insufficient consumption or absorption of these nutrients weakens the body's capacity to block pathogenic penetration. Various epithelial surfaces, including the squamous cells of the skin and the inner surfaces lining the lungs, the intestines, and the genitalia, by serving as a multilayer barrier, provide the first line of bodily defense against pathogens. Vitamin A deficiency impairs the epithelial cells that produce protective secretions, such as host defense peptide antibiotics like the β-defensins which, in addition to their direct role in combating bacteria, may also have immunomodulatory and antiviral functions (Agerberth & Gudmundsson, 2006).

Another way in which micronutrient deficiency suppresses immunity is by limiting cellular responses to pathogenic challenges, diminishing antibody production, for example, by such means as weakening natural T-cell mediated antibody responses and interfering with other critical enzyme activities (Chandra & Chandra, 1986). It is known that micronutrients like vitamins A, B6, B12, C, D, E, and folic acid and the trace elements iron, zinc, copper, and selenium, working synergistically, enhance cellular immunity. Tang, Graham, Chandra, and Saah (1997), for example, in a nine-year study of over 300 HIV-positive individuals, found that people with low serum B12 levels had a significantly shorter period following infection (four years) before conversion to AIDS than did those with normal B12 levels (eight years). In contrast, low serum concentrations of vitamin B6 and folate were not associated with either progression to AIDS or a decline in the CD4 lymphocyte counts of study participants. Other research indicates that inadequate intake of various vitamins, especially B6 and B12, folic acid, C, and E and also several trace elements, limits the ability of the body to mount the cytokine-mediated immune response needed to fight certain infections. **Cytokines,** hormones that are released by wounded or infected cells, are critical to immune response because they attract immune cells (that is, defensive white blood cells), like neutrophils and macrophages, to infection sites (Martin & Leibovich, 2005). Further, some micronutrients, like selenium (one of the most studied micronutrients), are critical to the proper functioning of a range of immune cells, including neutrophils, macrophages, natural killer cells, and T cells. Similarly, zinc has been shown to be crucial both for the development and expression of T-cell and B-cell immune functions (Good & Lorenz, 1992). A consistent finding of this line of research is the existence of a strong correlation between blood selenium status and the progression of HIV and HIV/AIDS mortality, with selenium-deficient AIDS patients exhibiting as much as a twentyfold increase in AIDS-related mortality (Baum, Shor-Posner, & Lai, 1997).

Iron deficiency also affects the immune system, although it probably has less effect on the production of antibodies than on the process of cell-mediated immunity that provides backup protection against antigens that successfully bypass even healthy antibody defenses. Macrophages are known to retain bodily iron as part of their normal functioning, and iron deficiency may diminish their effectiveness in engulfing foreign matter like pathogens (Tamura & Goldenberg, 1996).

A final issue in micronutrient deficiency is that the pathways of effect are not unidirectional. On the one hand, infection can exacerbate nutrient deficiencies by altering critical metabolic processes involved in nutrient intake and utilization. In the case of

HIV infection, suboptimal body levels of macro- or micronutrients may be due to inadequate diet or to metabolic disruptions caused either directly by HIV infection or by HIV-related opportunistic infections; they may even, in the case of people receiving highly active antiretroviral therapy, be a treatment side effect. On the other hand, chronic undernourishment weakens the body's immune response, leading to reductions in immune cell populations and competence. This debilitating process is magnified by the deleterious effects of HIV infection on the immune system (Cunningham-Rundles, McNeeley, & Moon, 2005).

Malnutrition and HIV/AIDS Comorbidity

The complex nature of the syndemic interactions that occur between malnourishment and HIV infection are suggested by a growing number of comorbidity studies in southern Africa, especially with reference to such subgroups as women and children. Assessment at baseline of the initial cohort of HIV-infected children to receive AIDS treatment in Botswana (Anabwani, 2003), for example, found that almost 60 percent were severely underweight, while 75 percent were severely stunted (that is, height for age was equal to or greater than two standard deviations below the median). These findings reflect severe nutrient insufficiency. Similarly, in a review of research on HIV-infected children in South Africa, Hendricks, Eley, and Bourne (2007) found that over 50 percent were underweight and exhibited body stunting and that more than 60 percent showed signs of suffering from multiple micronutrient deficiencies.

Among HIV-infected women, nutritional status before and during pregnancy has been found to affect health outcomes for both mothers and newborns. Biological changes during pregnancy create the need for greater than normal nutrient intake for mothers, both for adequate gestational weight gain and for normal fetal growth and development. Inadequate maternal nutritional status is associated with adverse birth outcomes including fetal growth retardation and death (Fawzi et al., 1998). Micronutrient studies have also affirmed the impact of diet on birth outcomes among HIV-infected mothers. In a controlled clinical study in Malawi involving almost 700 HIV-positive pregnant women, for example, Kumwenda et al. (2002) found that vitamin A was essential for neonatal growth. In the experimental arm of the study, women received daily doses of iron and folate, either alone (control group) or in combination with vitamin A (experimental group). The researchers found that among women in the experimental group, mean birth weights were significantly greater than they were among mothers in the control group; the percentage of low birth weight infants was significantly lower in the experimental group (14 percent versus 21 percent); the proportion of anemic infants at six weeks postpartum was 23 percent for the experimental group compared to 41 percent for the control group; and the respective cumulative proportions of infants who were diagnosed as HIV-infected at six weeks and twenty-four months of age were 26.6 percent and 27.8 percent (experimental) and 27.7 percent and 32.8 percent (control). In short, ingestion of vitamin A improved birth weight and neonatal growth and reduced anemia, but did not affect perinatal HIV transmission.

Wasting Syndrome

Severe weight loss is a common feature of advanced HIV infection. As indicated in its 1993 redefinition of AIDS, the Centers for Disease Control and Prevention considers unexplained weight loss of more than 10 percent that is accompanied by fever or diarrhea, a condition known as **wasting syndrome,** to be an indicator in an HIV-infected person of transition to AIDS. Significant loss of body mass can have several direct causes in HIV infection but is often a consequence of inadequate food consumption due to the adverse effects of opportunistic diseases (especially *Mycobacterium avium* complex infection, cytomegalovirus infection, *Pneumocystis carinii* pneumonia, and tuberculosis). Wasting syndrome is associated with a poor prognosis and more rapid disease progression (Williams, Waters, & Parker, 1999). In a study designed to determine the most frequent signs and symptoms of recently diagnosed HIV/AIDS patients at a teaching hospital in Nigeria (Akolo, Ukoli, Ladep, & Idoko, 2008), researchers found that the most common patient-reported symptoms were weight loss (65.5 percent), fever (41.5 percent), chronic cough (38.5 percent), diarrhea (32.0 percent), intense itchiness (13.0 percent), and body rash (12.5 percent). The major observable signs were pallor (25.0 percent), oral thrush (20.5 percent), wasting (20.0 percent), enlargement of the lymph nodes (18.0 percent), dermatitis (16.0 percent), hyperpigmented nails (13.5 percent), and finger clubbing (8.5 percent).

In some settings, wasting syndrome may be part of a larger set of interacting disorders that include drug abuse. In a Miami study of outreach-recruited street drug users, for example, the prevalence of HIV-related wasting was found to be 17.6 percent, with a much higher proportion of those who experienced wasting reporting periods during the previous month when they went for at least a day without eating compared with those who did not experience wasting (81 percent versus 57 percent). Participants who experienced wasting shared a number of drug-use characteristics, including being more likely to be heavy alcohol consumers and being cocaine users (Campa et al., 2005). As these studies in Nigeria and Miami suggest, in quite varied settings wasting is a regular feature of HIV infection linked both to social conditions and to disease interactions.

In sum, among impoverished populations AIDS and malnutrition "are locked in a 'vicious cycle' that worsens the impact of both" (Porter, 2006). Even when AIDS treatment reaches new patients in heavily affected areas, malnourishment becomes a factor because it diminishes the efficacy and increases the toxicity of antiretroviral drugs. With food prices rising throughout the world, the potential for this devastating syndemic to have even greater impact looms large.

CARDIOVASCULAR DISEASES AND HIV/AIDS

Various studies have addressed the relationship of HIV/AIDS to cardiovascular disease. Findings of a number of studies show that people with HIV/AIDS are at higher risk of developing cardiovascular problems than uninfected individuals, a vulnerability that may be related directly to HIV infection or may be the result of metabolic complications caused by highly active antiretroviral therapy (HAART).

HAART and Heart Disease

One study (Obel et al., 2007) that has looked at both the direct (patients are not receiving HAART) and indirect (patients are receiving HAART) effects of HIV infection on heart disease focused on risk for ischemic heart disease, a condition involving a decline in the flow of blood in the coronary arteries that supply the heart muscle. Ischemic heart disease not only can cause angina (chest pain during exertion), it can lead to a heart attack. The researchers in this study examined all patients with HIV infection admitted to Danish hospitals for the first time for ischemic heart disease between January 1995 and December 2004 and compared them with a matched sample (by age and sex) drawn from a population-based control group of people who were not infected with HIV. They found that HIV patients who had not begun HAART were slightly more likely to be hospitalized for ischemic heart disease than the controls were, but the difference was not statistically significant. For those on HAART, risk for heart disease was notably higher than among the controls and those on both HAART and AIDS medications were more likely to die within thirty days of being admitted to the hospital than those in the control sample were. HIV patients at highest risk for heart disease were those who had the more advanced cases of HIV infection, as indicated by a low CD4 cell count or high HIV load. The increased risk of heart disease for those on HAART was calculated by these researchers as being the equivalent of smoking one to four cigarettes a day.

Controversies in Heart Research with HIV Patients

Biomedical concern with the potential negative impact of HAART on cardiovascular disease has grown considerably in recent years. It began with a letter written by a clinical research group led by Keith Henry, professor of medicine at the University of Minnesota School of Medicine, to the British medical journal *Lancet*. In the letter the group reported two cases of heart attacks in young men being treated with protease inhibitors, a central component of the HAART cocktail. Subsequent review by the D:A:D Study Group (Friis-Møller et al., 2006) of 23,400 HIV-infected patients from eleven research cohorts, in Europe, Australia, and the United States, confirmed that exposure to protease inhibitors was associated with an increased risk of myocardial infarction. This finding attracted considerable attention because of the size and diversity of the research sample. Other linkages between cardiovascular disease and HIV/AIDS have also been reported. Mujawar et al. (2006), for instance, identified the existence of previously unrecognized dysregulation of intracellular lipid metabolism in macrophages that have been infected with HIV. These patterns suggest an association of HIV disease and atherosclerosis.

Findings from other research have not supported the HIV–cardiovascular disease link, however. To further test the relationship of HIV treatment to cardiovascular problems, Bernal et al. (2008) examined peripheral arterial disease in a sample of 91 Spanish HIV patients, 81 percent of whom were on antiretroviral therapy and 63 percent of whom had been treated with a protease inhibitor. Peripheral arterial disease was chosen because it is an indicator of hardening of the arteries and a strong predictor of an increased risk of death from heart disease and it is easy to assess using a blood-pressure cuff.

Unlike several other studies, this research found a low prevalence of peripheral arterial damage among its cohort of HIV-infected patients. Similarly, Grandominico and Fichtenbaum (2008) found no significant short-term (four to six weeks) changes in systolic, diastolic, or mean arterial pressures in a comparison of HIV patients in and not in HAART treatment.

These various studies have reported conflicting findings (a not uncommon occurrence in early stages of research, when many of the factors at play are not yet well understood), suggesting that the relationship of HIV/AIDS to the range of cardiovascular diseases that together constitute a leading cause of mortality in developed and developing countries is uncertain and that additional research is needed to clarify the existence of an HIV and heart disease syndemic.

EMOTIONAL AND COGNITIVE HEALTH AND HIV/AIDS

HIV-related syndemics involve not only infectious and chronic physical diseases but emotional, cognitive, and psychiatric illnesses as well (Baingana, Thomas, & Comblain, 2005). For example, in a cross-sectional study of the prison population under the jurisdiction of the Texas Department of Criminal Justice that focused on the association of six major psychiatric disorders with HIV alone and with HIV and hepatitis coinfection, Baillargeon et al. (2008) found that compared to inmates with HIV alone, inmates with HIV and HCV coinfection had an elevated prevalence of at least one of the six psychiatric disorders. Treisman, Angelino, and Hutton (2001) have classified the mental and behavioral health conditions linked to HIV into the following four categories:

- Brain diseases

- Problems that emerge from life circumstances (including stress and discrimination)

- Personality and temperament disorders

- Disorders of motivated behavior

The process of understanding the various entwinings of HIV/AIDS with psychiatric diseases and emotional, cognitive, and personality disorders is burdened by the complexities of the interactions that occur: emotional problems can lead to HIV risk behaviors (for example, risky sexual behaviors) that result in HIV infection; HIV infection can directly cause organic diseases of the brain and central nervous system and can contribute to various mental health diagnoses; and HIV infections, in combination with accusatory social constructions of HIV and the social stigmatization of HIV sufferers, can cause depression, anxiety, and other emotional disorders.

Organic Brain Diseases

Autopsies performed on people who died of AIDS-related causes have found that many (75 percent) exhibit neurological changes, and about 30 percent have multiple central nervous system lesions (Mamidi, DeSimone, & Pomerantz, 2002). Both HIV itself and other opportunistic infectious agents are believed to be involved in causing lesions. Common HIV/AIDS-related brain disorders are cryptococcal meningitis, cytomegalovirus encephalitis, progressive multifocal leukoencephalopathy, and AIDS dementia complex (ADC). The latter, which occurs in approximately 20 percent of people living with HIV/AIDS and is the most common dementia worldwide, is characterized by "marked impairment in cognitive functioning, involving the ability to observe, concentrate, memorize, and quickly and flexibly process information" (Gallego, Gordillo, & Catalán, 2000, p. 49). Neurochemical changes associated with ADC have been found to begin within a few months of infection (Koutsilieri, Scheller, Sopper, ter Meulen, & Riederer, 2002). The temporal progression of ADC appears to be slowed by HIV/AIDS treatment, however, with the majority of patients on HAART exhibiting an attenuated form of dementia (McArthur, 2004).

Mood Disorders

Mood disorders, such as depression, are twice as prevalent among AIDS patients as among the general population (Treisman et al., 2001), although diagnosis of depression is complicated by the fact that depression symptoms can be masked by their similarity to other HIV symptoms (such as significant weight loss and sustained fatigue). Nonetheless, the bulk of the psychiatric complications of HIV infection fall into the category of mood disorders. Notably, in HIV/AIDS patients mood disorders tend not to occur in isolation, but rather are commonly associated with other conditions, including psychiatric diseases and substance abuse. For example, Berger-Greenstein et al. (2007) examined a cohort of U.S. HIV/AIDS patients receiving care at two urban medical centers. Most participants (almost 75 percent) were people of color and most were unemployed. Structured clinical interviews found that over 70 percent of participants met established criteria for a major depressive disorder. Inadequate nutrition (for example, inadequate macronutrient intake) in HIV/AIDS patients may be a contributory factor in the development of mood disorders in this population (Isaac et al., 2008).

Life Circumstances and Emotional Health

Interviews with people living with HIV/AIDS in the United States show that they often complain of suffering more from the way they are treated socially than from the physical effects of the disease that they endure (Mosack, Abbott, Singer, Weeks, & Rohena, 2005; Romero-Daza, Weeks, & Singer, 2003). Stigmatization stems from fear of contagion, a perceived link between HIV infection and immoral behavior, and cultural presumption of infection among already marginalized populations. Discrimination, mistreatment, and physical abuse (including murder) have been reported for people living with HIV/AIDS in various countries (Castro & Farmer, 2005). It is for this reason that AIDS stigmatization has been referred to as the **third epidemic** (that is, HIV, AIDS, and stigma); it not only acts as a barrier to seeking testing and treatment and hampers the ability of a society to respond effectively to the epidemic, it also inflicts extensive, health-degrading suffering in its own right.

Motivated Behaviors

Motivated behaviors are actions undertaken to fulfill a need or craving or to seek a particular reward. In HIV/AIDS prevention research, drug use and sex risk taking are motivated behaviors of particular concern that are linked to underlying emotional or psychiatric conditions. The link between mental health problems and HIV risk has been extensively discussed in the literature; some of these analyses indicate that many people self-medicate their underlying mental health problems with alcohol and other drugs (Singer, 2006c). Abrams, Teplin, McClelland, and Dulcan (2003), for example, interviewed a group of over 1,800 adolescents incarcerated for various crimes and found that significantly more females (56.5 percent) than males (45.9 percent) met established criteria for two or more psychiatric disorders. Significantly, almost 14 percent of female and 11 percent of male participants had both a major mental disorder (for example, psychosis, manic episodes, or major depressive episodes) and a drug abuse disorder. Compared with participants with no major mental health illnesses, those with a major mental disorder had significantly greater odds (1.8 versus 4.1, respectively) of being a drug user. Approximately 30 percent of females and more than 20 percent of males who were drug abusers had major mental disorders and were at risk for drug-related HIV infection.

Various psychiatric conditions, including bipolar disorder, schizophrenia, and depression, have been linked to sexual risk behaviors for HIV. For example, Dyer and McGuiness (2008) report that most people with serious mental health problems are sexually active and participate in behaviors that place them at high risk for HIV infection. As a result this population has been disproportionately affected by the HIV/AIDS epidemic (Meade & Sikkema, 2005). In a study of twenty-four Latina women suffering from severe mental illness in New York City, for example, Collins, von Unger, and Armbrister (2008) found that in their effort to avoid stigmatizing labels concerning their mental health status, participants sought to achieve less stigmatizing social identities (for example, "good girls" and "church ladies") but were undermined by the vulnerabilities of being poor, being members of a marginalized ethnic minority group, having mental health problems, and having a low level of personal empowerment. As a result participants regularly engaged in sexual risk behaviors that placed them in harm's way for HIV infection.

Impact on Outcomes

A large body of literature on the mental health of people living with HIV infection indicates that comorbidity is associated with poorer clinical outcomes, including greater psychiatric severity and more frequent HIV risk behaviors. Illustrative of this pattern is a study by Gaynes, Pence, Eron, and Miller (2008) that assessed 152 consecutive HIV-infected patients at a southeastern medical center using a standard diagnostic tool (a modified structured clinical interview based on criteria in the American Psychiatric Association's *Diagnostic and Statistical Manual of Mental Disorders* (fourth edition). They found that during the month prior to testing, 21 percent suffered mood disorders, 17 percent suffered from anxiety, and 11 percent were involved in drug abuse. Forty percent of the total sample met DSM criteria for multiple diagnoses. Notably, psychiatric comorbidity was associated with greater HIV symptomatology. Similar rates of psychiatric comorbidity have been found by Adewuya et al. (2008) in Nigeria, indicating this interaction's cross-cultural expression.

The emotional, cognitive, behavioral, and psychiatric diseases connected to HIV/AIDS complicate help seeking, care and treatment, and overall health, and add significantly to the health burden of people living with infection. As a result these diseases constitute an important part of the syndemogenic profile of HIV/AIDS. As is evident from the role of life circumstances in mental disorders (as discussed earlier), sociocultural factors are critical to the development of HIV/AIDS syndemics. This issue is addressed in Chapter Six, but is preceded in the final part of this chapter by an examination of a silver lining to the cloudy domain of disease syndemics.

COUNTERSYNDEMICS

The discussion thus far of adverse disease interactions raises a question about the possibility of an opposite kind of disease interface: namely, are there **countersyndemics,** disease interactions that lower the burden of disease in a population below the sum effects of the individual diseases involved (that is, improve health)? The discovery of countersyndemics is important because these entities may suggest novel strategies for the prevention and treatment of disease.

Recent findings suggest that countersyndemics do occur and are part of the complex world of comorbidity. For example, William Moss et al. (2002; see also Garcia, Yu, Griffin, & Moss, 2008) at the Johns Hopkins Bloomberg School of Public Health found that human immunodeficiency virus is transiently suppressed during an acute measles infection. This finding was the product of a study of HIV-infected children living in Zambia. In the study, children who had measles, and reported various typical symptoms, including fever, rash, conjunctivitis, runny nose, and cough, had a significant drop in HIV levels detectable in their blood as compared to HIV-infected children who were not infected with measles.

Several mechanisms have the potential to be responsible for the temporary suppression of HIV replication early in the course of a measles infection. Morbillivirus (measles virus) infection is known to cause lymphopenia, a reduction in the number of CD4+ T lymphocytes circulating in the blood. The low point in lymphocyte levels occurs just prior to the onset of the distinct, red, circular skin rash (called rubeola) characteristic of a measles infection. Within a month of this nadir, the number of lymphocytes tends to return to normal levels. The drop in HIV may reflect a decrease in target CD4+ T cells needed for replication. Alternately, measles virus infection may stimulate the production of cells that are directly responsible for suppressing HIV replication. Several candidates have been suggested, including the ß-chemokines, the CD8+ cell antiviral factor, and the cytokines known as interleukin-10 and interleukin-16 (biochemicals that inhibit HIV transcription), but none has been confirmed as the source of HIV suppression. Additionally, Moss et al. (2000) found that median plasma levels of RANTES, a chemokine that attracts immune system components like eosino-phils (white blood cells that destroy parasitic organisms), monocytes (macrophage precursors), and lymphocytes were higher in HIV-infected children with measles than they were in those without measles. HIV suppression has also been identified in patients suffering tsutsugamushi disease, a mite-borne infection found in Asia and Australia and also known as scrub typhus, although how this occurs is not clear.

Another possible HIV countersyndemic involves coinfection with GBV-C, originally known as hepatitis G virus. First described in 1995 and related to HVC, GBV-C has not been found to be a cause of chronic hepatitis or any other clinical condition in humans. Hence it has been called "an 'orphan' virus in search of a role in human pathology" (Canducci et al., 2003, p. 191). Coinfection with HIV and GBV-C, Tillmann et al. (2001) found, is associated with significantly longer survival, lower HIV viral load, and slower HIV disease progression. This finding, which has been replicated by other (but not all) researchers who have investigated this relationship, suggests that the presence of GBV-C inhibits HIV replication, although the mechanism involved is not clear. Together the various studies discussed here affirm the existence of countersyndemics, an issue of potential clinical importance taken up further in Chapter Seven. It seems likely that other countersyndemics will be discovered as researchers find it useful to emphasize studies of syndemic processes and relationships.

SUMMARY

This chapter expanded the discussion of HIV/AIDS syndemogenesis launched in Chapter Four by considering the convergence of HIV/AIDS with several varied noninfectious diseases. It began by reviewing recent exploration of the role of infections generally in the development of noninfectious chronic diseases and then turned to the specific interactions of HIV with various chronic health conditions. The case of HIVAN, a disease involving the copresence of HIV and kidney disease, supported a review of the definitional boundaries of the syndemic concept. The chapter ended with discussion of countersyndemics, a set of disease interactions that have some beneficial consequences.

KEY TERMS

autoimmune disease
countersyndemics
cytokines
food insufficiency
macronutrients
micronutrients

motivated behavior
oxidative stress
third epidemic
wasting syndrome
zoonotic transmission

QUESTIONS FOR DISCUSSION

1. What are the reasons that the discovery of interactions between HIV/AIDS and various chronic diseases is alarming?

2. Explain why zoonosis is an important aspect of syndemics.

3. How was it discovered that stomach ulcers and gastritis can have a bacterial cause? Why is this discovery of importance to syndemics research?

4. Name and describe some of the biological pathways that can syndemically link acute infectious diseases and noninfectious chronic diseases.

5. Discuss the syndemic and nonsyndemic features of HIVAN.

6. Describe how nutrition and the immune system interact. Differentiate micro- and macronutrients. Where has the food insufficiency or malnourishment and HIV syndemic already become a major health problem? Why have women and children been at special risk because of this syndemic?

7. What is oxidative stress, and what is its adverse role in HIV/AIDS?

8. Highly active antiretroviral therapy (HAART) has been linked to cardiovascular diseases. Explain the nature of this linkage. Discuss current controversies in heart health research among HIV patients.

9. Identify the differences between syndemics and countersyndemics. Why is understanding countersyndemics an important public health challenge?

PART

3

SOCIETY, HISTORY, AND THE ENVIRONMENT

Chapters Six through Eight address the fundamental importance of social factors in the creation of syndemics, beginning in Chapter Six with the issue of social inequality and health disparity, followed in Chapter Seven with the impact of syndemics on human health and social history, and concluding in Chapter Eight with the role of the environment, and of the human impact on the environment, in shaping the nature of syndemics and their development, spread, and ultimate toll.

In assessing the social factors in syndemic formation, Chapter Six, "Inequity as a Cofactor, The Syndemic Impact of Social Disparities," links social disparity to health disparity, and both of these in turn to the disproportionate clustering and interacting of diseases among marginalized, subordinated, and otherwise disadvantaged populations. Through an exploration of structural violence, this chapter affirms the connection between social injustice and disease and shows how syndemics are an important part of this connection.

Chapter Seven, "Syndemics and the Worlds They Made," considers a set of syndemics that have played roles in shaping local, national, or even international cultural histories. The purpose of this chapter is to show that syndemics are not a narrow health topic of concern only to those with professional health interests but are often momentous social phenomena that have moved actors on the local, regional, and global stages of human history.

Chapter Eight, "A World Out of Balance: Emergent and Reemergent Ecosyndemics," examines the development and nature of a set of contemporary emergent syndemics in light of the changing environment. The title of this chapter—which deliberately echoes the title of science writer Laurie Garrett's 1994 book The Coming Plague: Newly Emerging Diseases in a World Out of Balance—*calls attention to the fact that significant changes in human societies and their interactions with the physical environment have created the opportunity for the rapid spread of new diseases but have also left most societies unprepared to respond effectively. The result, as argued in this chapter, is the appearance of a new group of multidisease syndemics, like those ushered in by HIV/AIDS as described in Chapter Four. Beyond HIV/AIDS, recent decades have witnessed the emergence or reemergence of numerous infectious diseases and rapid increases in the number of other health conditions. This development affirms Hans Zinsser's epidemiological axiom, expressed in his book* Rats, Lice and History (1935/2000): *"Nothing in the world of living things is permanently fixed."*

CHAPTER

INEQUITY AS A COFACTOR

The Syndemic Impact of Social Disparities

After studying this chapter, you should be able to

- Understand the reasons threats to health tend to congregate in particular populations at particular points in time and in particular places.

- Identify the ways social factors and diseases interact in specific syndemics.

- Differentiate micro- and macroparasitism.

- Explain the analytical process involved in identifying the underlying social causes of disease (that is, explain the "making social of disease").

- Explain the relationship of social and popular epidemiologies to the syndemic perspective.

- Explicate the nature of structural violence and physical violence and their roles in syndemics.

DISEASE IN THE TIME OF DISPARITY

As noted in a World Health Organization (WHO) report, there is a "growing body of evidence accumulated over the last 20 years which shows that people who live in disadvantaged social circumstances are more prone to illness, distress and disability and die sooner than those living in more advantaged circumstances. . . . Evidence from around the world points to an increase in the gaps in health status and health care by socioeconomic status, geographical location, gender, race, ethnicity and age group" (Currie et al., 2008, p. 2),

The kind of social disparity described in the WHO report is a primary social cause of syndemics, the topic examined in this chapter. Social inequalities that result in some sectors of a population living in overcrowded conditions; having significantly restricted access to adequate diets and clean water; lacking sanitary facilities; being subject to residential instability; being denied access to adequate medical care and public health promotion; enduring discrimination, social opprobrium, and related sources of stress; and being targeted for physical violence, often at the hands of representatives of the criminal justice system, produce optimal circumstances for disease spread, concentration, and interaction. Witness the Peruvian cholera epidemic of 1991.

Cholera in Peru

An epidemic outbreak came to the attention of the Peruvian Ministry of Health on January 19, 1991, when a report describing a mounting number of gastrointestinal and diarrheal disease cases arrived from Chancay, a coastal district north of Lima, the Peruvian capital. The causative agent was soon identified as *V. cholera*. Within a few days all of coastal Peru was involved, and then the cholera epidemic moved inland. By April, Dos de Mayo Hospital in Lima was admitting over 150 cholera patients a day. Typical was Oscar Quintana, a fourteen-year-old boy who was brought into Hospital de Apoyo, in one of the poorest sections of Lima, on a stretcher, emaciated from dehydration, curled in a fetal position, his eyes caught in a vacant stare.

> His mother, Juana Quintana, a tiny woman, stood outside the ward, holding a roll of toilet paper she had used to help clean her son. That morning at 10 o'clock, Oscar first started to vomit and have severe diarrhea. Doctors said she probably brought him to the hospital in time. . . . In the next ward, eight patients lay still, some unconscious, others staring into space. All were dehydrated, and they had the look of people starving to death. One man lying on a bed heaved repeatedly, struggling to breathe as doctors rushed to insert another intravenous catheter [Nash, 1999, p. 1].

Within the first year of the epidemic there were 34,000 cases and 265 deaths. Infection was characterized by symptoms of varying intensity, including capacious quantities of watery diarrhea, vomiting, severe dehydration, and shock (due to the loss of significant amounts of potassium ions). Untreated, an intense case of cholera infection can lead to death within eighteen to forty-eight hours. Assessment of diarrhea samples from Chancay and elsewhere revealed a cholera strain called *V. cholerae* O1 biotype El Tor serotype Inaba, which is known to grow in various foods and to persist in aquatic environments.

In all there are more than sixty serotypes or families of *V. cholera*, but only serogroup O1 causes human disease. The particular strain in that family that showed up in Peru had been seen in Calcutta, India, in 1989. Although less virulent than the classic strain, infection with El Tor lasts longer. It is of note that the outbreak in Peru represented the first time during the twentieth century that epidemic cholera had visited South America (Layseca, Parodi, & Carrasco, 1991), the last South American cholera epidemic having occurred in 1895. From Peru the new wave of deadly cholera spread to other countries of Latin America, which within a few years were reporting 1,300 cholera-related fatalities annually (Mata, 1994).

The nature of El Tor as a pathogen is only part of the story of the Peruvian cholera epidemic, however. Social conditions also were primary factors ushering in the outbreak. As Martinez (1999) points out, "Peru is characterised by extreme inequalities in income distribution, with 20 per cent of the population controlling over 54 per cent of national income. It is estimated that around 50 per cent of Peruvians live in poverty, and 20 per cent in extreme poverty" (p. 1). The income of the latter group is on average about one dollar per day. When the cholera epidemic began, the country had an infant mortality rate that was estimated to be almost 60 deaths per 1,000 live births. The first national health census of schools, conducted in 1993, had found that nationally, 48 percent of the children between six and nine years of age were suffering from chronic malnutrition. In 1996, only two-thirds of pregnant women received any form of prenatal care, ranging from 87 percent in the capital to about 45 percent in rural parts of the country. Social conditions outside of Lima are particularly harsh.

As a consequence, illicit cocaine production has attracted thousands of families fleeing extreme poverty in other parts of the country to coca growing regions. In the latter areas, growing coca is one of the few viable ways of making a living as the soil is not well suited to intensive agriculture. For families that get involved in coca growing, the illegal crop offers a means of staying one step ahead of household collapse and complete destitution; it offers a slim hope in what for South America's poor is a world of extremely limited options.

One of the primary forces that has pushed the poor of Peru to adopt the "coca option" was the **structural adjustment policies** (SAPs) developed by international lending institutions, like the International Monetary Fund, and imposed on developing countries in desperate need of development loans. When Alberto Fujimori, who had been a little-known university professor, became president of Peru in 1990, he readily adopted SAP policies, implementing an economic plan that came to be popularly known as *Fujishock*. As Kim, Shakow, Bayona, Rhatigan, and de Celis (2000) explain:

> During the campaign, Fujimori promised his supporters that any plan to reinitiate [international] debt payment would be gradual, and sensitive to the most vulnerable members of Peruvian society. Just after his victory, the president-elect flew with several of his top advisors to New York for a meeting with executives of the International Monetary Fund (IMF), World Bank, United Nations, and other multilateral agencies. When one of his economic planners laid out the new administration's sketch for a gradual approach to correct Peru's hyperinflation, those across the table put their collective foot down [pp. 129–130].

Fujimori bowed to the demands of the powerful international lending institutions and completely revised his economic plan. His radical new economic policies included the elimination of government subsidies on necessary household items like staple food items and fuel, coupled with dramatic cuts in public employment. As a result, from one day to the next, "fuel prices shot up by 2,000 to 3,000 percent" and "real wages for private sector employees . . . dropped to half their 1989 levels" (Joralemon, 1999, p. 48). The consumer price index climbed by 7,650 percent. Four to 5 million people were quickly thrust into extreme poverty, and mass starvation was only narrowly averted by a tripling of U.S. food donations. Unable to afford food and other necessities of life, many took the cocaine option. The choice between watching their families starve and surviving on drug money was not a moral one; it was a simple matter of feeding their children, of living through today in hope of a miracle tomorrow, of living in a harsh world of enduring threat, looming scarcity, and shrinking government support.

It is a world also known by people like Fernay Lugo and Blanca Ruby Pérez, two peasant farmers who were interviewed by *New York Times* reporters Juan Forero and Tim Weiner (2002) in nearby Colombia. When the illicit cocaine companies added heroin to their product line, they recruited people like Lugo and Pérez to grow the poppy plants that produce a resin that is the raw material that can be transformed into heroin (a product highly desired, especially by the poor, of developed nations).

> Here in rugged southern Colombia, a one-acre plot belongs to Fernay Lugo, rail thin and agile, who works, razor in hand, slicing open the pods of his blossoming poppies to collect the milky gum that is refined into heroin. He explained how—day after day, bit by bit, in mountains 7,000 feet up—he tries to accumulate a few pounds, enough to sell for the kind of profits his slumping coffee plants could never fetch. He does not ponder who his buyers are, the shadowy men who meet him at a distant roadside, or their ultimate customers. "When we harvest and sell, we do not even think where it goes," said Mr. Lugo, 29, the father of two girls. . . . Farmers also disperse their poppy crops, Mr. Lugo said, to make them harder to identify by satellite and reconnaissance aircraft. . . . Blanca Ruby Pérez, 39, said she and her family lived by poppies, which can be harvested twice a year and bring far more money than blackberries, corn, beans and lettuce. "It is much easier to grow than the other crops," she said, carefully tiptoeing around the small, green leaves. "Look, we have put no fertilizer on it, and look how pretty it is" [Forero & Weiner, 2002, p. 1].

A similar view is held by Mariana Almendro, who also grows heroin poppies on a small plot of rugged land:

Clinging to a steep hillside 9,000 feet high in the Andes, Mariana Almendro's tiny garden is a gorgeous blanket of red, violet and pink opium poppies. Profitable, too, producing a milky gum that brings about $115 a pound from buyers who turn it into heroin. A Guambiano Indian living on a reservation a half-hour drive from the nearest paved road, Almendro, 48, sees nothing wrong with her illegal crop. "It just brings in a little money for food," she said. . . . One acre of poppies yields about 11 pounds a year of milky gum that hardens into opium, worth about $1,250 . . . In comparison an acre of onions brings about $30. "No one is rich here. This is just to be less poor," said Almendro, a widow living with her three children in a one-room adobe hut up a steep and winding gorge [Tamayo, 2001, p. A1].

For families who did not move to the coca or opium growing areas, the last remaining alternative for most, as Fuchs (2007) describes, was to migrate to the capital city and "suffer through life in the shantytowns" (p. 13). Many of Peru's urban **shantytowns,** or *pueblos jovenes* ("young towns"), as they are popularly known, are "little more than rows of cardboard shacks, with no roofs, dirt floors and no electricity or running water. Children play in the streets alongside garbage. Dogs forage among piles of trash. The streets are full of dust and sand, prime breeding grounds for . . . [the El Tor] strain of cholera, health experts say. In these areas, cholera is striking with the greatest force" (Nash, 1991, p. 1).

The vulnerability to cholera among shantytown dwellers, as well as among other impoverished people in Peru, stems in part from lack of access to clean drinking water. Notes Marston (1998), "In 1991, there was little chlorination in Peru; even today [seven years after the epidemic began] the water system frequently shuts down and existing pipes don't reach all areas. Water pressure often drops, allowing pipes to take in sewage from lines nearby" (p. 1), An example is found in a settlement known as Pampas de San Juan de Miraflores. This neighborhood is inhabited by rural migrants who are new to Lima, "who live in houses without running water and use the outhouses that dot the hillsides above" (Marston, 1998, p. 1). Indeed, at the time of the cholera outbreak, 40 percent of Lima's 7 million inhabitants did not have access to potable, piped water (Brooke, 1991b). Families that lived in the Pampas in 1991 used one-tenth the water used by wealthier families with running water but were forced to pay nearly five times more for it. The cost of water became a major economic cause of health problems. Observes Robert Gilman, an epidemiologist, under such conditions "[s]anitation is always the first thing to go" (quoted in Marston, 1998, p. 1).

In his celebrated novel *Love in the Time of Cholera*, a universal tale of human passion and suffering set in an obscure South American town, Nobel Prize author Gabriel García Márquez (1989) provides a concise literary glimpse of the fateful relationship between health and social inequality: "The well-equipped colonial houses had latrines with septic tanks, but two thirds of the population lived in shanties at the edge of the swamps and relieved themselves in the open air. The excrement dried in the sun, turned to dust, and was inhaled by everyone along with the joys of Christmas in the cool, gentle breezes of December" (p. 109). In this brief encapsulation of contrasts, Márquez suggests why sentences like "cholera is caused by the bacterium *Vibrio cholera*" are incomplete at best and reductionist at worst. Although *V. cholera* is certainly the immediate source of the disease, the biological bullet that penetrates and damages the human body, the structure of social relations—and the resulting inequalities that negatively affect the ability to maintain good health (and hence the ability to respond to new health challenges), living conditions, vital resources, social status, and power—like the hand that holds the gun, determines who does and who does not get exposed to sickness, and once sick, who does and who does not get health care and of what quality.

The Fujimori government responded to the growing cholera epidemic by seeking to protect the reputation of Peru's corporate sector. Brooke (1991a) describes a part of this response:

> Evidently under pressure from Peru's powerful fishing industry, President Alberto K. Fujimori, his wife, Susana, and his ministers of fisheries and of agriculture went on television eating ceviche, a dish prepared by marinating raw fish in lemon juice. Trying to revive tourism, the President also played host to 20 foreign correspondents for a lunch of ceviche and sashimi at a beachfront restaurant. Within days, hospital admissions for cholera soared. One patient reportedly was the Fisheries Minister, Felix Canal, who spent a week in a military hospital. Through a spokesman, the minister denied that he had fallen ill with cholera, saying he had a bad case of laryngitis [p. 1].

The failure of the government to respond to the growing needs of the poor led Health Minister Carlos Vidal Layseca to resign in protest, declaring, "There is one ceviche for the rich, and another ceviche for the poor" (Brooke, 1991a, p. 1).

The importance of socioeconomic factors was underlined by the co-occurrence of a host of other health problems that beset the poorer sectors of the population. As Gall explains (1993): "In Peru, the cholera epidemic was preceded by decay of water and sewage systems and by secular increases in morbidity from diarrhoea, tuberculosis and other acute respiratory infections, meningitis, malaria and yellow fever, as well as surges of violence. . . . When cholera first struck on January 23, 1991, epidemiologists in Peru were struggling with an outbreak of dengue haemorrhagic fever (DHF) that has been spreading in the Americas over the past three decades" (p. 46).

In other words, while various socioeconomic factors, including rural to urban migration of the poor, intense urban crowding under the worst of hygienic conditions, a breakdown of the water and sewage systems owing to a lack of government investment, and the imposition of structural adjustment policies that significantly altered the quality of people's diet, the stressfulness of their living conditions, and their access to medical care, the impact of the cholera epidemic and its toll among the poor was promoted as well by multiple overlapping and interacting epidemics.

Cholera: An Ecosocial Case Comparison

The importance of social factors in the production of cholera and associated epidemics can be seen as well in a case comparison of two of the Marshall Islands carried out by Seiji Yamada and Wesley Palmer (2007). The Marshalls, a former trust territory of the United States, comprise twenty-nine atolls, each made up of many islets, and five islands scattered over 750,000 square miles in the central Pacific Ocean. The islands are inhabited by approximately 60,000 Marshallese people (as of 2005) who share a common cultural identity and language. From December 2000 through January 2001, a cholera epidemic broke out on the islet of Ebeye, resulting in 400 cases of the disease and six deaths. Three miles away, a short twenty-minute ride by ferry, lies Kwajalein Island, which, like Ebeye, is part of the Kwajalein Atoll. Unlike Ebeye, Kwajalein Island had no cholera cases. What factors accounted for this epidemiological difference?

In answering this question Yamada and Palmer first dispelled any paradisal images their readers might have of a white sand–beached Shangri-la populated by indigenous people leading a traditional and harmonious way of life. The Marshall Islands are named for John Marshall, the British captain who happened upon the area in 1788 on a return trip from ferrying prisoners to Australia and whose only contact with the islanders was to fire his ship's guns at some of their approaching canoes. The Marshalls have been under colonial control by one distant country or another for most of the time since. It was at the close of World War II that the islands came to be a U.S. trust territory, after the United States captured the Japanese military base on Kwajalein. From 1946 to 1958, the U.S. military turned that facility into an operations headquarters for testing nuclear and thermonuclear weapons, conducting sixty-seven atmospheric atomic and hydrogen bomb tests in the Marshall Islands. The tests left Bikini and Enewetak islands uninhabitable and exposed populations on other nearby islands to radioactive fallout and resulting radioactive sickness. In 1954, the indigenous people of Rongerik Atoll, who had been evacuated, were "returned to their atoll to live in what was known to U.S. scientists to be a heavily contaminated environment" but were not informed of the risk until 1982 (Johnston, 2007, p. 39). Some of the people displaced by the testing were moved to Ebeye. In 1961, the United States built the Ronald Reagan Ballistic Missile Defense Test Site in the Kwajalein Atoll. As Yamada and Palmer (2007) emphasize, "U.S. strategic policies of maintaining global military superiority, manifested by the development of a nuclear arsenal in the post-World War II period can be thus identified as a fundamental cause of the conditions under which the people of the Marshall Islands live" (p. 84).

Ebeye is now the second largest population center of the Marshall Islands, and its social order is largely a creation of the U.S. military. At the time of the Japanese census of 1930, only nine people lived there. The jump in population began in 1951 when 559 people were moved there from Kwajalein Island to provide a workforce for the military. Poor planning resulted in inadequate preparation for the natural growth of this population and for the maintenance of the desalination and electrical plants. An influx of people displaced by military testing added to the growing problem of overpopulation and inadequate facilities. Homes were built of plywood with corrugated iron or aluminum roofs and no running water. Traditional foods were generally not available, and people were forced to rely on imported canned and processed foods. Although comprising only seventy-eight acres, Ebeye came to be populated by over 10,000 people, giving it one of the highest density populations in the world and earning it a designation as "the worst slum in the Pacific" (Ridgell, 1995, p. 82). Overcrowding has destroyed the limited natural resources to be found on Ebeye, including potable water. Malnutrition among children raised on nonnutritious imported foods has been reported. Resistance to change, however, comes from U.S. maintenance and reinforcement of traditional island chiefdom and landowning patterns, a strategy that has resulted in some individuals becoming extremely wealthy from U.S. rent payments while the majority of the population remains poor and dependent.

In his historical novel *Melal: A Novel of the Pacific*, Marshallese author Robert Barclay (2002) graphically describes the unhealthy conditions on Ebeye, as seen through the eyes of his main character, Rujen Keju:

When the sewage pump was not working, people still had to go—no stopping it, no saving it for another day—so they had to find someplace outside. With more than eight thousand people living on one-tenth of a square mile, finding a private place to go took some work. . . . The sewage pump always broke if there was diarrhea going around . . . and when that happened, those afflicted emptied their guts where they had time to get to, sometimes very close to their homes. . . . Rujen also knew that spilling raw sewage into the lagoon was unhealthy, the cause of skin infections, and it spread sickness through the fish people caught (he and his household never ate fish from Ebeye) [pp. 91–92].

In contrast with Ebeye, the population of Kwajalein Island is between 2,000 and 4,000, with a much lower population density. The island is under military command but is run by private contractors. Kwajalein has broad streets, markets stocked with fresh fruits and vegetables (because it is home to expatriate Americans who work for U.S. corporations on the island), and clean drinking water (obtained by catchment from the island's airport runway). Further, note Yamada and Palmer (2007): "Most of Kwajalein's long-term residents are civilian employees of defense contractors and members of civil society such as school or hospital workers. While there is some racial diversity among the workers on Kwajalein, their U.S. citizenship sets them apart from the Marshallese, particularly in that their living conditions are privileged in stark comparison to the residents of Ebeye. The demand for security on a military base effectively keeps Americans apart from Marshallese" (p. 81).

It was under these contrasting living and social conditions that cholera arrived, perhaps from the bilge water of an ocean tanker. The people living on Kwajalein were not the only ones spared infection; on Ebeye, too, various social factors were linked to who got sick and who did not. Ebeye residents who could not afford their own facilities to catch rainwater were at higher risk of contracting cholera. Those who lacked access to fresh fruits and vegetables and depended completely on imported food, including alcohol, bleached white rice, and high-fat and high-sodium processed foods, were more likely to have diabetes, and those with diabetes were at heightened risk of cholera infection. Vitamin A deficiency, also linked to the poor quality of the diet, is also known to be associated with poor outcomes in cases of diarrheal disease. Frequent bouts of diarrheal disease among children leads to their being underweight and having poor resistance to subsequent infection. All of these factors, including the nuclear testing and the creation of a refugee population, the social and geographical separation between expatriate Americans and indigenous people, the significant differences in living conditions and resources, and the preexisting, socially generated distribution of other diseases that interacted with cholera, helped to create the pattern exhibited by the 2001–2002 cholera epidemic in the Marshall Islands.

The central role of social inequality in the production of ill health is by no means restricted to infectious epidemics but, as discussed with reference to obesity-related diseases in the following section, is a critical factor in chronic health problems as well.

Obesity and Poverty

Obesity in the United States has been described as a national crisis. It is estimated that one-third of Americans are overweight and that this percentage is climbing. Only four of the forty-five states that participated in the Centers for Disease Control and Prevention's 1991 Behavioral Risk Factor Surveillance System annual survey had obesity prevalence rates of 15 to 19 percent, and not a single one of these forty-five states had obesity prevalence rates of 20 percent or more. Nine years later, all fifty states had obesity prevalence rates of 15 percent or more, with thirty-five states having obesity prevalence rates as high as 20 percent or more (Centers for Disease Control and Prevention, 2001). Meanwhile, the National Health and Nutrition Examination Surveys conducted in 1999–2000 and 2003–2004 (using stratified, multistage probability samples of the civilian, noninstitutionalized U.S. population) found an increase in the prevalence of overweight among female children and adolescents from 13.8 percent in 1999–2000 to 16.0 percent in 2003–2004, and an increase in the prevalence of overweight in male children and adolescents from 14.0 to 18.2 percent. Among adults the prevalence of obesity among men increased significantly, from 27.5 percent in 1999–2000 to 31.1 percent in 2003–2004, while among women there was no significant increase in obesity between 1999–2000 (33.4 percent) and 2003–2004 (33.2 percent). The prevalence of extreme obesity in 2003–2004 was 2.8 percent in men and 6.9 percent in women (Ogden et al., 2006). In these studies, body fatness was assessed indirectly by using the **body mass index** (BMI), a formula-based number calculated from a person's weight and height (weight(kg)/[height(m)]^2). Adults with a BMI score between 25 and 29.9 are defined as overweight, those with a BMI between 30 and 39.9 are considered obese, and those with a BMI of 40 and higher are extremely obese.

Overweight and obesity are significant health issues because they are linked with over thirty diseases, many of which have been described in prior chapters in terms of their syndemic interactions with other diseases and which include type 2 diabetes, heart disease, cancer, high blood pressure, and depression. Approximately half a million people in North America and Western Europe die from obesity-related diseases every year. It is estimated that the direct health care costs of obesity exceed $100 billion in the United States alone (Seth, 2005). Yet like food itself, obesity is not evenly or equitably distributed across all sectors of U.S. society: it is disproportionately a disease of the poor and of marginalized ethnic minorities, as seen in Table 6.1.

TABLE 6.1.　Prevalence of Obesity: Adults Twenty Years Old and Older

	Male	Female	Total
Ethnicity			
White, non-Hispanic	20	24	22
African American	21	38	30
Hispanic or Latino	24	35	29
Family income			
<130 percent of poverty level	21	35	29
>130 percent of poverty level	20	23	21

Source: Adapted from U.S. Department of Health and Human Services, 2000, table 19-2.

The patterns described in Table 6.1 have continued in subsequent years. In 2003–2004, for example, the National Health and Nutrition Examination Survey found a continued significant difference in obesity prevalence by ethnicity. Approximately 30 percent of non-Hispanic white adults were found to be obese as were 45.0 percent of non-Hispanic black adults, and 36.8 percent of Mexican Americans (Ogden et al., 2006).

As Seth (2005) states, "there is reason to believe that the relationship between poverty and obesity is causal." A review of the available literature by Drewnowski and Specter (2004) concluded that a likely mechanism causally linking poverty and obesity is the tendency of the poor to select foods high in energy density, a category colloquially referred to as *junk food,* so as to acquire the greatest amount of food energy for the lowest cost. This selection pattern may be reinforced by the high sugar and fat content of these foods. Sugars and fats have been found to trigger high levels of pleasure when consumed, to be the most frequent objects of food cravings, and to have broad and possibly innate taste appeal (Birch, 1999; Levine, Kotz, & Gosnell, 2003; Yanovski, 2003). A study of over 350 low–income women who participated in the Expanded Food and Nutrition Education Program found that a $10 to $20 per month drop in the family food budget correlated with a net increase of 300 kilocalories per day in energy intakes (Burney & Haughton, 2002), suggesting that people respond to worsening poverty by increasing their consumption of energy-dense foods if they are obtainable. In the United States, where energy-dense foods are both widely available and heavily advertised as desirable by the food and restaurant industry, the consequences are disproportionate overweight and obesity among the poor and other marginalized populations, with resulting health consequences. Seth (2005) similarly argues that the available research supports a *food choice constraint model.* "In this model, one's ability to purchase healthy foods declines as income falls (or as economic constraint increases) in a standard budget constraint shift fashion because healthy foods (non-energy-dense foods) are relatively costly. In this way, consumption of an energy-dense diet is a strategy of the poor to consume more energy at a lower cost. This strategy is reinforced by a biological preference for energy-dense foods."

The U.S. pattern just described is being increasingly replicated around the world, in both developed and developing countries. The World Health Organization (WHO) estimates that more than 1 billion adults worldwide are overweight and at least 300 million are clinically obese. According to WHO (2006b), although once "considered a problem only in high-income countries, overweight and obesity are now dramatically on the rise in low- and middle-income countries, particularly in urban settings." Writing of the poor in Buenos Aires, Argentina, for example, Patricia Aguirre (2000) observes: "The comparative advantages of carbohydrates and fatty foods are evident: not only are they less expensive but they produce a feeling of being full. The poor do not choose this group of products because they do not know better but because they cannot afford to eat other more expensive foods" (pp. 14–15). As a result, "the poor are malnourished because they do not have enough to feed themselves and they are obese because they eat poorly, with a significant energy imbalance" (p. 11).

THE MAKING SOCIAL OF DISEASE

As seen in the previous examples of the social origins of disease and ill health, a fundamental aspect of the syndemic perspective is its focus on the reasons threats to health tend to congregate in particular populations at particular points in time and place. Disease clustering, as the cholera epidemics in Peru and the Marshall Islands suggest, commonly arises out of the noxious effects of oppressive social relations, directly or as mediated by environmental conditions, diet, and related factors, all of which put socially and economically disadvantaged groups at heightened and often grave risk. Syndemics theory, in other words, is rooted in a social epidemiological approach to conceptualizing health issues.

Social epidemiology is an approach to the study of health issues that builds on the classic epidemiological interactive triangle of host, agent, and environment and that involves investigation of the distribution of health outcomes and their social determinants (Poundstone, Strathdee, & Celentano, 2004). In contrast, most traditional epidemiological work focuses on individual factors. For example, the initial epidemiological studies of HIV/AIDS adhered to traditional epidemical patterns and focused on individual characteristics and behaviors in determining risk for infection (Fisher & Misovich, 1990). Fee and Krieger (1993) label this traditional approach *biomedical individualism.* In contrast social epidemiological research seeks to transcend the individual level and to understand how people come to be exposed to risk or protective factors, under what social conditions individual risk develops, and to what degree behaviors that put people at risk are responses to pressing demands and challenges of the unequal or exploitive social structure. As Rhodes, Singer, Bourgois, Friedman, and Strathdee (2005) point out with reference to HIV transmission among injection drug users (IDUs):

> A synthesis of global evidence over the past decade emphasises that HIV prevention interventions among IDUs which focus solely on individual behaviour change are likely to result in only a partial reduction of HIV transmission risk, perhaps in the order of 25 percent to a maximum of 40 percent. . . . Effective HIV prevention not only comprises targeted interventions fostering changes in individual behaviour, but also interventions creating local environments conducive to, and supportive of, individual and community-level behaviour change. This inevitably necessitates a focus in bringing about changes in the physical, social, economic, legal and policy environments influencing HIV risk and HIV prevention [p. 1027].

Linked to social epidemiology is a community-based, activist approach that Brown (1992) has labeled **popular epidemiology,** namely the efforts of communities to document the social origins of the health problems they suffer. Typical are struggles to show how diverse health symptoms among community members are the consequence of potent environmental pollutants given off by industrial manufacturers (Dietrich, 2008).

As in social and popular epidemiologies, in the syndemics approach it is causative social factors that are a primary object of initial investigation and analysis (Gehlert et al., 2008). Only once these have been eliminated as critical factors shaping disease clustering are alternative (including more individual-level) variables considered.

As Paul Farmer (1996), Presley Professor of Medical Anthropology at Harvard University and cofounder of Partners in Health, has written with regard to the spread of AIDS, the "only well-demonstrated cofactors are social inequalities, which have structured not only the contours of the AIDS pandemic, but also the course of the disease once a patient is infected" (p. 264). Living in poverty, for example, has been found to increase individuals' likelihood of exposure to a range of diseases, including HIV. Given the impacts of (1) enduring stress associated with poverty, unemployment, stigmatization, marginalization, residential instability, and population density; (2) diet insufficiency (especially early in life) and malnourishment; (3) frequent exposure to street crime and violence; (4) demoralization associated with living in a deteriorating social environment; (5) exposure to man-made toxins produced by aging and ill-repaired housing structures; and (6) the adoption of behaviors such as abusive drinking and illicit drug use in order to cope with and medicate the emotional injuries of deprivation, the physical capacity of the poor to ward off new diseases can be significantly diminished. At the same time, social disparity tends to be associated with disparities in health care access and in possession of the resources that facilitate adherence to treatment plans. The resulting concentration of multiple, debilitating, and potentially lethal diseases in impoverished populations significantly increases the likelihood that disease interactions will occur, exposing the poor to the added health burden of syndemics. It is the argument of syndemics theory that efforts to account for changing health patterns (including the rise of new epidemics) that fail to consider the fundamental importance of social conditions and the structure of social relations are overlooking critical determinants of health, indeed the most critical determinants.

Microparasitism and Macroparasitism

From the vantage of syndemics theory, there is value in invoking historian William McNeil's differentiation, in his classic book *Plagues and Peoples* (1976), between **microparasitism** and **macroparasitism,** and just as important, in drawing attention to the interaction of the two. *Microparasites* are the pathogens, like HIV or the many other tiny organisms discussed in Part Two of this book, that find resources for sustaining their vital processes or, if they are viruses (which straddle contemporary definitions of life), their genetic codes and their reproduction in human tissues and fluids and that in the process of gaining access to and taking these resources for their own use trigger disease. For example, the human immunodeficiency virus, as we have seen, requires certain human cells to make copies of it, causing the destruction of the human immune system in the process. *Macroparasites* are the larger organisms that prey on other organisms. The chief macroparasites that humans face are other human beings. Again, the goal is the acquisition of resources from the prey, including labor, raw materials, and other items of value. In the course of human history, macroparasites, in part through their impact on microparasites, have become ever more important. With the emergence of class structures of inequality, according to McNeil, a form of institutionalized macroparasitism was established. As a consequence of such macroparasitism, some human beings, primarily those with less power and fewer resources, are put at greater risk than other human beings are for microparasitism and other threats to health.

McNeil came to recognize the relationship between microparasitism and macroparasitism as he attempted to fathom how in the sixteenth century Hernán Cortés and his relatively small band of Spanish soldiers overcame the vast, complex, and quite militaristic Aztecan empire in the Valley of Mexico. Although the Spanish had certain technological advantages, these in and of themselves could never have tipped the balance of power away from the Aztecs, given the latter's vastly superior numbers, home court advantage, and considerable military experience. Even the support given to Cortés by enemies of the Aztecs (other Indian peoples the Aztecs had been extracting resources from through military dominance), though important, became decisive only when it came to appear to these enemies that the Spanish could win and that it made good military sense to side with them. Ultimately, what McNeil came to realize was the fundamental role microparasites—those the Spanish carried across the ocean in their bodies and for which the Aztecs had no prior immune experience—played in carrying the day for the macroparasitic Europeans: "No wonder, then, that once contact was established, Amerindian populations of Mexico . . . became the victims, on a mass scale, of the common childhood diseases of Europe and Africa" (McNeil, 1976, p. 178), including measles and mumps, whooping cough, and diphtheria. McNeil also speculated that dietary deficiencies, born of a corn-based diet low in protein and overpopulation, and ecological strain in the Valley of Mexico may have had an impact on the immune systems of indigenous people that increased their susceptibility to foreign diseases.

Debilitated and disorganized by disease (for example, the death of the Aztec military leader assigned to drive the Spanish out), the Aztec fell in great numbers to the superior Spanish steel swords, were pounded underfoot by the powerful horses on which the Spanish rode into battle, and were battered by old foes with a renewed sense of the possibility of victory over the mighty Aztec. In the end, it was a historic unification of micro- and macroparasitism that was decisive.

Since the publication of McNeil's book there has been some controversy about the origin of the disease that befell the Aztecs following the arrival of the Spanish. This controversy is based on the work of Rudolfo Acuna-Soto (Acuna-Soto et al., 2000) of the Department of Microbiology and Parasitology in the School of Medicine at the National Autonomous University of Mexico, but in fact, Acuna-Soto's research focuses not on the initial period of conquest but on later epidemics that undisputedly nearly wiped out the Aztec population. These later epidemics the Aztecs attributed to a disease that in their Nahuatl language was known as *cocoliztli*. This "illness was characterized by an acute onset of fever, vertigo, and severe headache, followed by bleeding from the nose, ears and mouth; it was accompanied by jaundice and severe abdominal and thoracic pain as well as acute neurological manifestations. The disease lasted three to four days, was highly lethal, and attacked mainly the native population, leaving the Spanish population almost untouched" (Acuna-Soto et al., 2000, p. 733). After examining this reported symptomatology and other data, Acuna-Soto argued that rather than being smallpox, which dating to the time of the Spanish conquest has been the usual assumption, this disease was in fact a hemorrhagic fever of indigenous but unknown animal origin.

A problem with existing interpretations of the source of these symptoms almost five hundred years after they occurred is the traditional tendency to presume that these symptoms are the consequence of a single disease rather than considering the possibility of multiple interacting diseases (for example, smallpox interacting with one or more introduced diseases, such as measles, mumps, whooping cough, or diphtheria) when the latter was very likely the case in the original epidemic soon after the arrival of the Spanish in Mexico. Without doubt the symptoms described do not precisely fit either of the two major types of smallpox, variola major (the more lethal of the two) and variola minor, which tend to be characterized by the acute onset of fever, chills, headache, nausea, vomiting, and severe muscle aches, followed by flushing of the skin and the appearance of a distinctive skin rash. There is, however, another expression of smallpox called purpura variolosa, which is in fact a hemorrhagic-type disease characterized by severe loss of blood into the skin and internal organs. This form of the disease was seen during the Boston smallpox epidemic of 1901–1903 (Albert, Ostheimer, Liewehr, Steinberg, & Breman, 2002). Smallpox is a highly syndemic disease and may be associated with encephalitis, pneumonia, and other conditions. As Heymann (2004), maintains, smallpox "provides a striking example of the complex interaction of infectious diseases, and a justification for sustainable multi-disease surveillance mechanisms" (p. 70).

Three Needed Processes in Health Analysis

The discussion so far underlines the importance of a differentiation made by British medical anthropologist Ronald Frankenberg (1980) between three needed processes in health analysis. The first process is what he calls the *making of disease,* which entails the doctor or other health care provider detecting and assembling signs and symptoms and constructing from them a biological (or psychiatric) diagnosis. Rather than following an unambiguous, clear-cut path that leads directly from recording signs and symptoms to the pronouncement of a diagnosis (as expressed in the ideal biomedical account of this process), doctors must engage in a highly constructive activity involving the social construction of a disease from a welter of clear and not-so-clear evidence.

The second process in Frankenberg's schema involves the *making individual of disease.* This consists of the development of patient consciousness about and experience with being sick. Part of biomedicine involves helping patients to conceptualize their symptoms (or even lack of symptoms) as a biomedically verified disease (or lack of disease). At the same time, recognition of *illness* (defined as the patient's emic conception and experience) as different from *disease* (defined as the doctor's perception and conception) allows analysis of disjunctions in the doctor-patient relationship.

The third and ultimate process is the *making social of disease,* which entails both the revelation of the structure of social relationships that shape the making of disease and the social roles, behaviors, locations, and messages involved in the making individual of disease. Further, the making social of disease involves a critical deconstruction of the making individual of disease, using the lens of social contextualization to identify relevant disparities in health care and in society generally. Moving from biological to social etiology, the making social of disease includes assessment of the social conditions (including features of the physical environment such as pollution of the air or water that reflect social conditions) that directly or indirectly put individuals at heightened risk for disease, the social differences in health care quality and access (differences based on social class or ethnicity, for example), the biology of inequality (lifelong malnutrition leading to low stature, for example), and the social construction of biomedicine as practice, as institution, and as social ideology. Frankenberg's schema is harmonious with the concept of social epidemiology (and of social medicine, as discussed in Chapter Nine).

BIOLOGIZING EXPERIENCE

Inherent in Western culture and as a consequence built into the worldview of biomedicine as well is a traditional dualism that separates the seemingly incorporeal mind (and all that that implies in terms of cognitive and emotional experience) and the undeniably physical body in which that mind, in some sense, is housed. As a result, biomedicine has a tendency to draw a bold line around the fuzzy box of so-called psychosomatic causes of illness, such as individuals' expectations and emotions, separating the contents of that box from the material causes of organic diseases, including identifiable pathogens, other components of the physical environment (for example, living near a natural underground source of radon gas or drinking water or breathing air polluted by the waste products of industrial production), and genetic defect or predisposition.

Kirmayer (2003) effectively illustrates this division—and the problematic assumptions it entails—by citing a passage from the book *Dreams of a Final Theory,* by Nobel laureate and physician Steven Weinberg (1992). Weinberg describes a hypothetical situation in which a medical journal carries two articles, each reporting a different cure for the disease of scrofula (lymphoid tuberculosis). The first article reports the efficacy of chicken soup; the second reports the efficacy of the king's touch (an allusion to an ancient belief that TB could be cured by the touch of a king). Which article, he asks, would the medical community and everyone else find most credible? He confidently asserts that the chicken soup cure would produce the greatest interest because something in chicken soup could be effective against the mycobacterium that causes scrofula. In contrast, "readers would tend to be very skeptical" of the ability of the king's touch to exert curative power over an unambiguously organic condition "because they would see no way that such a cure could ever be explained reductively" (p. 63) and, further, they would not believe that the mycobacteria would care about the social status of the person doing the touching. Comments Kirmayer (2003), in this scenario,

"Weinberg misplaces the causal action in infectious disease, privileging the mycobacterium as the locus of infection. But the proximate 'cause' of a disease is not simply the virulence of bacteria—it includes the host organism's immune response" (p. 282).

In short, what is critical is the relationship between a pathogen and the immune system. A healthy immune system overcomes most bacterial, viral, fungal, or other infections. However, a compromised immune system—damaged by, for example, poor diet, drug use, or a prior or co-occurring infection (in other words, by syndemic interaction)—may not be able to ward off a mycobacterium leading to disease. Hence, in assessing healing capacity, whether of the king's touch or of an antibiotic, it is necessary to know the status of the host's immune system and what things are having beneficial or detrimental impacts on that system.

The king's touch, or any other culturally constituted therapeutic activity, need not have a direct effect on an infectious agent like a mycobacterium to have real effect on health. Rather, it can have an indirect influence on the mycobacterium through the impact it has on the body of the host, a body that is entwined in emotions, cognitions, memories, and experiences in ways that are evident if not fully understood.

Traditionally, mechanical models of the human body have been dominant in biomedicine (Engel, 1977), and this has led to the kind of privileging of reductive explanations seen in Weinberg's discussion. However, as an extensive body of research on the placebo effect, psychophysiological responses, psychoneuroimmunological processes, and related phenomena confirms (Wilce, 2003), these mechanical models overlook the ways in which human bodies, although machine-like in many ways (in having order, being composed of parts, and constituting interactive systems, for example), are far more complicated than machines. Most important with regard to the healing capacity of the king's touch, human bodies have the ability to *biologize experience.* They have the capacity to incorporate or embody events as they are experienced, that is, in light of the meanings and emotions individuals attach to them. Childhood sexual abuse can have lifelong effects on health, as discussed in Chapter Two, because people's bodies biologize trauma. The same is true of positive experiences or the fulfillment of expectations; their impact, mediated by emotions (Lyon, 2003), can beneficially affect health. As a result, "[s]ymbolic, meaningful acts in a medical context can have a substantial effect on the sick person's experience of illness; they can have a substantial effect on actual physical lesions, and, indeed, on mortality" (Moerman, 2003, p. 221). In short, if a person believes in the healing capacity of the king's touch, the king's touch can have healing capacity. The disinclination of Weinberg's imagined medical readers to fully recognize this is a consequence of their culturally and medically informed tendency to "dematerialize social symbols and relationships—which are in fact quite solidly material in their manifestations and consequences" (Kirmayer, 2003, p. 283).

This discussion provides a context for assessing the impact structural violence can have on the appearance of syndemics in subordinated populations, as illustrated in the following section.

Structural Violence and Direct Mediators of Its Disease Effects

The term *structural violence* was defined in Chapter Two as relations of social inequality that increase human suffering to a level that merits their being seen as a form of socially sanctioned brutality. Like physical violence, structural violence is an important source of human injury and ill health. Unlike physical violence, which is often (although not always) visible when committed against whole populations, structural violence commonly is socially invisible (except to its victims), as it is embedded in the day-to-day workings of dominant institutions. As contrasted with street violence or intimate partner violence, forms of physical harm that are criminalized and often punished by pulling violent offenders out of the community and warehousing them in prisons, structural violence generally is legal or at least overlooked and tolerated and hence usually unpunished; indeed, perpetrators, if they are corporate heads, may be rewarded with stock options and other perks that boost their salaries to astonishing levels relative to the prevailing wage system in society generally. Further, structural violence is rarely publicly presented as a form of direct assault on the health of victimized populations; indeed, health care access, access to housing, and even access to food are not legal rights in many countries. As a result the effects of structural violence often are normalized and made to seem failures on the part of its victims.

The term *structural violence* was first introduced by Johan Galtung (1969), a Norwegian scholar and one of the founders of peace research, and was adopted first by liberation theologians and later by social and health scientists. Galtung used the term to label socially imposed constraints on human potential generated by prevailing political and economic structures, such as unequal access to resources needed to sustain life or to provide a reasonable quality of life (for example, adequate nutrition), restraints on the acquisition of political power, denial of equal opportunity for education and the acquisition of helpful information, unequal legal status, and discrimination in housing or other spheres of daily life. For example, in their analysis of the role of structural violence in the spread of HIV among women of color in the United States, Lane et al. (2004) identify this set of macrolevel risk factors as expressions of structural violence: disproportionate incarceration rates of African American men, residential segregation, constraints on access to sexually transmitted disease prevention and treatment services, an African American sex ratio in which women outnumber men (as a result of both high rates of incarceration and mortality among African American males), and the commercial promotion and sale of douching products. Further, as Farmer, Nizeye, Stulac, and Keshavjee (2006), maintain, "The idea of structural violence is linked very closely to *social injustice* and the social machinery of oppression." In addition to assessing health and social consequences and varied mechanisms of enactment, investigation of structural violence includes analysis of "the complicity necessary to erase history and cover up the clear links between the dead and near-dead and those who are the winners in the struggle for survival" (Farmer, 2004, p. 307).

Discussion of the issue of **social injustice** brings up important distinctions made in the literature about social differences in health status and health care access internationally. In their discussion of the concepts and principles involved in responding to social inequalities in health, Whitehead and Dahlgren (2006) define **health inequalities** as a set of measurable differences in health experiences and health outcomes between different population groups based on socioeconomic status, geographical location, age, disability, gender, or ethnicity. As they use the term, inequality is about objective differences between groups and individuals, differences measurable in terms of mortality and morbidity. In much of the health literature in the United States, the term *health disparities* is used as an equivalent term. In contrast to health inequalities are *health inequities,* which Whitehead and Dahlgren define as differences in opportunity among population groups that lead to unequal life chances and inadequate access to health services, nutritious food, and appropriate housing. Health inequities, some of which are measurable, are perceived as being unfair and unjust. One way to see structural violence, then, is as a pernicious expression of health inequity.

The effects of structural violence on health and well-being have been thoroughly documented, and many examples have been mentioned in the previous pages. Although the specific expressions of structural violence overlap (for example, the effects of poverty and of ethnic discrimination are commonly interconnected), for purposes of analysis it is useful to first assess them individually before considering their cumulative and interactive effects. The term *structural violence* lumps together quite different configurations of domination, an inclusiveness that has been identified as one of the weaknesses of the concept (Wacquant, 2004). Its value as an analytical concept, however, lies in the attention it calls to diverse, structurally imposed (and often crisscrossing) pathways to a common outcome: poor health and social suffering. The following sections examine two prominent (and interlocked) expressions of structural violence, poverty and racism, and also discuss the effect of cumulative structural violence of many kinds.

Poverty As Grace Budrys (2003) points out in her book *Unequal Health: How Inequality Contributes to Health or Illness,* from a health standpoint, "being at the top of the [social class] heap is a lot better than being on the bottom. . . . There has been an explosion of research indicating that social class is a powerful, and arguably the most powerful, predictor of health" (pp. 179–181). For example, writing about the city of Boston in light of the groundbreaking epidemiological work of Harvard professors Nancy Krieger and Pamela Waterman, Drexler (2006) poignantly observes:

> If you live in Beacon Hill's Louisburg Square, which sits in the federal census tract with the third highest median family income in Suffolk County—$196,210—you're sitting pretty. Your risk of dying before the age of 65 is about 30 percent less than if you live on Pleasanton Street in Roxbury, about four miles away, where the median family income is $30,751, and where one-third of residents live (or more accurately, survive) below the poverty line. . . . Pleasanton Street and its environs—home to dilapidated Victorians and untended maple trees, abandoned lots and overflowing dumpsters, shards of automobile glass and billboards that say "Looking to Re-Establish Credit? We Finance Anyone"—in effect act like a potent risk factor for a spectrum of ills.

Health disparity is not a problem peculiar to the United States or to the Western world, it is a global structural problem. Internationally, it has two expressions: disparities between wealthier and less wealthy countries and disparities within the population of each nation around the world. With regard to the first of these, the United Nations Development Programme (2008) reports that over the last several decades the number of people in the world living on less than $2 per day has grown to almost 3 billion. Further, income disparities between the rich and the poor around the world are getting wider. Whereas the income of the richest 20 percent of the population in the world was thirty times that of the poorest 20 percent in 1960, today it is eighty-two times greater. Moreover, as summarized by Smith, Wentworth, Neaton, Stamler, and Stamler (1996), "The continuous association between socioeconomic position and mortality risk is a robust finding that has been demonstrated for many populations, both historical and contemporary" (p. 502). Critical findings on the relationship of poverty and health (Smith, 2003) are that

■ Poverty is accompanied by poorer health status while people are alive.

■ Poverty is associated with heightened mortality from multiple causes, varying by social and geographical location but consistent across time and space.

■ The longer people spend in both poverty and in poor places, the earlier they tend to die.

■ Deprivation in childhood influences disease patterns in adulthood.

Racial and Ethnic Discrimination   Like social class, racial and ethnic discrimination is another expression of structural violence known to have significant health consequences. In Brazil, for example, even though race-based oppression is denied officially as well as at the popular level, research indicates that "the structures of racism are present in everyday experience" (Goldstein, 2003, p. 105). Consequently, writing of **internalized racism** in Brazil, Neusa nir Souza (1983) observes that darker skinned Brazilians often feel inferior and ugly because of the steady if subtle flow of reminders they receive each day from various sources that whiteness equals superiority and beauty. The term *internalized racism* describes what results when a member of an ethnic minority group accepts the racist stereotypes the dominant group expresses about that minority, and internalized racism, no less than open color-based discrimination, has been linked with heightened levels of HIV risk and infection (Baer, Singer, & Susser, 2003).

Similarly, Tull et al. (1999) found that internalized racism in African Caribbean individuals was associated with increased levels of depressed mood and abdominal obesity independent of body mass index. In a follow-up study Tull and Chambers (2001) investigated the relationship of internalized racism on glucose intolerance, using a nested case-control research design as part of a larger study of diabetes risk factors on Saint Croix in the U.S. Virgin Islands. This substudy compared the internalized racism scores of newly diagnosed type 2 diabetes patients with matched nondiabetic control subjects and found a significant association between internalized racism and glucose intolerance in their study population. These researchers hypothesized that internalized racism may be a marker for a cascade of metabolic abnormalities. This finding supports Björntorp's (1988) hypothesis that some individuals are prone to respond to stressors by exhibiting a dysfunctional hypothalamic-pituitary-adrenal (HPA) reaction that leads to abdominal obesity and metabolic abnormalities, including glucose intolerance.

Another issue is how a person is treated socially by others with negative racial attitudes. For example, it is well known from a considerable body of research that hypertension plays a significant role in lowering the life expectancy of people of African descent in the New World. Moreover, among African Americans those with darker skin color have typically been found to have higher blood pressure than those with lighter skin color, leading to the hypothesis that a genetic predisposition for higher blood pressure might exist. To test this hypothesis, Gravlee, Dressler, and Bernard (2005) conducted a study in Guayama, a town in southeastern Puerto Rico, in which they used a narrow-band reflectometer to objectively determine each participant's color. An automatic blood pressure monitor was used to measure each participant's blood pressure three times during the course of an hour-long interview. The researchers found that skin color was not associated with blood pressure. The culturally defined color group a person was assigned to, however, was associated with blood pressure, with those labeled *blanco* or *trigueño* (lighter-skinned racial groupings) having statistically lower blood pressure than those labeled *negro*. In other words, the key factor associated with blood pressure, they found, was not one's actual skin pigmentation but rather how people in the community culturally defined someone's "racial" heritage. This study provides support for the idea that being perceived as having darker skin subjects individuals "to racial discrimination, poverty, and other stressor related to blood pressure" (Gravlee et al., 2005, p. 2191). These and many other studies and reviews of the literature (Dressler, 2004) affirm the negative health consequence of racism as an expression of structural violence.

Cumulative and Interactive Effects   From a **life course perspective,** it is evident that a *cumulative effect* of various expressions of structural violence occurs, in which childhood poverty contributes to poor nutrition, repeated exposures to malnutrition, repeated exposures to infections, and enduring exposure to stress resulting in heightened adult risk for chronic disease. Moreover, the life circumstances of childhood may lead to circumstances in adulthood that affect adult health. Education offers an example of this kind of *pathway effect*. Pressures that lead to dropping out of school also affect some health factors, in part because dropouts are likely to have low levels of health literacy. Cumulative and pathway effects can interact and multiply the health challenges faced by the poor in adulthood (Marmot & Bell, 2006). Inequalities at birth, in effect, reiterate biological inequalities in susceptibility to disease throughout the life course. Subsequent structural deprivations only add to the burden of risk, producing significant health deficits among the poor (Ben-Shlomo & Kuh, 2002).

Structural Violence and Indirect Mediators of Its Disease Effects

The various impacts of structural violence on health are not always direct. Many are mediated through mechanisms involving interfaces between the internal and external environments of the human body, including stress, exposure to noxious environmental substances, and diet, as discussed next.

Stress Chapter Five discussed stress, or life circumstances, as a factor in the emotional health and HIV/AIDS syndemic. Beyond HIV/AIDS, stress is one of the primary pathways through which the structural violence of social inequality affects health. Short-term stress responses (for example, fight-or-flight changes in the body that release energy to the muscles in times of perceived threat) evolved as survival resources that help the body respond rapidly to perceived danger; however, enduring stress responses, caused by prolonged exposure to such social stressors as discrimination or other mistreatment, are highly destructive and can lead to immune system damage, including suppression of T-cell-dependent cellular immune capacity. As a result, stressed populations, especially those that endure multiple threats over an extended period, have a heightened vulnerability for disease clustering, disease interaction, and one or more lethal syndemics.

One example of this pattern is seen in the mortality rates of African Americans. African Americans are at significantly greater risk of death, including premature death, than whites are, with most existing studies showing a 30 percent higher age-adjusted risk of mortality. A higher prevalence of several threats to well-being, including diseases known to be highly interactive, such as HIV, hypertension, infection, ischemic heart disease, stroke, and cancer, account for the higher death rate of African Americans. Much though not all of the disparity in this burden of disease is explained by differences in the socioeconomic status (SES) of African Americans as compared to whites. Health-related expressions of African American versus white differences in SES include a number of indicators of well-being tracked by the Annie E. Casey Foundation. The foundation's 2008 annual report found that (1) the infant mortality rate for the African American population (13.7 per 1,000 live births) is more than double the non-Hispanic white rate (5.7); (2) deaths among one- to fourteen-year-olds are significantly higher among African Americans (29 per 100,000 population) than they are among non-Hispanic whites (18 per 100,000 population); (3) deaths among those fifteen to nineteen years of age are higher among African Americans (84 per 100,000 population) than they are among non-Hispanic whites (60); and (4) the percentage of African American children living in poverty (that is, with an income below $20,444 for a family of two adults and two children in 2006) (35 percent) is more than triple the rate among non-Hispanic white children (11 percent) (Annie E. Casey Foundation, 2008). Moreover, in an analysis of several national studies, Franks, Muennig, Lubetkin, and Jia (2006) found that "African-Americans experience about 67,000 more deaths than they would have had their mortality rates been similar to whites. This translates into 2.2 million more YLL [years of life lost]. After adjusting for SES, these numbers drop to about 38,000 lives and 1.1 million YLL.

Thus, roughly 29,000 of the lives lost and 1.1 million years lost annually may be attributable to differences in income and education between the groups" (p. 2472). The additional burden of morbidity and mortality among African Americans after statistical adjustment for SES is believed to be a consequence of the health damage done by the biochemical changes suffered by a socially stressed population.

Stress due to experiences of racism, for example, is believed to contribute to adverse birth outcomes among African American women. Nationally, the percentage of low birth weight children born to African American mothers (13.6 percent) is almost double the percentage born to non-Hispanic white mothers (7.3 percent) (Annie E. Casey Foundation, 2008). Given that babies born weighing less than 5.5 pounds have a higher probability of suffering developmental problems, experiencing short-term and long-term disabilities, and dying in the first year of life than babies with a higher birth weight do, this is a critical health indicator. To test the idea that this marked difference in birth weights is at least in part due to racism, Rosenberg, Palmer, Wise, Horton, and Corwin (2002) used data from the Black Women's Health Study, a follow-up study of African American women that began in the mid-1990s, and follow-up questionnaires. They compared the mothers of over 400 babies born three or more weeks prematurely with the mothers of over 4,500 babies of longer gestation. They found an increase in preterm birth among women who reported enduring experiences of racism, especially women with lower levels of education. Similarly, Dominguez, Dunkel-Schetter, Glynn, Hobel, and Sandman (2008) found that perceived racism and several indicators of general stress predicted birth weight independently of medical and sociodemographic control variables in both African American and non-Hispanic white women.

Following in this line of research linking stress, disease, and social inequality, Culhane, Rauh, McCollum, Elo, and Hogan (2002) investigated the contribution of chronic social stressors to ethnic differences in rates of bacterial vaginosis in pregnant women. Bacterial vaginosis refers to a reduction of benign or helpful bacteria in the vagina combined with an increase of such harmful bacteria as *Gardnerella vaginalis, Mobiluncus, Bacteroides,* and *Mycoplasma.* It is a condition that has been linked with premature delivery and low birth weight newborns as well as heightened vulnerability to sexually transmitted diseases including HIV. Culhane and coworkers found that the African American women in their sample had significantly higher rates of bacterial vaginosis (64 percent) than the white women did (35 percent). Further, their research showed that exposure to chronic stressors at the individual level differed by ethnicity. For example, 32 percent of the African American women reported threats to personal safety compared with 13 percent of the white women. Similarly, at the community level, African American women were more likely to live in a stressful environment. Thus 63 percent of the African American women lived in neighborhoods with aggravated assault rates that were above the citywide mean whereas only 25 percent of the white women lived in such areas. Given these findings these researchers concluded that exposure to higher levels of stress is positively associated with bacterial vaginosis during pregnancy.

Environmental Conditions A second way in which inequality acts as a cofactor involves environmentally mediated conditions, such as parasitism or toxic exposure. For example, the poor have been found to have high rates of parasitic infection owing to unequal access to hygienic facilities and clean water. Research by Giovanna Raso et al. (2006) in the village of Zouatta II in rural Côte d'Ivoire illustrates this point. In a study of intestinal infections, they found that high numbers of community members suffered from various disease-producing parasites (from 40 percent of the population to over 75 percent depending on the parasite being measured). These parasites included *Schistosoma mansoni* (a helminth that is one of the major agents of the disease schistosomiasis), hookworms (a leading cause of maternal and child morbidity in lesser developed countries), *Plasmodium falciparum* (the protozoan that causes malaria), *Entamoeba histolytica* (a tissue-destroying microbe that causes amoebic dysentery) and several other intestinal protozoa. Suffering from multiple parasites, a condition known as **polyparasitism,** was found to be very common among villagers, with fewer than 2 percent of the 500 individuals who were tested in the study having no infections, and 75 percent being infected with three or more parasitic species.

Polyparasitism is the norm rather than the exception in many sectors of the developing world, reflecting North-South disparities in living conditions around the world and raising the possibility of disease interaction and heightening the health burden among the poor. As Hotez (2006) states, "Polyparasitism has a number of consequences for children and pregnant women in the developing world. . . . Chronically infected children suffer from deficits in physical growth, physical fitness, intelligence, cognition, school attendance and performance, and iron status; pregnant women are at risk for higher maternal and neonatal mortality" (p. 251). With reference to just one helminth, hookworm, Stoll (1962) observes that "[n]ot with dramatic pathology . . . but with damage silent and insidious," it produces severe social consequences, including impaired learning ability, increased school absence, and decreased future economic productivity (p. 242). Chronic infection with hookworm "promotes long-term disability and increases the likelihood that an afflicted population will remain mired in poverty" (Hotez, Bethony, Bottazzi, Brooker, & Buss, 2005).

As this discussion suggests, poverty and its negative impact on the availability of hygienic living conditions commonly provide the social and environmental contexts for disease interactions that increase the misery of populations and serve as barriers to national development, especially in resource-poor nations.

Another example of environmentally mediated disease interaction was described by David Greenberg et al. (2006) in their study of pathogens associated with exposure to secondhand tobacco smoke among mothers and children. Secondhand smoke exposure, a consequence of living or working in an environment with a smoker, is estimated to affect over 125 million people each year in the United States alone. Nonsmokers exposed to secondhand smoke have a 30 percent greater chance of developing heart disease and cancer than do those who are not exposed. Components of the chemical compounds that make up secondhand tobacco smoke, including nicotine, carbon monoxide, and a number of tobacco-specific carcinogens, have been detected in exposed nonsmokers' body fluids (U.S. Department of Health and Human Services, 2006). Greenberg et al. (2006) examined the nasopharynx (the cavity that lies behind the nose and above the soft palate) and associated tissue areas in a sample of 208 children under five years of age and in their mothers. They also recorded data on tobacco exposure and medical history. Their findings showed that 76 percent of the children exposed to secondhand smoke had pneumococcus infections, compared with 60 percent of those not exposed. Among the mothers, rates of pneumococcus infections for those who smoked, those who did not smoke but were exposed to secondhand smoke, and those in neither category were 32 percent, 15 percent, and 12 percent, respectively. Although the study did not find differences in rates of infection with pathogens like *Haemophilus influenzae,* other research with children under five years of age has found that exposure to secondhand smoke is a significant risk factor for *H. influenzae* infection (Vadheim et al., 1992). Moreover, *H. influenzae* and *Streptococcus pneumoniae* are among the most common bacteria found in the middle ear fluid of children suffering from acute otitis media, a condition that can result in perforation of the eardrum. Further, these two bacteria have been found to be the most common bacteria involved in viral and bacterial coinfections associated with respiratory diseases in children (Korppi, Leinonen, Koskela, Mäkelä, & Launiala, 1989). Although additional research is needed, there is sufficient evidence to suggest the possibility that exposure to secondhand smoke is a factor in bacterial syndemics associated with respiratory and middle ear infections in children.

Exposure to secondhand smoke is also linked to socioeconomic status. The British anti-tobacco organization ASH (Action on Smoking and Health), for example, has produced a set of maps showing the correlation of local rates of smoking and poverty in the United Kingdom. According to Deborah Arnott (2006), director of ASH, these maps "show . . . the iron chain that links smoking and deprivation. Smoking is the biggest killer in England, and it kills more people in poorer communities than in richer ones. This project shows . . . why smoking must be top of the list of concerns for everyone who cares about tackling poverty and social exclusion." Despite drops in parental smoking in the presence of children in recent years, "approximately one third of smokers—about 4 million people in the UK—continue to smoke in the presence of children" (Action on Smoking and Health, 2006, p. 4). Similar patterns are found in the United States. A study of smoking in Iowa, for example, found that "[a]dult Iowans who smoke [and who live] in a household at or below the poverty guidelines were two and one-half times more likely than Iowans with incomes above this level to currently smoke cigarettes (prevalence of current cigarette use: 44% versus 17% respectively)" (Center for Social and Behavioral Research, University of Northern Iowa, 2007, p. 3).

The relationship of children's health to environmental risk goes far beyond heightened risks for respiratory or ear infection. The condition of the environment in which they live, including the quality of the air they breathe, the water they drink, the food they eat and the areas in which they play, is a primary influence on children's health worldwide. Children are at particular risk from environmental toxins because their brains, nervous systems, and immune capacities are still developing and exposure to environmental poisons can cause lifelong damage and chronic disadvantage. Air pollution, for example, both outdoors and in the home, is a primary cause of acute lower respiratory infections in children, especially pneumonia. Such infections are among the biggest sources of mortality among young children, causing more than 2 million deaths each year, the vast majority in resource-poor nations (WHO, 2006a). Similarly, lack of access to clean water is common in poor countries. Each year, diarrheal disease, a consequence in part of unclean drinking water, takes the lives of 1.5 million children. Moreover, WHO (2006a) estimates that 2.5 billion people, most of them in poor countries, lack access to adequate sanitary facilities.

Even in developed countries, environmental toxins are an important source of illness, especially among children. Valent et al. (2004), for example, assessed the role of environmental toxins in the disability-adjusted life years (DALYs) and deaths among European children. They found that among children under four years of age, between 1.8 and 6.8 percent (varying by region) of deaths were primarily the result of outdoor air pollution. Acute lower respiratory tract infections attributable to indoor air pollution accounted for 4.6 percent of all childhood mortality in this age group, as well as 3.1 percent of DALYs. Mild mental retardation caused by lead exposure accounted for 4.4 percent of DALYs. Among children under fourteen years of age, diarrhea linked to inadequate water and sanitation accounted for 5.3 percent of deaths and 3.5 percent of DALYs.

The children most at risk for environmentally related morbidity and mortality are those from poor families (Krieger et al., 2003), as seen in an epidemic of lead poisoning in France. Although concern about childhood lead poisoning in the United States has been ongoing for decades, it was not until the1980s that the first case was identified in France (Cordier et al., 1981). The reaction of the medical establishment and policymakers to early public health reports of encephalopathy caused by lead poisoning among children of African origin in France was denial. This denial was characterized by intense subsequent questioning of the accumulating evidence that children were the main group at risk; that identified cases were not scattered and isolated but part of an epidemic among more than 85,000 French children; that disintegrating wall paint in old, dilapidated apartments and a resulting layer of lead dust on floors was the source of contamination; and that poor housing conditions, and not exotic cultural practices (for example, pica and geophagy), were responsible for the high incidence in immigrant African families. This questioning was part of a concerted resistance to recognizing lead poisoning as an expression of structural violence against a marginal minority group (Fassin & Naudé, 2004). According to Fassin (2004): "The Paris municipal housing authorities dragged their feet when it came to rehousing, and balked at participating in inquiries on old buildings. National health authorities were reluctant to recognize prevention of lead poisoning in children as a health priority" (p. 170).

Investigations were launched to identify potentially dangerous cultural objects and practices in the homes of African families, including analysis of the composition of the ink used by self-identified folk healers to write prescriptions and prayers, the contents of traditional eye shadow, the makeup of craft pottery used in cooking, and the ingredients of home cures given to children. Even once lead paint emerged as the undeniable source of the poisoning, victim-blaming explanations were unfurled to account for the epidemic: African children "lacked toys and stimulations, they were bored and spent their time on the floor or in front of a window, left to themselves; the mothers were mostly uneducated and ill-informed, they failed to watch their children or to check their deviant appetites" (Fassin, 2004, p. 172). At work in these interpretations was a "form of practical culturalism that essentializes culture and makes it a last resort interpretation of . . . inequalities" (Fassin, 2004, p. 175). Denied in the enactment of such cultural explanations were the economic and social realities facing African migrants in France. The country was suffering from an economic slump leading to massive unemployment. Recent African immigrants, most of whom were from former French colonies, were unable to find work, denied access to social housing, and subjected to intense discrimination. They were forced to move into dilapidated housing, sometimes as squatters and sometimes as renters paying high prices in a scarce housing market. Overcrowding in inner-city and other underprivileged areas soon followed. It was this set of factors, expressions of structural violence, that was the primary source of lead poisoning and other health problems suffered by at-risk children and their families. Lead poisoning is known to cause a host of neurological, hematological, endocrinological, and other maladies, including damage to the immune functions of the spleen, interference with the metabolism of calcium and Vitamin D, and high blood pressure, and hence it can play an important role in the syndemics of structural violence. Although the interactions of lead poisoning and other diseases have not been extensively studied (except in water fowl that consume lead shot fired by hunters), there is evidence that lead poisoning interacts with a range of other conditions including sickle-cell anemia, dietary deficiencies, and infectious diseases (Loueiro, Spinola, Martins, & Berreto, 1983; Suk & Collman, 1998).

Diet   As seen in the case of malnutrition and AIDS, discussed in Chapter Five, a third interface between structurally generated social conditions and health is the mechanism of diet and nutrition and such deficiencies as inadequate macro- and micronutrients, protein or calorie insufficiency, and poor diets (that is, with high levels of carbohydrate and sugar consumption, as discussed earlier in this chapter). The number of undernourished people in the world is estimated to be close to 900 million, the vast majority (95 percent) in developing countries. The Food and Agriculture Organization of the United Nations (2008) has identified thirty-seven countries that are facing a food crisis and in need of external food assistance: twenty-one in Africa, ten in Asia, five in Latin America, and one in Europe. The World Health Organization (1995) has found that in developing countries, one-third of children under five years of age have stunted growth as a result of long-term cumulative inadequacies in both nutrition and health generally and that 30 million babies are born each year with impaired growth stemming from poor in utero nutrition. In Latin America, for example, the Pan American Health Organization (2004) reports rates of malnutrition-related severe growth retardation among school-age children of 14.5 percent for Guatemala and 15.2 percent for Honduras. In eastern Africa, among preschool children the prevalence of stunting and being underweight are estimated at 48 percent and 36 percent, respectively, and in South and Central Asia the estimated prevalence of stunting was 44 percent in the year 2000 (United Nations Administrative Committee on Coordination, Sub-Committee on Nutrition, 2000).

Malnutrition in all its forms increases the risk of disease and early death, and, as Arthur Kwena et al. (2003) found among preschool children in a rural area of western Kenya, "the interaction between infectious diseases and malnutrition is likely to augment case fatality rates" (p. 98), placing children three to twenty-four months of age at high risk of premature death. The impact of malnourishment on the immune system can affect the body's ability to protect itself against infection but also plays a role in a range of noninfectious diseases as well:

> Individual nutritional status depends on the interaction between food that is eaten, the overall state of health and the physical environment. Malnutrition is both a medical and a social disorder, often rooted in poverty. Combined with poverty, malnutrition contributes to a downward spiral that is fuelled by an increased burden of disease, stunted development and reduced ability to work. Poor water and sanitation are important determinants in this connection, but sometimes improvements do not benefit the entire population, for example where only the wealthy can afford better drinking-water supplies or where irrigation is used to produce export crops [WHO, 2001].

With regard to the relationship between diet and structural violence, a telling aspect of the world food profile is "the difference between progress in availability of food and the lack of progress in access to food" (Pingali, Stamoulis, & Stringer, 2006, p. 3). The export of food from poorer to wealthier nations, even in the midst of food insufficiency, for example, is a not infrequent expression of structural violence. The production of food that was shipped to England, for instance, was a significant factor in the Irish potato famine (the Great Famine) of the 1840s. As historian Cecil Woodham-Smith (1992) notes in his book *The Great Hunger: Ireland 1845–1849,* "In the long and troubled history of England and Ireland no issue has provoked so much anger or so embittered relations between the two countries as the indisputable fact that huge quantities of food were exported from Ireland to England throughout the period when the people of Ireland were dying of starvation" (p. 69). In fact, Irish exports of various foodstuffs, including grain, livestock, and bacon and ham, increased during the five years of the famine. Exported food was shipped under armed guard from the most famine-stricken areas of the country with the approval of the government.

A more recent nutrition-related expression of structural violence is that an ever-growing percentage of food plants (for example, corn and soy), previously exported to countries facing food shortages, is now being converted into biofuels for use in the ever-growing number of private vehicles in wealthy and fast-developing nations. By 2008, one consequence of this pattern, in conjunction with the structural adjustment policies of global lending institutions and the effects of a changing climate, was a significant global rise in the price of food and food riots among the poor in several nations. A number of nutrition advocates began to express concern about the potential for a world food crisis. Supporting this concern, Jacques Diouf, director-general of the Food and Agriculture Organization, has warned that the "problem is very serious around the world due to severe price rises, and we have seen riots in Egypt, Cameroon, Haiti and Burkina Faso. . . . There is a risk that this unrest will spread in countries where 50 to 60 percent of income goes to food" (quoted in Evans-Pritchard, 2008).

Typical is the experience of the laid-off Haitian factory worker in her fifties who told Mark Schuller (2008) of the Americas Program of the Center for International Policy:

> The thing that destroys the country is that you can't buy anything. This high cost of living is killing us in Haiti. . . . If you used to buy a sack of rice for 1,000 goud, you have to buy it at 1,500 goud ($37.50). Only now, a cup of sugar costs 25 goud, a cup of rice costs 18 or 19 goud, a cup of beans costs 25 goud. Even if you work for 70 goud per day (minimum wage), you buy a gallon of gas for 150 goud ($3.75) . . . you see? Here you can work two whole days and you can't even buy a gallon of gas.

The response of the Haitian government to the growing cost of food was limited and ineffectual. The now defunct interim regime of Gérard Latortue, in power from 2004 to 2006, did not implement any helpful policies or programs intended to arrest the rapidly rising costs of food, housing, and fuel. Rather, in his role as interim prime minister, Latortue withdrew the demand of the former president, Jean-Bertrand Aristide, for $22 billion in restitution payments from France, broke off diplomatic ties with CARICOM (the Caribbean community) nations, and granted a three-year tax exemption for large importers (the traditional Haitian elite who control the country's foreign trade). Further, the Latortue government agreed to the implementation of neoliberal plans that included privatization of state-run enterprises, lower tariffs for imported rice, and an export-oriented agricultural and industrial plan that proved highly detrimental to local production. As a result, when my colleagues and I conducted a 2008 door-to-door community survey on pressing needs in Cité Soleil, an impoverished sector of the Haitian capital city of Port-au-Prince, we found that people listed hunger as the primary concern they faced in their lives (Interuniversity Institute of Research and Development, 2008).

Overall in Haiti—the poorest country in the Western Hemisphere—80 percent of the population live on less than $2 a day, with half earning $1 a day or less. Yet the country also has the most millionaires per capita in the Caribbean region (Jadotte, 2006), suggesting the role of structural violence across class lines. In the aftermath of food riots in Haiti in April 2008, the government of Prime Minister Jacques-Édouard Alexis also collapsed and the president was forced to get business interests to take a smaller profit and lower the price of rice, a dietary staple.

Self-Destructive Responses   Structural violence takes an even greater toll on human life and well-being than is described on the preceding pages owing to some of the strategies people adopt in coping with the social suffering this violence inflicts. These strategies, including alcohol and drug abuse, obsessive gambling, and risky sexual behaviors, offer immediate relief but are ultimately self-destructive. Addressing this issue requires recognition of structural violence as a component of *lived experience*. Studies of health status among the poor by physical location, for example, show that the *sociophysical environment* in which people live—that is, their day-to-day, lived experience of their surrounding community, including their awareness of threats, danger, stress, discomfort, and alienation from their local social environment—is a critical determinant of their behavior (Budrys, 2003; Singer, 2007). Feelings of hopelessness and powerlessness in a community have been found to be good predictors of health risk practices and the appeal of psychotropic drugs (Bourgois, 2003; Waterston, 1993). All of these adaptive strategies have been analyzed as **self-medication** of the emotional injuries of structural violence. Their adoption—given their ultimate costs (which are often evident, to varying degrees, in the lives and miseries of people in local communities)—suggests the lack of options for those subjected to various expressions of structural violence and the appeal of even short-term reprieves from them.

Edward John Khantzian, a clinical professor of psychiatry at Harvard Medical School, introduced the concept of drug use as a form of *self-medication* in the mid-1980s (Khantzian, 1985). This idea developed out of three decades of clinical work with drug-abusing patients as well as a series of studies he conducted. Khantzian noticed that drug-addicted patients often had histories of difficulties with aggression, including problems of rage and depression, that long preceded their involvement with drugs. He also found that many of these patients reported that the use of heroin gave them relief from dysphoric feelings of restlessness, anger, and rage. Khantzian (1990) argued that there are two key factors in drug abuse: human suffering and problems with self-regulation. The primary urge driving the continued use of drugs, he asserted, is not a search for euphoria or even simple pleasure but rather for relief from the burden of personal suffering. It is in this context, and while moving from the level of intrapsychic pain to structural sources of suffering, that Cameron and Jones (1985) coined the term *drugs of solace*. The poor use drugs like alcohol, tobacco, heroin, and cocaine, Cameron and Jones maintain, because they provide solace, even if for a short time, from the daily social stress of perceived personal failure and associated feelings of damaged self-worth in the context of structural violence. In other words, to Khantzian's initial conception of drug use and addiction as self-medication of individual-level emotional suffering, other researchers have added coping with social suffering linked to structural causes. In this view, heavy substance use or other abusive behavior is not seen as deviance from society but is understood as a tortured effort to adjust to suffering caused by society.

The longer-term consequences of drug use, of course, tend to add to the miseries of structural violence. The consumption of both legal and illegal mood-altering substances significantly contributes to the overall poor health of groups subjected to domination. The prevalence rates for various drug use–related diseases, including AIDS, heart disease, and stroke, tend to closely reflect social inequalities (Smith et al., 2003). In the United States, for example, across all age levels, although whites have higher rates of alcohol use than African Americans, the negative consequences of alcohol abuse, including alcohol-related death, are more prevalent among African Americans. Among Latinos, the rate for alcohol-related cirrhosis of the liver is double the rate for non-Latino whites (Arias, Anderson, Kung, Murphy, & Kochanek, 2003). Alcohol and tobacco use threaten the health of ethnic minorities disproportionately partly because of the role they play in the development of cancer, cardiovascular diseases, stroke, and tuberculosis, and because of their impact on vehicle-related and other accidental injury. Illegal drugs also cause considerable harm in groups oppressed by structural violence. For example, Latinos, especially Puerto Ricans and Mexican Americans, suffer the highest level of injection drug-related HIV/AIDS infection in the United States (Singer, 1999).

Behaviors like drug abuse have another relationship with structural violence beyond their role as immediate coping strategies. As described by Michael Agar (2006): "Drugs are great for what I call chemical scapegoating. The anthropologist Levi-Strauss once described totemism by saying 'animals are good to think with' [that is, they provide readily available symbols to use in organizing concepts]. Drugs . . . are good to blame with" (p. 20).

At the same time, the ready availability of drugs among the poor and oppressed, quite literally on every corner in many poor neighborhoods (be it in the form of legal alcohol outlets, stores that sell cigarettes, street dealers of illicit drugs, or after-hours illicit alcohol sellers), helps to create a condition Friedrich Engels long ago called "social murder" because both legal and illegal drug sales are facilitated by mainstream social institutions and fiscally benefit dominant social strata, which itself constitutes an additional expression of structural violence (Singer, 2006b, 2007).

SUPERSYNDEMICS

The increasing prevalence of emergent and reemergent diseases and the accelerated spread of infectious diseases as a result of globalism, global warming, and degradation of the environment—all factors that involve the same structures of inequality that perpetuate structural violence—raise the possibility that **supersyndemics,** involving synergistic interactions among two or more previously independent syndemics, might develop. Such "perfect storms" of disease would affirm both the importance of addressing the health needs of highly vulnerable populations (in which such extreme disease events are most likely) and the likelihood that the world of disease, already moving toward periodic multidisease global syndemics, will continue to remain a constantly moving target for public health and biomedical interventions.

The term *supersyndemic* might well be applied, for example, to the disease multiplex known as metabolic syndrome and found in the context of industrial societies. Metabolic syndrome, which in many countries affects 20 to 30 percent of the adult population, involves an interacting cluster of conditions: obesity, high cholesterol levels, high blood pressure, diabetes and insulin resistance, and elevated triglyceride (fatty acid) levels in the bloodstream (Grundy, 2008). Having this set of interacting, life-threatening conditions puts people at high risk for heart disease and stroke. This entire complex, moreover, has been tied to carbon dioxide emissions and global warming, in that exercise levels, which help people to prevent metabolic syndrome, have decreased during "the past 50 years [as] we have discovered how to substitute fossil-fuel energy for human muscular work—from occupational work to modes of transport, and from domestic tasks to leisure pursuits" (Prentice & Jebb, 2006, p. 2197).

HEALTH AND HUMAN RIGHTS

Recognition of the roles of structural violence and social inequality as global threats to health has led to efforts to define health as a basic human right. An active proponent of this initiative prior to his untimely death in 1998 was Jonathan Mann, who had served as the director of the World Health Organization's Global Program on AIDS (a position from which he resigned when the United Nations failed to respond aggressively to the AIDS pandemic). Mann argued that health and human rights are integrally connected, and pressed for a unification of the public health and human rights movements. According to Mann et al. (1999): "Exploration of the intersection of health and human rights may help to revitalize the health field as well as contribute to broadening human rights thinking and practice. The health and human rights perspective offers new avenues for understanding and advancing human well-being in the modern world " (p. 18).

Recognizing "the synergy between human rights and public health" (Gostin, 2000, p. 107) is harmonious with the biosocial understanding of the syndemic perspective on health and disease because (1) government regulations that restrict personal freedom limit people's health-seeking behavior; (2) discrimination and the resulting stigmatization are also disincentives for effective health-seeking efforts; and (3) the denial of social, economic, and political rights impedes people's ability to protect their health and safety. All of these, in turn, increase the likelihood of syndemic exposure.

SUMMARY

In assessing the social factors that contribute to syndemic formation, this chapter linked social disparity to health disparity, and both of these in turn to the disproportionate clustering and interaction of diseases among marginalized, subordinated, and otherwise disadvantaged populations. An exploration of structural violence affirmed the connection between social injustice and disease and showed how syndemics are an important part of this connection. Expanding on this examination, the chapter concluded with a discussion of the ways in which an understanding of syndemics contributes to the health and human rights discourse.

KEY TERMS

biologizing experience
biomedical individualism
body mass index
ecosocial
health inequalities
internalized racism
life course perspective
macroparasitism
microparasitism

polyparasitism
popular epidemiology
self-medication
shantytown
social epidemiology
social injustice
structural adjustment policies
structural violence
supersyndemics

QUESTIONS FOR DISCUSSION

1. Why are social conditions and the structure of social relationships critical to syndemic formation? Discuss the role of social and related environmental conditions in the Marshall Islands cholera outbreak of 2000–2001. Relate this discussion to William McNeil's (1976) differentiation in *Plagues and Peoples* between microparasitism and macroparasitism.

2. Why is health disparity a critical concept in syndemics research?

3. How does poverty contribute to the obesity in highly developed nations? How does obesity interact syndemically with other diseases? Explain the food choice constraint model.

4. What is meant by the "making social of disease"? Relate this idea to the development of syndemics. Similarly, what is meant by the "biologizing of experience"? Why is this concept relevant to understanding syndemics?

5. Define structural violence. What are the direct mediators of its effects on disease?

6. How does the sociophysical environment in which people live, including their day-to-day lived experience of their local social environment, play a role in syndemics?

7. What is a supersyndemic? Can you name a potential supersyndemic that could develop in the future?

8. In what ways is the threat of syndemics related to the broader global discourse on health and human rights?

CHAPTER

7

SYNDEMICS AND THE WORLDS THEY MADE

After studying this chapter, you should be able to

- Understand why the occurrence and importance of syndemics in human health was not often recognized in the past.

- Identify the role of specific syndemics in shaping past events.

- Recognize that wars and syndemics have been commonly entwined events in human history.

BEFORE NOW

In his book *The Healthy Body and Victorian Culture*, Bruce Haley (1978) offers the following account of syndemic disease patterns in the United Kingdom during the year 1847:

As had happened a decade earlier, typhus occurred simultaneously with a severe influenza epidemic, one which carried off almost thirteen thousand. There was also a widespread dysentery epidemic, and as if all this were not enough, cholera returned in the autumn of 1848, assailing especially those parts of the island hardest hit by typhus and leaving about as many dead as it had in 1831. . . . Diseases like cholera, typhus, typhoid, and influenza were more or less endemic at the time, erupting into epidemics when the right climatic conditions coincided with periods of economic distress. The frequency of concurrent epidemics gave rise to the belief that one sort of disease brought on another; indeed, it was widely believed that influenza was an early stage of cholera [p. 34].

As a result of such experiences, Haley argues, Victorians were more concerned with health than with almost all, if not all, other issues in their lives, including politics, religion, and their emergent ambivalence about change and modernity. The imprint of entwined epidemics on Victorian culture may be seen in that era's romantic poetry, utopian and other literature (novels like *The Mill on the Floss, The Egoist,* and *Tom Brown's School Days,* for example), views on spiritual perfection and virtue, commitment to hiking and other athletic recreation (such as calisthenics), ideas about the benefits of dieting and bathing, use of architectural tiling depicting plants and flowers, and resurgence of interest in the ancient Greek and Roman cultures, especially the embrace and celebration of Hygeia, the Greek goddess of health. Exemplary is John Ruskin's *Unto This Last* (1877), a set of essays in which a healthy Britain is likened to a human body after exercise: "Thus the circulation of wealth in a nation resembles that of the blood in the natural body. There is one quickness of the current which comes of cheerful emotion or wholesome exercise; and another which comes of shame or of fever. There is a flush of body which is full of warmth and life; and another which passes into putrefaction" (p. 140).

Similarly, John Kay, a leading figure during this era's emergent public health movement, wrote that "the moral leprosy of vice [is] capable of corrupting the body of society, like an insidious disease" (quoted in Adams, 1999, p. 175). This frequent cultural linking of the health of the social body to the health of physical bodies (Scheper-Hughes & Lock, 1987) draws attention to an important component of the social nature of sickness.

Although the rate at which new syndemics develop has accelerated over time as human populations have became larger and more concentrated (consider, for example, the growing number of megacities around the world), as the speed of transportation (carrying people, animals, commodities, and pathogens) has increased through new technologies, and as the human impact on the earth's climatic and other environmental systems has grown, syndemics are not a new phenomenon. The title of this chapter is borrowed from medieval historian Norman Cantor's book *In the Wake of the Plague: The Black Death and the World It Made* (2002). In this book (which is enlivened, if somewhat scientifically diminished, by its serious consideration at one point of the notion that the Black Death might have had an extraterrestrial origin), Cantor questions the received wisdom about the cause of the epidemic. Its metaphorical designation, the Black Death, is often attributed to the dark skin blotches that characterized victims, but that name more likely was intended to convey the devastating social impact of this epidemic, which swept through Europe in the mid-fourteenth century and killed at least a third (if not far more) of the total population. Epidemiological and history texts usually assert that the outbreak was caused solely by the rat-borne pathogenic bacterium *Yersinia pestis.* Cantor, however, picking up an idea introduced by British zoologist Graham Twigg, cogently argues that the engine driving the Black Death was a syndemic uniting the effects of *Y. pestis* with anthrax, an acute animal and human disease caused by a different microorganism, the spore-forming bacterium

Bacillus anthracis. Similarly, in his book *A History of Bubonic Plague in the British Isles,* J.F.D. Shrewsbury (1970), a bacteriologist with a keen interest in disease history, argued that the Black Death was the consequence of a co-epidemic involving yersinial plague and louse-borne typhus.

More recently, DeWitte and Wood (2008) used skeletal remains of 490 Black Death victims (from the East Smithfield Black Death cemetery in London) to test the assumption that the Black Death was so virulent its victims were killed indiscriminately. Using the methods of paleodemographic age estimation and a multistate model of selective mortality, these researchers counted bone lesions suggestive of prior infections and other health problems on the skeletons of the individuals in their sample. They also assessed dental development to determine approximate age. These findings were then compared with data for 291 individuals buried in cemeteries in the medieval Danish towns of Viborg and Odense shortly before the Black Death epidemic began. As would be expected, findings from the Danish sample suggested that bone lesions were associated with earlier death (that is, those with more health problems had died at a younger age). Significantly, this was also true of the Black Death victims from London, indicating that the epidemic tended to take the lives of those who were already in poor health. In particular, the lesions found on the London skeletons DeWitte and Wood examined appeared to have been caused by malnutrition. This suggests that the Black Death was a syndemic caused by diet-related immune system damage and infection with *Y. pestis.*

Whichever of these various explanations of the virulence of the Black Death prevails (and they are not mutually exclusive, multiple infections and malnutrition may have been involved), it is evident that syndemics have had an impact on the course of history, have helped to shape the world as we know it, and will continue to do so in the future. As the multiple disease entwinements of HIV/AIDS, the largest syndemic in human history, make clear, the impacts of disease interactions on human life can be profound. If, as Marx suggested, the goal is not merely to understand the course of history but to change it, then the lessons learned in the study of syndemics may be equally profound.

Although a worthy endeavor, researching syndemics of the past is hampered on the one hand by the limited availability and quality of health records and on the other hand by a less than complete level of disease knowledge. The further back in time one goes, the more problematic the quality of the health records, from the standpoint of both systematic data collection and precision of terminology. When one considers the symptom descriptions provided by ancient Latin authors such as Celsus (25 B.C.–37 A.D.) and Aretaeus of Cappadocia (circa 200 A.D.), for example, it is evident that they were applying the disease term *elephantiasis* to cases of leprosy and not to the helminth infection that now bears that label. Moreover, although epidemics have been recorded since the beginning of writing, the tendency has been to focus on periodic outbreaks that were seen as being caused by a single disease. The result is year-by-year listings of a small, rotating set of diseases, implying that only one disease was present in any given year. However, as Herring and Sattenspiel (2007) observe, "The historical record documents epidemic after epidemic of newly introduced diseases, but these diseases did not occur in a vacuum; rather, they interacted with those already present" (p. 200). Thus Sallares (2002) has suggested that the cases of typhoid fever described in the *Epidemios* volumes of the Corpus Hippocraticum (see Chapter Two) "could very easily have been infected with malaria as well, but this would not be apparent from the description given in the ancient text" (p. 127). Similarly, in commenting on the national mortality statistics for Italy toward the end of the nineteenth century, a malaria researcher noted that "medical science shows that for each death attributed to malaria there are several other deaths, which are attributed to other causes, but nevertheless are directly linked to malaria or indirectly caused by the debilitating effects of malaria infection" (Bonelli quoted in Sallares, 2002, p. 119).

Evidence of unrecognized disease interactions of the past does in fact appear in malaria data from rural Italy. Prior to the 1930s, the Italian hill town of Sermoneta, on the edge of the Pontine Marshes, for example, was recorded as having a crude death rate of 41 per 1,000 population, and 8 percent of these deaths were attributed to malaria. Eradication of mosquito breeding sites in the marshes, however, halved the annual death rate (Hackett, 1937), suggesting a synergistic interaction between malaria and the diseases that were recorded as the cause of death. The same pattern is seen in pre-independence British Guyana, where malaria is assumed by modern researchers to have been the cause of death at a level almost four times the number of deaths actually attributed to it (Jones, 2000). Overall, the use of death records to assess disease interaction is hampered, as Noymer and Garenne (2000) observe, "because even if contributory causes are listed on the death certificate [which they often are not], a unique cause of death is recorded" (p. 573).

Syndemics in the past were not often recognized as such by physicians or public health officials of the day. An example of this is what was once called *typho-malarial fever*, a disease label dating to the period before the pathogenic etiology of malaria was determined in the late 1800s. Patients exhibited typhoid's gastrointestinal symptoms and malaria's debilitating effects, but the medical experts of the time saw these as symptoms of a single disease. The existence of two separate but interacting diseases was not realized. Such confusion is understandable given the tendency for diseases of diverse origin to generate similar symptoms. Adding to the difficulty of identifying syndemics is the atypical disease expression that sometimes occurs when diseases interact.

Despite these challenges, it is possible to discern from the existing archival records the critical or at least influential role disease interaction has had on history. It is the argument of this chapter that attention to the issue of disease interface—which includes an analytical focus on the array of both local and wider social conditions that foster disease spread, clustering, and exchange—contributes to an improved understanding of the history of diseases and the diseases of history. The syndemics concept, in other words, is of value to both history and historical epidemiology.

The remainder of this chapter examines a number of past syndemics in their historical and social contexts:

- The Irish famine syndemic of 1741

- The Gibraltar cholera syndemic of 1865

- The Massachusetts scarlet fever syndemic of the 1800s

- The global influenza syndemic of 1918

- The syndemics among Native Americans on the American frontier

- The syndemics of the Mormon migration

- The syndemics of war

IRISH FAMINE SYNDEMIC OF 1741

On December 27, 1739, temperatures across Ireland fell below freezing; they felt even colder because of bitter easterly gales. Thus began the Great Frost, the most severe period of extreme freezing cold on record for Ireland and beyond. Although much of Europe was hit, the resulting crisis was particularly severe in Ireland. The blast of Arctic weather, a parting nod from the last ice age, hung on for almost two months, followed by an erratic spring that saw no rainfall. As a result, both cereal and root crops failed, and stored potatoes froze and became inedible; meanwhile, domestic animals died in great numbers, ill-preparing people for a snowy winter and continued drought the following year.

What followed was the first great Irish famine, characterized not only by the loss of the staple food sources but also by a painful economic recession tied to the breakout of war between Britain and Spain and a resulting loss of overseas trade. Tens of thousands of Irish were reduced to begging and to the consumption of famine foods like nettles, seaweed, and dock leaves. Rising malnutrition and unhygienic living conditions stemming from the faltering economy and a breakdown of the social infrastructure led in the later months of 1740 to a series of overlapping epidemics: typhus (caused by the louse-borne bacteria *Rickettsia prowazekii*), dysentery (caused by unsanitary drinking water containing various microorganisms), and relapsing fever (a tick- and body lice–borne infection caused by *Borrelia recurrentis*).

Soon mortality rates began to rise, peaking the following year. Although the records are seriously inadequate for establishing the actual death rate thrust upon the Irish by the famine, Lee (1989) draws on various sources to suggest a rate of mortality similar to that of the better known Irish potato famine of the 1840s, during which 10 percent of the population succumbed. As Clarkson and Crawford (2001) comment: "We can only guess at how many died, but on the basis of contemporary accounts and burials recorded in parish registers, there may have been between 300,000 and 480,000 famine-related fatalities in the two years 1740–1741, the majority of them in the south and east of the country" (p. 126).

The Irish people's experience of the catastrophe is expressed in the folk name given to the deadly famine: *bliain an áir,* or "year of the slaughter" (Post, 1977). According to one eyewitness: "Multitudes are daily perishing. . . . I have seen the labourer endeavouring to work at his spade, but fainting for want of food and forced to quit it. I have seen the aged father eating grass like a beast . . . the helpless orphan exposed on the dunghill, and none to take him in for fear of infection . . . the hungry infant sucking at the breast of the already expired parent" (BBC, 2008). Another observer commented: "We have a great mortality among the poor people, who die in great numbers from fevers and fluxes. One poor man buried eight of his family in a few days" (BBC, 2008). In even starker terms a third witness, the Reverend Philip Skelton, curate of Monaghan parish, recorded the demise of "whole parishes in some places . . . the dead have been eaten in the fields by dogs for want of people to bury them. Whole thousands in a barony have perished, some of hunger and others of disorders occasioned by unnatural, unwholesome, and putrid diet" (BBC, 2008).

In sum, the Irish famine syndemic of 1741 began with a mix of both environmental factors and political and economic factors that led to a radical drop in available food sources and a breakdown of the social and hygienic infrastructure. Malnutrition ushered in and united with several diseases of poverty to possibly kill one of every ten people in Ireland, with the poor disproportionately shouldering the brunt of the disaster. Although unique in its particular array of events and conditions, this syndemic shares many features of others that were to follow on the local or global stage of subsequent history. Unlike the well-known famine that was to strike the Emerald Isle 100 years later, this earlier crisis caused no migration to distant shores, a factor that has obscured popular awareness of it even within Ireland. On the summit of Killiney Hill, in Dublin, overlooking the wealthy neighborhood that sports the expansive mansions owned by people like Van Morrison and Bono, however, there is a an obelisk that commemorates the famine and the relief program that carried many families through the harshest days of the crisis.

GIBRALTAR CHOLERA SYNDEMIC OF 1865

Cholera possesses the dubious distinction "of being one of the most fatal diseases in history" (Sawchuk & Burke, 2003, p. 199). The earliest known reference to this deadly ailment dates from fourth-century B.C. India, a land where cholera has been endemic since ancient times. The world, of course, came to know cholera not as a distinctly Indian or even Asian disease, although it still sometimes is referred to as Asian cholera, but rather as a Grim Reaper making periodic sweeps of the planet. People outside of India began witnessing pandemic undulations of cholera in the 1800s, a century in which there were six great waves, each of which, "[l]ike a forest fire . . . pushed along a rough direction and sparked blazes sporadically in its way" (Auyang, 2003, p. 12). The first of these waves began in 1820 and spread across India and up into China to the east and to the Caspian Sea to the west, leaving in its wake a trail of death and suffering. Military movements during the Russian, Persian, and Turkish wars (1826–1829) and the crushing of the 1831 Polish revolt helped to spread the disease during this outbreak. Twenty years later a second cholera pandemic broke out and ultimately became a world affair, with a significant number of deaths recorded in Europe and North America. John Snow (1855) described the arrival of cholera in London during this second epidemic wave:

> The first case of decided Asiatic cholera in London, in the autumn of 1848, was that of a seaman named John Harnold, who had newly arrived by the Elbe steamer from Hamburgh, where the disease was prevailing. . . . He was seized with cholera on the 22nd of September, and died in a few hours. . . . Now the next case of cholera, in London, occurred in the very room in which the above patient died. A man named Blenkinsopp . . . [suffered] rice water evacuations [profuse diarrhea]; and, amongst other decided symptoms of cholera, complete suppression of urine from Saturday till Tuesday morning; and after this the patient had consecutive fever [p. 1].

A third pandemic commenced in the 1850s and took its major toll primarily in Russia. The fourth pandemic began in 1863 and raged across Europe and Africa, hitting Gibraltar in 1865. It is its impact on Gibraltar, or the Rock as it is known colloquially, that is of concern here.

From the researcher's point of view, there is an excellent reason for focusing on this tiny European country of 3.6 square miles, with a population that even today does not surpass 30,000. Larry Sawchuk, a professor of anthropology at the University of Toronto, and his colleagues and students have pored over historical archives to assess the country's social history of health and disease, including syndemically related diseases. These records (Sawchuk 2001), which are linked to Gibraltar's status since 1713 as a British military garrison and colonial outpost (though physically connected by a small thread of land to Spain and 1,000 miles from Britain), include the Gibraltar Police Death Registry, the Gibraltar Government Census of 1868, and the Colonial Blue Books (a record of death counts). An important finding of careful examination of this archival material is that cholera had the single greatest impact of any disease on the life expectancy of people on the Rock during the mid-1800s and was responsible for reducing the average duration of life by twelve years.

A particular configuration of social conditions and social relations formed the context for health on Gibraltar in the mid-nineteenth century. The local "medical topography" was summarized by Hennen (1839), a British physician who subsequently died in an epidemic on the Rock, as being strongly influenced by a population that was "overcrowded, perhaps, beyond any community in the world" at the time (p. 71). The dwellings of the poor were described as being small, dirty, and poorly ventilated, places at high risk, Hennen believed, for febrile miasmas, a view in keeping with the prevailing ideology of disease causation at that time. The cause of these conditions, as Sawchuk and Burke (2003) observe, "was the fact that landowners were more concerned with making large and quick profits than with providing proper accommodation for the poor working classes" (p. 178). Further, as a garrison town Gibraltar had come to be a temporary home to several thousand military families. The regular relocation of troops from Gibraltar to sites across Britain's dispersed empire offered a ready mechanism for population mixing and the continual arrival of infectious diseases. Additionally, access to clean water was minimal, with the purity of the well water continually sabotaged by the poor disposal of sewage and refuse. At the same time, adequate nourishment was also a problem, especially during the hot summer months. Finally, maintenance of domestic animals in close proximity to dwellings resulted in additional pollution. For the poorer families of Gibraltar, susceptibility to disease "was not simply the result of a lack of wealth or lax hygiene, but, rather, a constellation of factors that were experienced together in a 'poverty complex'" (Sawchuk & Burke, 2003, p. 203).

Within this social environment, the people of Gibraltar were regularly beset by what Sawchuk and Burke refer to as the **pathogens of everyday life.** By this they mean a cluster of persistent endemic infections that routinely ensured significant rates of morbidity and mortality. During the first years of the colony, years in which the residents' lives were fragile at best, diarrheal diseases—"the product of synergy between enteric infections, malnutrition, repeated insults by infectious disease, and a poor weaning diet that [set] up a vicious cycle of gastroenteritis/malnutrition lowering overall disease resistance"—resulted in considerable and consistent sickness and death among children (Sawchuk, Herring, & Waks, 1985, p. 619). Moreover, "even infants who survived the infection were prone to other opportunistic infectious diseases" as well as to "the periodic outbreak of synergistic infectious diseases such as measles" (Sawchuk & Burke, 2003, p. 188). In adulthood, respiratory tuberculosis, another endemic condition, was the primary cause of death of Gibraltarians during this era. Records suggest a high annual rate of TB infection, with virtually everyone being infected by age twenty. In addition, an array of respiratory conditions formed a "disease cluster" that included pneumonia, bronchitis, and other inflammations of the lungs (Sawchuk & Burke, 2003, p. 189).

This overall description suggests important components of the local medical topography (to borrow Hennen's term again) on Gibraltar at the time of the arrival of cholera in the summer of 1865, thrusting Gibraltarians from high but normal levels of mortality from various diseases into an episode of what is referred to in demography as *crisis mortality*. During this brief period, almost 600 people died. Mortality was not equally distributed in the population, however. Simply put, "poverty put some Gibraltarians at greater risk than others" (Sawchuk & Burke, 2003, p. 203). It was among the poor that cholera—as a result of its syndemic interaction with debilitating social conditions, malnutrition, and various other infectious diseases—wreaked the greatest havoc and took the steepest toll.

MASSACHUSETTS SCARLET FEVER SYNDEMIC OF THE 1800S

In her classic novel *Little Women*, Louisa May Alcott uses the expression "castle in the air" metaphorically to refer to the gap that commonly emerges between one's dreams and lived reality. First published in 1868, the book describes the lives and relationships of four sisters growing up in Massachusetts during the Civil War. One of the sisters, Beth, the second youngest, a shy but charitable girl, experiences the death of a neighbor's baby in her arms. Soon she too develops symptoms of the disease that took the baby's life. She explains to her sister Jo what happened when the baby died: "I just sat and held it softly till Mrs. Hummel came with the doctor. He said it was dead, and looked at Heinrich and Minna, who have sore throats. 'Scarlet fever, ma' am. Ought to have called me before,' he said crossly. Mrs. Hummel told him she was poor, and had tried to cure the baby herself, but now it was too late, and she could only ask him to help the others and trust to charity for his pay" (Alcott, 1872, p. 166).

Realizing that she too has been infected, Beth tries to convince her sister that she will be all right: " 'Don't be frightened, I guess I shan't have it badly. I looked in Mother's book, and saw that it begins with headache, sore throat, and queer feelings like mine, so I did take some belladonna, and I feel better,' said Beth, laying her cold hands on her hot forehead and trying to look well" (p. 166). At first, it appears that Beth will survive her bout with scarlet fever, but she develops rheumatic fever and ultimately dies of congestive heart failure, affirming the metaphor around which the book is constructed.

During the time that Alcott was writing *Little Women,* the world was in the midst of a pandemic of scarlet fever that ran from 1820 to 1880. Notes Krause (2001):

> [S]carlet fever most likely occurred for centuries either as an endemic disease or as localized epidemics. And then, in the early part of the 19th century, a pandemic of often fatal scarlet fever appeared suddenly and swept through Asia, Europe, and the United States. . . . Physicians in 1830, reflecting on their past experience, noted a striking increase in mortality not seen previously, and fatality rates of up to 30% were often reported. Scarlet fever became the most common fatal infectious childhood disease, more fatal than measles, diphtheria, or pertussis, a fact that is difficult to comprehend today [p. 15].

One of the places hit by the pandemic, in 1858–1859 and again in 1867–1868, was the Connecticut River Valley of western Massachusetts. Anthropologists Alan Swedlund and Alison Donta (2003) of the Connecticut Valley Historical Demography Project have studied archival records of this segment of disease history, focusing their research on the population of a fertile agricultural valley at the onset of the industrial revolution and especially on four towns spread across the valley. These towns, Deerfield, Greenfield, Montague, and Shelburne, varying in their level of dependence on agriculture, commercial, and industrial economies, form a natural laboratory. Although all these towns had doctors when scarlet fever arrived, there were no effective medical treatments at the time for the disease. (Indeed, even after *Streptococcus pyogenes* was identified in the third quarter of the nineteenth century as the immediate pathogenic cause, no effective treatment became available until the emergence of antibiotic pharmacology.)

The 1858–1959 epidemic in the Connecticut River Valley was severe. Throughout the state of Massachusetts this first scarlet fever epidemic caused over 2,000 deaths, 95 percent of which were among children. In the four towns studied by Swedlund and

Donta, there were over 89 deaths among children that were tied to scarlet fever in 1858–1859 and 1867–1868. In Deerfield, for example, twelve households lost children to scarlet fever in 1859. The average age of those who died was three years and eleven months. In examining cases of scarlet fever in the target towns, it was not evident to research team members that nutritional or socioeconomic characteristics were significant risk factors for scarlet fever infection. They note, however, the importance of "the close and perhaps synergistic interrelationship between nutrition and infection that . . . can be influential not so much in who becomes infected, but in who survives" (Swedlund & Donta, 2003, p. 171). As noted in Chapter Six, nutrition plays an important role in immune health, including the ability of mothers to pass temporary immune protection to newborns.

GLOBAL INFLUENZA SYNDEMIC OF 1918

A world-shaping syndemic was sparked by the global influenza pandemic of 1918, which epidemiologists estimate was responsible for the deaths of between 40 and 100 million people worldwide, making it one of the most deadly events in human history. More people died during the 1918 pandemic, which lasted two years, than during all four years of the Black Death outbreak (although of course the world population was by 1918 far larger than it had been during the Middle Ages). Arriving during the closing phase of World War I, the pandemic had a significant impact on mobilized national armies. Half of the U.S. soldiers who died during the Great War, for example, were victims of influenza, not of enemy bombs and bullets. It is estimated that almost three-quarters of a million Americans died during the pandemic. Its impact was so harsh that the average life span in the United States fell by ten years in the second decade of the twentieth century. Among those struck was President Woodrow Wilson, who became ill early in 1919 while in Versailles negotiating the treaty to end the world war (Tice, 1997). The pandemic was truly global in its impact, showing up in almost all heavily populated areas but in sparely populated Arctic settlements and in remote Pacific islands as well. In this respect the pandemic exposed the early stages of the most recent wave of globalism and its reconstruction of the modern world as a socially smaller, more integrated place.

The lingering if muted presence of what has been called the **forgotten pandemic** (Crosby, 2003) is captured by Restifo (2000):

There is a cemetery in a small railroad town in northern Ohio where I grew up that tells a sliver of the story of the great 'Spanish' influenza pandemic of 1918. One section of the cemetery is full of simple, rough, limestone markers that tilt willy-nilly in the perpetually damp sod of the graveyard. These unembellished memorials mark the graves of unfortunate souls who died one week during the fall of 1918 from the flu. In other towns all over the country there are similar hastily prepared grave sites. At least 10,000 people died in the city of Philadelphia during one three-week period during the month of October, overwhelming doctors, hospitals and undertakers [p. 12].

Moreover, as the panicked reaction to the recent SARS outbreak suggests, perhaps the 1918 epidemic is not such a forgotten pandemic after all.

An important part of the death toll in 1918 and 1919 was caused by viral pneumonia characterized by extensive bleeding in the lungs and resulting in suffocation. Many victims died within forty-eight hours of the appearance of the first symptoms. In fact it was not uncommon for people who appeared quite healthy in the morning to have perished by sunset. Historian Adolph Hoehling (1961), for example, relays the remembrances of Henrietta Burt, a secretary, who visited a friend's home to play bridge during the epidemic: "We played until long after midnight," she recalled. "When we left we were all apparently well. By eight o'clock in the morning I was too ill to get out of bed, and the friend at whose house we played was dead" (p. 163). Eino Hautala, a child of eleven living on his family's farm in Minnesota, remembered a local barn that was pressed into use as a morgue. Because it was a particularly brutal winter and the ground was frozen, inside the barn the bodies of flu victims were "stacked like cordwood until the spring came" ("Personal Histories," 2006).

The devastating impact of the 1918 pandemic on the U.S. military during World War I led the nation's surgeon general to establish the Pneumonia Commission in July of 1918 to investigate the nature and cause of the disease outbreak. Among the five members of the commission was Captain Francis G. Blake. In letters that he wrote while on the commission, Blake poignantly described the misery caused by the 1918 pandemic on U.S. army bases. On September 25, for example, he wrote from Camp Pike: "You ought to see this hospital tonight. Every corridor and there are miles of them with a double row of cots and every ward nearly with an extra row down the middle with influenza patients and lots of barracks about the Camp turned into emergency infirmaries and the Camp closed" (quoted in Pettit & Bailie, 2008, p. 92). A few days later, after another round of new cases, Blake wrote, "I am getting too tired to write about anything that is going on here. There is only death and destruction anyway" (p. 96).

Even before the 1918 pandemic, researchers were confused about what caused the *grippe,* as the disease was then known. Some thought that the source might be a bacterial infection. At the time, virology had not emerged as a discipline, but bacteriology was already a flourishing field. As Crosby (2003) notes, at autopsy, "By far the commonest microorganism in the lungs of influenza victims was found to be Pfeiffer's bacillus [*Bacillus influenzae*]" (p. 40), and hence this microbe was at one time proposed as the source of the pandemic. Subsequent research, however, showed that it was not present in every case, provoking caution about its role. Writing during the second year of the pandemic, John Ruhräh (1920), a professor of diseases of children at the University of Maryland, summarized what the scientists knew:

In 1892, Pfeiffer announced his discovery of the influenza bacillus and since that time to the present this has generally been credited with being the cause. These statements have not, however, passed entirely unchallenged and Rosenthal, in 1900, and others, have questioned the role of the Pfeiffer bacillus in influenza. In 1910, Vincent suggested that epidemics of grippe might be due to a filtrable virus. In the epidemic of last year the bacillus of influenza was reported in large numbers by certain observers and in smaller numbers by others, and sometimes it was not found at all. . . . The Conference of Bacteriologists at the British War Office under Leishman believed that the influenza bacillus played a part of great importance in the epidemic, although they were not sure of its being the primal cause [p. 160].

Ultimately, it was confirmed that the pandemic was caused by a virus, specifically an influenza A virus of the H1N1 subtype (Taubenberger & Morens, 2006). By way of a virological or epidemiological pathway that is not yet fully understood, the virus had successfully "jumped" the species barrier (presumably through a genetic mutation that allowed infection of human cells). The origin species was likely avian, as ducks and geese appear to be the primary animal reservoirs for all known influenza viruses (although horses, pigs, and even marine mammals can be infected). Although in humans (and bird species like chickens) influenza is a respiratory infection of varying degrees of intensity, in waterfowl the infection targets the gastrointestinal tract and tends to produce subclinical infection.

Among people who survived the first several days of infection during the pandemic, however, many subsequently died of secondary conditions. Most notable among these was bacterial pneumonia, and it was this tendency to promote secondary complications that made the 1918 influenza so deadly. As summarized by Morens and Fauci (2007), individuals suffering from viral infection during the 1918 pandemic were at risk for the development of "aggressive bronchopneumonia featuring epithelial necrosis, microvasculitis/vascular necrosis, hemorrhage, edema, and widely variant pathology in different parts of the lung, from which pathogenic bacteria could usually be cultured at autopsy. . . . In a few autopsies, severe bronchopneumonia was seen without evidence of bacteria, but studies generally showed a close correlation between the distributions of pulmonary lesions and cultured bacteria...identifying the major bacteria as the organisms now known as *Streptococcus pneumoniae, S. pyogenes*, and, less commonly, *Haemophilus influenzae* and *Staphylococcus aureus*" (p. 1020).

In other words, the bacteria found in the lungs of many victims that at first were thought to be the source of the influenza were actually evidence that a syndemic interaction involving a virus and one or more strains of bacteria was an important factor in the lethality of the 1918 pandemic. This interpretation is supported by research with animal models that identified a lethal synergism between influenza virus and *Streptococcus pneumoniae* (McCullers & Rehg, 2002). This research showed that if influenza infection precedes bacterial infection, there is a 100 percent rate of mortality. If the reverse occurs and bacterial infection precedes viral infection, a countersyndemic reaction occurs that confers protection from influenza and leads to improved rates of survival.

Moreover, it has been argued that countless numbers of those who expired quickly from the disease were coinfected with tuberculosis, which would explain the plummet in TB cases after 1918; many carriers of the disease may have perished during the pandemic. Noymer and Garenne (2000), who believe that "[t]uberculosis and influenza very likely interacted in 1918" (p. 573), analyzed a data set of 1918 influenza cases originally developed by Raymond Pearl, a well-known biologist and statistician long affiliated with Johns Hopkins University, who exhibited an early interest in disease interactions (for example, Pearl, 1919, 1928). Although Noymer and Garenne (2000) noted the limitations of the data set (for example, a lack of controls for age, sex, and socioeconomic status, a focus only on white households, and the inclusion only of households with at least one case of tuberculosis), their regression analysis led them to conclude that "many influenza deaths in 1918 took place among the tuberculous— persons with clinical disease or latent infection with *Mycobacterium tuberculosis*. That the 1918 influenza virus, known to be atypical, should interact pathologically with *M. tuberculosis* seems likely" (p. 573). It is this syndemic interaction, they assert, which accounts for various features of the 1918 epidemic, including both its extreme mortality rate and the age group (twenty-five- to thirty-four-year-olds) that was hardest hit (tuberculosis being a disease of adulthood, not old age). The significant drop in tuberculosis cases after 1918 (likely due to the high fatality rate during the epidemic) can in this light be interpreted as a countersyndemic outcome, although one with a high initial cost in human lives.

SYNDEMICS AMONG NATIVE AMERICANS ON THE AMERICAN FRONTIER

An example of a consequential syndemic from the nineteenth century can be found on the reservations on which indigenous peoples were confined with the closing of the U.S. frontier. For example, the Sioux (a term derived from the French spelling of an Ojibwa word for "little snakes" that was officially applied to the Lakota, Dakota, and Nakota peoples in 1825) are known historically for their abilities as mobile foragers and fierce warriors, but were militarily forced by the U.S. government onto a series of small reservations, including Rosebud, Pine Ridge, Lower Brule, Crow Creek, Cheyenne River, and Standing Rock, where they could not practice their previous subsistence patterns (for example, the last bison hunt occurred in 1882, by which point not a single wild bison remained in Lakota territory) and were treated as a conquered population. The Rosebud Sioux, for example, descendants of the Sicangu Oyate of the Tetonwan Division of the Lakota people, had their broader tribal homeland recognized by treaties signed in 1851 and 1868 but then watched it being reduced by the U.S. Congress to its current boundaries in south central South Dakota as part of the Great Sioux Agreement of March 2, 1889. Moreover, the U.S. government reneged on its promises to adequately provision Sioux reservations; such failures to respect treaty terms with Native Americans were typical. Food that was provided was often of low quality. Living under extremely stressful conditions and having inadequate diets, as well as being the victims of overt racism on the part of the registration agents appointed to oversee their reserves, the Sioux suffered exposure to various infectious diseases transmitted by contact with whites.

One source for the Sioux experience with European disease is indigenous records. The Sioux subgroups or bands traditionally documented their histories using a calendrical system known as the *waniyetu wowapi*, or "winter count." These pictorial calendars, produced by designated tribal historians, or "keepers" (each affiliated with a subgroup or band maintaining its own records), consisted of drawings on muslin cloth or hide that recorded defining events during each year. The images used and name of the year were selected by the tribal historian in consultation with band elders. Some of these calendars are held by the Smithsonian Institution. A record in the Smithsonian collection for the year 1849–1850, for example, depicts a man suffering from stomach pains and diarrhea and is named "Many died of the cramps." For the following year, 1850–1851, another winter count drawing portrays a rough human shape covered with spots and is named "Many died of the smallpox." For the year 1873–1874, a drawing of a man covered with blotches is named "Measles and other sickness used up the people in winter" (Greene & Thornton, 2007). As these examples suggest, winter count records indicate a series of epidemics that took many lives and caused much illness among reservation residents.

During the closing years of the nineteenth century, the Sioux endured a number of particularly lethal epidemics. Charles Alexander Eastman (1936/1977), a Sioux physician and writer who worked on the Pine Ridge Reservation during this period, recorded his observations and reactions to the events he witnessed: "Rations had been cut from time to time; the people were insufficiently fed, and their protests and appeals were disregarded. Never was more ruthless fraud and graft practiced upon a defenseless people than upon these poor natives by the politicians! Never were there more worthless 'scraps of paper' anywhere in the world than many of the Indian treaties and Government documents! Sickness was prevalent and the death rate alarming, especially among the children" (p. 99).

Black Elk, a noted Sioux folk healer, told his biographer: "There was hunger among my people before I went across the big water [to Europe in 1886], because the Wasichus [whites] did not give us all the food they promised in the Black Hills treaty. . . . But it was worse when I came back [1889]. My people looked pitiful. . . . We could not eat lies and there was nothing we could do" (Neihardt, 2004, p. 177). James Mooney (2006), an anthropologist and representative of the Bureau of Indian Affairs sent to investigate a possible Sioux rebellion, described the health situation on the reservations similarly in 1896: "In 1888 their cattle had been diminished by disease. In

1889, their crops were a failure. . . . Sullenness and gloom, amounting almost to despair, settled down on the Sioux. . . . The people said their children were all dying from the face of the earth, and they might as well be killed at once. Then came another entire failure of crops in 1890, and an unexpected reduction of rations, and the Indians were brought face to face with starvation. Thus followed epidemics . . . with terrible fatal results" (pp. 826–827).

During this period, the Sioux endured epidemics of measles, influenza, and pertussis in rapid succession. Tuberculosis and skin-based TB diseases like scrofula were also frequent. Other common diseases among those living on the reservations were bronchitis, pneumonia, and pleurisy. As this list of clustered health conditions suggests, it is likely that during this period the Sioux were victims of a syndemic that combined a number of interacting infectious diseases, malnutrition, self-medicating alcohol abuse, and stressful and extremely disheartening life conditions. As a result, while the official annual mortality rate on the Sioux reservations was between 1 and 2 percent, the actually death rate is believed by a number of historians to have been probably closer to 10 percent, a devastatingly high toll that helped to shape the final phases of frontier history.

SYNDEMICS OF THE MORMON MIGRATION

The Western frontier and the mid-nineteenth-century westward migration have long been seen as compelling influences in U.S. cultural development, giving rise to the so-called frontier mentality that has often been proposed as the source of everything from a core cultural emphasis on individualism and self-reliance to high rates of interpersonal violence, an enduring social restlessness and geographical mobility, a profound automobile obsession, and a distinctive exuberance and action orientation. Tempering the optimistic aspects of the frontier experience, however, were persistent epidemic cycles and overlapping lethal diseases that cut life short and left lonely grave sites all along the migration pathways (McNeil, 1980).

Among the thousands of migrants from European and East Coast points of origin were those who headed west to Zion as members of the Church of Jesus Christ of Latter-day Saints (LDS). The Mormons, as church members came to be known, moved westward in droves, some 70,000 between 1840 and 1869 (the year the transcontinental railroad was completed), in one of the largest organized migrations in American history. As Black et al. (1998) report, the migration presented both emotional and physical challenges: "The long journey was filled with the natural fears of fatigue, possible illness, concern for food and water, questions about the durability of their wagons or handcarts or their domestic animals, the potential dangers of Indian attacks—indeed, all the fears that go with the unknown. Adding to these fears was the sorrow many felt as they left extended family members behind, most never to be seen again" (p. 40).

Although it would be impossible to calculate actual morbidity rates during the migration, LDS historians, using the vast genealogical and other archival data collected and maintained by their church, estimate that between 4,600 and 6,000 Saints (6.6 to 8.6 percent of their total migrant flow) died en route, either while crossing the ocean from Europe or on one of the land trails leading to their final destination in Utah or contiguous areas (Black et al., 1998). The immediate causes of death included violence, accidents, and acute diseases. Among the latter cholera was particularly significant and was responsible for many deaths among the European Mormon immigrants who landed in New Orleans between 1849 and 1854. A major epidemic of yellow fever also hit New Orleans in 1853, resulting in the deaths of one of every fifteen people and leading city folk to say that since so many people were dying "soon people will have to dig their own graves" (Louisiana State Museum, 2007). To limit exposure to epidemics along the way, Brigham Young, head of the Mormon church after the death of founder Joseph Smith, was forced to send messages to European migrants instructing them to avoid disembarking in New Orleans.

In addition to acute diseases, other health factors played important roles in contributing to Mormon migrant mortality; as Baker (2002) observes: "Malnutrition, intestinal parasites, or other chronic disease conditions made a person more susceptible to disease. Insufficient food, combined with inadequate sanitation, represented the greatest factor that led to serious outbreaks among Mormon immigrants at sea" (p. 86). Kimball (quoted in Baker, 2002) adds: "Injury, sickness and death were commonplace. Emigrants suffered cuts; broken bones; gun wounds; burns; scaldings; animal, insect and snake bites; stampedes; overturned wagons; shifting freight; drownings; quicksand; black scurvy [acute fever with hemorrhagic skin lesions]; black canker (probably diphtheria); cholera; typhoid fever; ague [malaria]; quick consumption (tuberculosis); headaches; piles [hemorrhoids]; mumps; asthma; inflammation of the bowels; scrofula; erysipelas [streptococcal skin infection]; diarrhea; small pox; itch; and infections of all kinds, including puerperal fever" (p. 86). Similarly, Mormon church records (Church of Jesus Christ of Latter-day Saints, 1996) note that conditions at longer term encampments set up by the Mormons before moving on to Utah were also characterized by multiple threats to health: "Life in these settlements was almost as challenging as it had been on the trail. In the summer they suffered from malarial fever. When winter came and fresh food was no longer available, they suffered from cholera epidemics, scurvy, toothaches, night blindness, and severe diarrhea" (p. 60).

As these accounts suggest, the significant toll taken by synergistically related diseases, disorders, and injuries was a critical aspect of the Mormon migration to Zion, and likely not one of minor historical significance for the survival of the Mormon church. Enduring sickness, death, and other hardships and sacrifices provided the survivors with important "faith promoting experiences" (Kimball, 1995) that no doubt helped to increase Mormon resolve and contributed to group solidarity and organization in the face of subsequent challenges, including, ultimately, open conflict with the U.S. government over the practice of polygamy and, more important, control of the Western territories, conflict that led to federal arrest of group leaders, military occupation of Salt Lake City, and the temporary confiscation of church property. In response to the health and other challenges faced during the migration, the Mormon church developed an internal system of support and welfare that continues to serve its members.

SYNDEMICS OF WAR

War and other forms of physical conflict rival infectious disease as global causes of morbidity and mortality. Moreover, they are breeding grounds of syndemics. Since the bloody end of World War II, there have been at least 160 wars around the world with as many as 25 million (and probably many more) people killed, most of them civilians. Directly or indirectly, war touches the lives of most people on the planet, often with enduring and costly impact. Preparation for war takes a further toll by diverting a people's resources from the health sector and other social needs. Further, because war destroys housing, disrupts social institutions, and displaces persons, it creates impoverished and highly vulnerable refugee populations (currently totaling 12 million people worldwide, as well as 20 to 25 million internally displaced persons) who often face severe problems of adequate nutrition, exposure to contagious diseases, and substandard health care.

In a famous passage about the intimate relationship of war and disease, the renowned bacteriologist Hans Zinsser (1935/2000) observed, "Soldiers have rarely won wars. They more often mop up after the barrage of epidemics" (p. 153). In the defeat of New World empires, for example, European diseases such as smallpox and measles were far more deadly than European weapons. Similarly, during the American Civil War, even though the average soldier might have feared the dreadful minié ball as his greatest threat to life and limb, "disease was the biggest killer of the war" (Civil War Society, 2002). In the federal army roughly three out of five died of disease, and among Confederate soldiers two out of three deaths were caused by disease (Bollet, 2004). Typhoid, dysentery, and malaria, often in some combination, were the primary pathogen-generated enemies on the Civil War battlefield. Together they have been called the third army that participated in the war. Similarly, despite the enormous firepower of modern warfare, in World War II's Pacific theater casualties were greater from diseases like malaria than they were from actual combat.

Usually an unintended consequence, disease also has been used intentionally as a weapon of war. This is not a new strategy; for example, during the fourth century B.C. Scythian archers covered the tips of their arrows with animal excrement to cause wound infections; during the Middle Ages the corpses and feces of individuals who had died of bubonic plague were catapulted over castle walls onto besieging armies; and more recently, during World War II, Winston Churchill at one point contemplated an anthrax attack on German cities. Indeed, in modern times biological warfare has come to be a grave threat.

Twin Scourges: War and Disease

The nature of the connection between war and disease, two of the greatest sources of human suffering, is complex; disease can trigger human conflict but it can also so decimate armies (as HIV/AIDS has done in the case of several African armies) that it forces a suspension or even an end to fighting. In either case, soldiers and civilians on both sides of the battlefield have endured often terrible health consequences (Smallman-Raynor & Cliff, 2004). Further, war has played a role in creating new diseases, reactivating old ones, and significantly elevating the impact of others, and, as a result the popular names of a long list of diseases reflect their close association with the battlefield environment: for example, trench fever, an infection caused by the louse-borne pathogen *Bartonella quintana*; trench foot, a condition characterized by blisters, open sores, and swelling and caused by prolonged exposure of the feet to a damp, unsanitary, and cold environment; trench mouth, a severe form of infected and bleeding gums; soldier's disease, an old term for opium addiction stemming from the use of opium to treat the pain of war wounds; and combat stress reaction (also called battle fatigue, shell shock, war neurosis, and soldier's heart, a lexical proliferation suggesting its frequency), an intense and usually short-term stress reaction to war experiences that impairs mental functioning (and which in prolonged form is now called posttraumatic stress disorder).

Additionally, down through the ages, as seen in the global transmission of cholera during the nineteenth century and the influenza pandemic of 1918 (which was first observed in the United States at Fort Riley in Kansas, a site so severely hit by the outbreak that the army ran out of coffins to bury the many victims), war has been a handmaiden of syndemics in many if not all regions of the world. By directly causing massive death and injury on the one hand, and by disrupting trade and destroying social infrastructure, including subsistence, hygienic, and medical systems, on the other, war has often set the stage for famine and epidemic diseases, or as often as not both at once as syndemically interacting sources of illness and death. Further, as soldiers are moved about the landscape of shifting battlefields, war has been a major spreader of disease, and consequently it has also brought diseases into contact that were previously isolated by geographical distance or topological barriers. War, in short, has been a powerful syndemogenic force in world history. As a result, the nexus of war and syndemics has played a major role in shaping the world as we know it.

Darfur: Physical Violence, Social Suffering, and Syndemics

A particularly grim and disturbing expression of the impact of war on health is the toll conflict takes on the lives of children. Countries that have been ravaged by internal wars, such as Sierra Leone, Angola, Afghanistan, Liberia, and Somalia, tend to have the highest child mortality rates in the world. In Sierra Leone, for example, over 250 out of every 1,000 children die before reaching five years of age, compared to 8 per 1,000 in the United States, according to UNICEF (Machel, 1996). Since 1990, 90 percent of conflict-related deaths have been among civilians, and of these 80 percent have been among women and children. UNICEF reports that in a typical war the death rate among children under five years of age goes up by 13 percent. The causes are multiple and usually entwined and include accidental or intentional violence (for example, military bombardment of civilian residences, gang rape by soldiers of women and girls, and ethnic cleansing); the spread of diseases facilitated by the destruction or chaos-driven breakdown of societal infrastructure; and the creation of vulnerable populations like refugees, who often wind up in overcrowded camps with inadequate or polluted water, lack of adequate food supplies, unhygienic living conditions, and limited health care. Moreover, many children are left orphaned, while others are abducted to be used as compliant soldiers.

The emotional scars children bear from exposure to violence, loss of family members, dislocation from their homes, their resulting impoverishment, and other **social suffering** can be lifelong. Typical is Sumaya, a fifteen-year-old girl from the Sudan, whose village was attacked in 2005 by an Arab tribal militia called the Janjaweed. Sumaya, one of over 2.5 million Sudanese refugees, was interviewed by UNICEF workers in the Kalma refugee camp in South Darfur:

> "I was at school when they attacked us," says Sumaya. My sisters ran back to the village, and I ran with some friends. My cousin Mona was running ahead of me when she was shot. I stopped and held her hand. When she died, her hand slipped out of mine. Some boys came and told me that I had to run, so I did." Along the way Sumaya found her grandmother and her 4-year-old brother, Mozamel (whom everyone calls Baba). She took the little boy in her arms and started running. "We ran and ran until I felt that I couldn't go on any longer," remembers Sumaya. "I thought about throwing my brother in the grass because he was so heavy, but my grandmother took my hand and told me that we should all stay together." Two agonizing weeks went by before Sumaya and Baba were reunited with the rest of the family. Together, they walked 147 kilometres to Kalma Camp [along with 70,000 other refugees] [UNICEF, 2006].

By the time the refugees of Darfur reached refugee camps, many children had been pushed to the brink by a combination of trauma, lack of food and water, and disease. Exemplary is Mukhtar, a one-month-old child treated by physician Sayid Obeid Bakhiet at his small clinic in the camp at Zam Zam in the Sudan.

> The boy's legs were limp. Folds of skin hung loosely from his bones, easily holding the shape of the doctor's pinch—a telltale sign of dehydration. His face glowed with fever, and his narrow chest heaved and fluttered. His milky eyes darted desperately around the dim tent. He was a month old but weighed less than five pounds. Dr. Bakhiet knew immediately that Mukhtar needed attention at once. His mother, Mariam Ahmed, a fire of panic burning in her eyes, urgently pressed the tiny child into the doctor's arms. "He vomits everything," she said. "It looks like he cannot breathe." Dr. Bakhiet listened to the boy's laboring chest and shook his head. "Pneumonia," he said. He felt the soft spot on top of Mukhtar's still-forming skull. It was sunken. "Dehydration," he added. . . . Dr. Bakhiet grew nervous. He had lost one little boy 10 days earlier to a deadly combination of disease just like Mukhtar's and could not bear to see it happen again [Polgreen, 2006].

Labeled by many observers as an act of genocide by the central Sudanese government against the impoverished and restive people of the Darfur region, and deemed the "world's worst humanitarian crisis" by the United Nations in 2004 (BBC, 2004), the tragedy in Darfur largely escaped world attention until tens of thousands of people (ultimately 450,000 in some estimates) had already fallen victim to the deadly syndemic that united war, gastrointestinal diseases, malaria, other infectious diseases, dehydration due to lack of water and to intestinal infection, and malnutrition. The government's announcement in 2005 that the ABCO corporation had begun drilling for oil in Darfur prompted some humanitarian workers to conclude that the government's brutal scorched-earth policies were intended to drive people off the land to open it to drilling by transnational oil companies.

SUMMARY

This chapter has examined a set of syndemics that played major roles in shaping local, national, or even international social histories. The purpose was to show that syndemics can dramatically alter individual lives, the course of social events, and the character of human experience in the world. Consequently, understanding syndemics is of importance not only to the health, social, and physical sciences and to public health and health care but also to comprehending the unfolding of human social worlds and human social suffering over time.

KEY TERMS

forgotten pandemic
pathogens of everyday life
social suffering

syndemics of history
syndemics of war

QUESTIONS FOR DISCUSSION

1. What are the challenges in assessing the role of syndemics in shaping the course of human history? Why were syndemics in the past often not recognized as disease interactions?

2. Discuss the role of syndemics in the Irish famine of 1741, the deterioration of health among Native Americans following internment on reservations, the health problems faced by Mormon migrants to Utah, the cholera epidemics in Gibraltar in 1865, and the scarlet fever epidemics of the nineteenth century.

3. The global influenza pandemic of 1918 has reemerged as an issue of keen public health interest because of the growing recognition that we are at significant risk for future influenza pandemics. How did syndemic disease interaction play a key role in the health impact of the 1918 pandemic? Discuss the countersyndemic aspects of the 1918 global influenza with regard to tuberculosis.

4. How does war contribute to the development of syndemics?

CHAPTER

A WORLD OUT
OF BALANCE

Emergent and Reemergent
Ecosyndemics

After studying this chapter, you should be able to

- Recognize the reasons for the rapid rise in the number of emergent and reemergent diseases and the resulting rapid rise in the potential for novel syndemics to form.

- Understand the role of the environment and environmental change in disease interactions and syndemic development.

- Be familiar with studies that explicate the role of animal populations as reservoirs for future syndemics.

- Define and work with the concepts of superinfection and the iatrogenic syndemic.

- Appreciate the potentially significant ability of global warming to produce ecosyndemics.

EMERGENT SYNDEMICS OF A TROUBLED WORLD

The capacity of various **emergent diseases** to spark new, environmentally based syndemic interactions is exemplified by the sudden 1993 outbreak of cryptosporidiosis in Milwaukee, which infected as many as 400,000 people. Cryptosporidiosis has also become a life-threatening syndemic complication in AIDS patients. In the last thirty years, many new infectious agents and the diseases they cause have been identified, including (in addition to HIV) *Rotavirus* (infantile diarrhea), ebola virus (ebola hemorrhagic fever), *Legionella pneumophila* (Legionnaires' disease), *Hantavirus* (pulmonary disease), *Escherichia coli* (hemorrhagic colitis), *Borrelia* (Lyme disease), *Helicobacter pylori* (gastric ulcers), and hepatitis C virus (hepatitis), all of which hold potential for new, possibly deadly comorbid interactions.

Also of concern is the syndemic formation of treatment-resistant pathogenic species, as seen in the earlier discussion of tuberculosis in Chapter Four. It is now of only historical interest that in 1969 U.S. Surgeon General William Stewart testified before Congress that advances in medical research made it possible to "close the book on infectious disease." Needless to say, this pronouncement proved premature. In the five-year period from 2003 to 2007, the World Health Organization (2007) recorded more than 1,100 infectious disease epidemics. Although new antibiotics have been identified, the constant processes of mutation and natural selection and also the misuse of pharmacological resources are reducing the capacity of the existing arsenal of antibiotics and other medical weapons to control disease-causing microbes. By the close of the twentieth century it had become painfully clear that antibiotics would not be the hoped-for panacea they were once envisioned to be. Indeed, new medical technologies are playing a growing role in disease evolution. Each advance in medical science, from the development of immunosuppressive drugs to transplant surgery, has created new opportunities for infection. As the Global Infectious Diseases and Epidemiology Online Network (GIDEON) (2008), an electronic system designed to assist physicians in diagnosing and treating infectious disease, reports, "each breakthrough in the prolongation of human life and ability to treat heretofore fatal diseases is inevitably followed by an interesting list of Infectious Diseases challenges."

At the same time, there has been a new life for old scourges. Although just a few years ago some opera aficionados might have assumed that the appearance of tuberculosis in the West was now limited to the stage performance of *La Bohème,* this dreaded affliction is not only raging in developing countries but is once again a menace of urban life in developed nations as well, especially among the poor, who are more likely to live in crowded, poorly ventilated, and inadequately maintained buildings. The World Health Organization has placed a number of reemergent infections on its international watch list, including diphtheria, cholera, dengue fever, yellow fever, and bubonic plague. As a result of such reemergences, infectious diseases seemingly gone today are back again tomorrow, and as a result the opportunities for disease interaction continue to mount.

Finally, the world is out of balance in another and more fundamental way, as seen in accelerated patterns of global warming. The various alterations that are restructuring the physical environment, not only global climate change but other pollution-driven transformations as well, have significant implications for disease clustering and synergistic exchange and are thus also issues of concern to this chapter. Inherent in this discussion is the idea that there is a need to adopt an ecohealth model that reconceptualizes human health (and ultimately animal health as well) in terms of environmental health. A deteriorating and disrupted environment, characterized by extreme weather, rising seas, species loss, and shrinking biodiversity, bodes poorly for human health.

Influences on Emergent Syndemics

The term *emergent syndemic* refers to a newly recognized, adverse interaction among diseases or other disorders, or the appearance of a syndemic known from one geographical area in a new area where it had not been seen previously. Syndemic emergence is affected by a number of factors:

- Changing political and economic conditions that significantly decrease the quality of the living conditions or the diet of a population or that significantly increase its exposure to and experience of violence, stress, malnutrition, or other noxious conditions

- Shifting ecological and environmental conditions (for example, deforestation, droughts, floods, storms, declining air and water quality, and climate change)

- Altering demographics and changing social behaviors (for example, population migration, urbanization, shifting social networks and practices, emergent sexual patterns, and other forms of human mixing)

- Rapidly developing technology that brings about the occupation of new geographical areas or new occupational risks

- Expanding patterns of globalization (for example, increasing international trade in exotic animals for pets and as food sources, drug flows, and global distribution of toxic or other harmful commodities)

- Ongoing microbial adaptation (for example, development of drug resistance and transfer of resistance among microbial species through gene mixing)

- Breaking down of public health protective measures (for example, decreases in sanitation policies and practices, vaccination programs, well-child programs, and nutrition supports) and treatment access

HIV, for example, appears to have begun spreading in Africa in the years after World War II, following large-scale human penetration of forested environments (that is, human occupation of new areas) and a zoonotic jump across the species barrier, through a microbial adaptation of a form of the simian immunodeficiency virus to the human biological environment. The subsequent global dissemination of the now-human disease HIV/AIDS was fostered by changes in transportation technologies and patterns, intensifying processes of globalization, and shifting forms of social interaction and sexual and drug-related practices, and this led to its consequent contact and interface with a multitude of other microbial and nonmicrobial threats to health. The end result has been the global HIV/AIDS syndemic.

A Local Example: Dhaka, Bangladesh

Sitting on the eastern banks of the Buriganga river, the city of Dhaka is the political, economic, and cultural hub as well as the capital of Bangladesh, a country of over 150 million people founded in 1971. Although its infrastructure is the most advanced in the country, the city faces severe challenges from a variety of sources.

Prominent among these problems are levels of air and water pollution that rank among the worst in the world (from such sources as an increasingly congested road system and increasing quantities of human and industrial waste). Almost 10 million tons of solid wastes are produced in Dhaka each year, much of which is dumped untreated in nearby low-lying areas and in several bodies of water, including the Buriganga, Turag, and Balu rivers and the Tongi canal. There are, for example, numerous tanneries in Dhaka, and they dump their waste directly into the Buriganga, one of the city's sources of drinking water. Tanning waste contains a number of dangerous chemicals, including sulfuric acid, chromium, ammonium sulfate, chloride, and calcium oxides. During the 1970s, tube wells became a popular source of drinking water in Dhaka. In recent years, it has become evident that millions of people are being exposed to arsenic through this water source. Exposure to arsenic from contaminated wells is projected to double the number of cancer deaths in Bangladesh over the next two or three decades (Van Geen et al., 2005).

The air in Dhaka has lead levels and greenhouse gas emissions, due to a growing number of motor vehicles, that are higher than the levels found in many other urban areas around the world. The average ambient concentrations of suspended particulate matter (SPM) and airborne lead are ten times higher than the amounts set by World Health Organization guidelines for safe air quality (Medical Information Group, 1998).

Another threat to public health in Dhaka is poverty. Pushed from the countryside by various forces, people have migrated to the capital in ever growing numbers. Unable to find jobs, many of these refugees have contributed to the significant rise in the homeless population living on the streets of the city, referred to sometimes as *pavement dwellers*. Other urban poor live in squatter settlements. Typical is Abul Alim, a teenager who begs for coins outside the Dhaka Sheraton Hotel, telling passersby, "I am hungry. God will bless you" ("Bangladesh Capital Hosts at Least 50,000 Beggars," 1999). Abul reports that he earns the equivalent of $1 a day through begging, out of which he must pay someone who takes him to the hotel each day, someone who brings him food during the day, and someone who allows him to sleep under a shed at night. He saves nothing and must beg every day or starve. One study has characterized the poor of Dhaka as, in varying degrees by subgroup, "roofless, rootless, and resourceless" (Ghafur, 2004; also see Speak, 2004), suggesting the magnitude of human suffering and vulnerability seen in this population.

Already boosting a population density among the highest in the world (876 people per square kilometer), Dhaka is projected to continue its rapid growth, reaching a population of 18 million by 2010. In 2000, Bangladesh ranked 145th out of 174 nations on the Human Development Index, a measure of human achievement or misery (depending on the end one is looking at) based on per capita income, literacy, and longevity (Bangladesh Institute of Development Studies, 2001).

Together, these ecological, economic, and demographic factors are having a growing adverse impact on health and the quality of life in Dhaka. Consequently, the city has one of the highest mortality rates from infectious diseases among Asian urban centers. Street dwellers, in particular, have been found to have extremely high levels of various health problems associated with severe poverty. As part of a World Bank development project, for example, Marr and Dasqupta (2008) assessed the impact of pollution on health in Dhaka and found a significant correlation between water pollution and diseases such as jaundice, diarrhea, and skin problems. In another study, carried out through the International Centre for Diarrhoeal Disease Research, Tarleton et al. (2006) assessed cognitive function in a group of 191 children who ranged from six to nine years of age. Scores were compared to health surveillance data on incidence of diarrhea, *Entamoeba histolytica* infection, and nutritional status. These researchers found that malnutrition during the school-age years (although not diarrhea or *E. histolytica* infection) was associated with a lower level of cognitive ability. Moreover, a study by the Centre for Health and Population Research (2005) found a significant level of "interaction between poverty, nutrition problems, failing sanitation and vector-borne infectious diseases." The destitute sectors of the population of Dhaka, in short, are at severe risk of a poverty-based syndemic that unites the mutually enhancing effects of food insufficiency and malnourishment, regular exposure to polluted water and air, and various infectious diseases, a lethal combination that threatens the health of a growing number of people in the megacities of the developing world.

FROM EMERGENT INFECTION TO EMERGENT SYNDEMIC

One abundant source of new and future syndemics is the continual emergence of new infectious disease among human populations. As displayed in Table 8.1, the discovery of new pathogens, some of which are widespread by the time they are recognized, is occurring at a rapid pace. On average, three new human diseases are identified every two years, with a new pathogen being described in the health literature every week. As of 2008, over 1,500 pathogens were known, although there is much still to learn about all of them.

Increasing Disease Understanding

Some of the diseases listed in Table 8.1 (for example, Lyme disease, legionellosis, cyclosporiasis) are not really new, but only in recent years has the development of scientific technology allowed a clearer understanding of them. This caveat applies as well to many emergent diseases, in that the pathogen that triggers their development could only be discovered with the introduction of new technologies in microbiology, virology, bacteriology, and cognate fields of research. For example, it was only in recent years that *Dientamoeba fragilis,* first described in 1918, came to be recognized as a frequent

TABLE 8.1. Major Infectious Diseases Discovered between 1972 and 2003

Year	Pathogen	Disease
1973	Rotavirus	Rotavirus disease
1975	Parvovirus B19	Fifth disease
1976	Cryptosporidium parvum	Cryptosporidiosis
1977	Ebola virus	Ebola
1977	Legionella pneumophila	Legionellosis
1977	Hantavirus	Hemorrhagic fevers
1977	Campylobacter jejuni	Campylobacteriosis
1980	T-lymphotrophic virus	T-cell leukemia
1981	Toxigenic S. aureus	Toxic shock syndrome
1982	E. coli O157:H7	Hemorrhagic colitis, HUS
1982	HTLV-II	Hairy cell leukemia
1982	Borrelia burgdorferi	Lyme disease
1983	HIV	AIDS
1983	Helicobacter pylori	Peptic ulcer disease
1985	Enterocytozoon bieneusi	Microsporidiosis
1986	Cyclospora cayatenensis	Cyclosporidiosis
1988	Human Herpes 6	Roseola infantum
1988	Hepatitis E virus	Hepatitis E
1989	Ehrlichia chaffeensis	Ehrlichiosis
1989	Hepatitis C virus	Hepatitis C
1989	Guanarito virus	Venezuelan hemorrhagic fever
1992	Bartonella henselae	Cat scratch disease
1993	Sin nombre virus	Hantavirus pulmonary syndrome
1994	Sabia virus	Brazilian hemorrhagic fever
1995	Human herpesvirus 8	Kaposi sarcoma
1999	Nipah virus	Nipah virus disease
2003	SARS Coronavirus	SARS

Source: Global Infectious Diseases and Epidemiology Online Network, 2008.

cause of diarrhea, abdominal pain, cramping, and various other abdominal discomforts. Since it was first identified as a pathogen, this unusual organism (originally thought to be an amoeba but now reclassified as a flagellate even though it lacks a flagellum) has been isolated from patients around the world. Despite the recentness of its "discovery" as a pathogen, a stool-sample review at the Cadham Provincial Laboratory in Winnipeg found that the incidence of this organism was greater than other better and longer-known intestinal microbes (Lagacé-Wiens, VanCaeseele, & Koschik, 2006). One point of uncertainty about *D. fragilis* is its route of transmission. Given its frequent coinfection with *Enterobius vermicularis* (pinworm) and the demonstrated development of *D. fragilis* infection following the ingestion of the eggs of the pinworm, the latter organism (which infects about one-third of the U.S. population) may serve as the vehicle of diffusion of *D. fragilis* to new hosts (Johnson, Windsor, & Clark, 2004), an example of one pathogen syndemically facilitating the transmission of another. After mating, the female pinworm migrates to the human anus, where 10,000 to 20,000 eggs are deposited. In addition, the pinworm secretes a chemical that causes a strong itching sensation. Scratching can transmit the microscopic eggs—and possibly *D. fragilis* with them—to the fingers, and from there to new hosts.

Animal Reservoirs of Disease

Diverse animal populations serve as reservoirs of many current and future human infections, suggesting why it is ultimately impossible to, as was once hoped, eliminate all contagious human diseases. Even when a wild pathogen is eliminated from every human population (as has occurred, for example, with variola major and variola minor, the microbial causes of smallpox, through a worldwide eradication effort by the World Health Organization), others pathogens will continue to jump from animals to humans, and some of them will adapt to the cells and structures of their new human hosts and trigger infections never seen before by the human immune system (Fauci, 2005). Thus smallpox may be gone (from everywhere but the laboratory), but the monkeypox virus, a member of the same *Orthopoxvirus* genus that the smallpox virus belongs to, appeared in the Midwestern United States in 2003 as an emergent source of human disease (that is, it was the first detection of this ailment in a new geographical area, the Western Hemisphere). A number of people contracted monkeypox that year following contact with infected pet prairie dogs (probably as a result of the exposure of pet trade prairie dogs to an imported exotic animal). Although causing a self-limiting febrile rash in some patients, it brought on severe neurological infection in others (Sejvar et al., 2004).

In Central and West Africa, there are a large number of rodents as well as some non-human primate species that serve as animal reservoirs of monkeypox. This virus was discovered in 1958 (in laboratory monkeys), and the first human cases of infection were reported in the early 1970s. In 1996, seventy-one cases of monkeypox, including six deaths, occurred in thirteen villages in the Kasai-Oriental region of central Zaire (now the Democratic Republic of Congo). Since then, reports of monkeypox virus infections in humans have escalated, including outbreaks involving direct human-to-human transmission

(Parker, Nuara, Buller, & Schultz, 2007). Human infection with other orthopoxviruses, such as the cowpox virus, is also occurring. Indeed, the term *vaccine* derives from the Latin word *vacca*, which means "cow," a reference to the fact that the first smallpox vaccine was made from the contents of a cowpox sore on the skin of Sarah Nelmes, a British dairymaid, after physician Edward Jenner discovered that people who get cowpox are immune to smallpox, an example of cross-immunity to related species of pathogens.

REEMERGENT DISEASES AND EMERGENT SYNDEMICS

In addition to the regular appearance and discovery of new human pathogens, old infections that had been on the decline are reemerging as threats to human health. Natural genetic variations, gene recombinations, and microbial adaptations allow new strains of known pathogens to appear as unfamiliar entities to the immune system. Increased availability and also misuse of antimicrobial drugs such as penicillin have contributed to the development of resistant pathogens, allowing diseases like tuberculosis to become renewed threats to human populations. Diminishing adherence to vaccination policies, as a result of economic crisis in fragile developing nations and deteriorating public health systems, has also contributed to the reemergence of various older diseases, such as measles and pertussis, that previously were largely controlled. Further, infectious diseases that have long posed significant threats to health in developing countries are emerging as new diseases in novel contexts (as has, for example, West Nile virus in the United States).

All of these new and renewed diseases have the potential to interact with other diseases (for example, HIV and TB) as they spread, sparking emergent syndemics.

SUPERINFECTION: INTRAGENUS SYNDEMICS

The term **superinfection** is used to refer to coinfection and disease interaction between two or more genetically different strains of the same pathogen or related pathogens, especially after immune response to the first infection has begun. The terms *coinfection* and *superinfection* may also be used to differentiate cases where two strains coexist (coinfection) from those where the most virulent strain becomes dominant (superinfection). Superinfection occurs, for example, in both HIV disease and dengue, as well as in other infections, with significant deleterious results. HIV-1, for example, is classified as existing in various subtypes (labeled A-D, F, G, H, J, and K), as well as in several circulating recombinant forms (CRFs) that are the product of coinfection with two or more HIV strains and subsequent gene mixing. Recombination of the genomes of different HIV strains has the capacity to link resistance mutations that developed in distinct viral populations, contributing to the appearance of viruses with enhanced drug resistance. HIV-1 superinfections are associated with accelerated disease progression in some patients, although not all. Superinfections have in fact even been detected in people whose immune systems are successfully controlling their HIV infections without antiretroviral treatment (van der Kuyl & Cornelissen, 2007).

Superinfection need not involve only two strains of HIV or any other pathogen, as cases of infection with three different strains have been reported.

Superinfection Among MSM

To determine the incidence of clinically significant HIV superinfection in men who have sex with men (MSM), Sidat et al. (2008) examined the hospital files of HIV-infected MSM patients who were not on antiretroviral treatment. In this group, they identified cases of sudden, unexplained, and sustained declines in CD4 T-cell counts and increases in HIV RNA serum levels, and these patients were assumed to be super-infected. Patients without these clinical characteristics were recruited as controls (four controls per possible superinfected case). Despite the considerable involvement of all of these men in unsafe sexual practices, their incidence of clinically significant HIV superinfection was found to be no more than 4 percent per year. Leontiev, Maury, and Hadany (2008) have suggested the intriguing notion that HIV may play a role in allowing superinfection. It is their hypothesis that superinfection is most likely in cases where an HIV infection is failing (as a result of AIDS treatment). In these cases, super-infection by a strain that is drug resistant (and subsequent gene mixing) can provide a distinct advantage to the original viral strain in adapting to the presence of anti-HIV drugs. A more successful HIV viral strain, they argue, will block superinfection of cells that are already infected. From an evolutionary perspective, in other words, super-infection can confer adaptive advantage on a less successful viral strain.

Dengue Superinfection

As with HIV, there are multiple strains of the virus that causes dengue. Similarly, coin-fection with more than one of the four identified strains can cause superinfection, which in the case of dengue produces a significantly more severe condition, known as dengue hemorrhagic fever (DHF). The incidence of DHF has increased dramatically in recent decades (Centers for Disease Control and Prevention, 2006a). For example, endemic in India for over two centuries as a relatively benign and self-limited disease, in recent years dengue infection has been more dramatic in that country and the preva-lence of DHF has gone up considerably (Gupta, Dar, Kapoor, & Broor, 2006).

Dengue has been spreading rapidly in South America as well. During the first nine months of 2007, over 625,000 cases of dengue were reported in Latin American coun-tries, especially Brazil, Venezuela, and Colombia, including over 12,000 cases of DHF that produced 183 fatalities. Mexico, in particular, has seen an alarming increase in the number of DHF cases; these now account for approximately one in four of the dengue cases in that country. The Mexican government has reported that the number of cases of DHF may currently be double what it was in 2006 (Melia, 2007).

Enterovirus Superinfection

In 2008, the People's Republic of China reported an outbreak of the enterovirus infec-tion known as hand-foot-and-mouth disease. Enteroviruses (which include the pathogen that causes polio) are a widespread group of single-stranded RNA viruses, commonly seen in infant and childhood gastrointestinal illness. Although many cases are asymptomatic or relatively mild, on par with a summer cold, they can contribute to the production of a wide range of more serious diseases. In the Chinese outbreak the specific pathogen was ultimately identified as enterovirus 71 (EV-71), a microbe first described in 1974. In China it began spreading in the city of Fuyang, in the eastern province of Anhui, in early March, resulting in over 3,000 infections of children and at least 40 deaths (mostly of pulmonary edema) by May (World Health Organization, 2008b). Why might this (or any) virus produce a range of responses from asymptomatic infection to the development of a deadly pediatric condition? One reason might be superinfection with another enterovirus. During an outbreak of EV-71 in Taiwan in 1998 (which led to the deaths of 71 individuals), it was suggested that some people developed severe infection because they currently or previously had been infected with another enterovirus, coxsackievirus A16. Superinfection, in other words, may be a key factor in enterovirus virulence (Ho et al., 1999). Further, superinfection may not require coinfection but may be a consequence of enduring effects of sequential infection among individuals in the sample population.

IATROGENIC SYNDEMICS

The term *iatrogenesis* means "brought forth by a healer" (*iatros* being the Greek word for "healer") and is almost always used to refer to adverse health conditions caused by medical treatment (such as unwelcome side effects). These adverse conditions may involve syndemics, as the following examples illustrate.

Iatrogenesis in Egypt

In his novel *The Constant Gardener* (later made into a major motion picture), John le Carré tells the story of a fictional multinational pharmaceutical company conducting clinical trials for a tuberculosis drug among the poor of Kenya. When the drug produces severe side effects and a number trial participants die, the company engages in an iniquitous cover-up and fiercely fights to avoid public exposure. The degree to which the book is an accurate portrayal of modern pharmaceutical companies and the clinical trial process is a hotly debated issue. Le Carré's position on the issue is expressed in the Author's Note at the end of the book, in which he states that as he conducted background research for the novel, "I came to realize that, by comparison with the reality, my story was as tame as a holiday postcard" (le Carré, 2005, p. 490). During the making of the movie, the film crew were so shocked by the poverty they encountered in Kenya that they established a charity, the Constant Gardener Trust, to provide water and educational services in several villages.

A far less malicious although tragically nonfictional case involving drug distribution is playing out in another part of Africa. For several decades after World War II, as part of economic development efforts, the Egyptian Ministry of Health implemented a control campaign using intravenous tartar emetic with the intention of protecting people living in the vicinity of the Nile River from schistosomiasis, a parasitic infection spread by freshwater snails (discussed briefly in Chapter Four). Infected snails regularly release the larvae from one of the several flatworm species that cause schistosomiasis into the water, where they swim until they detect the presence of certain chemicals given off by human skin. The larvae attach themselves to the skin, release an enzyme that dissolves skin protein, and penetrate the body surface. In this way the parasite gains access to the blood system and eventually the liver, causing an array of symptoms whose expression depends on the flatworm species and the health of the human host but that can include abdominal pain, fever, fatigue, diarrhea, and anemia. In the effort to stem this debilitating condition, individuals were given as many as sixteen injected doses of tartar emetic over a period of several months. Subsequently, people began to develop hepatitis C infections, and it is believed they were infected through the use of unsterile syringes by rural public health workers during the anti-schistosomiasis campaign (Frank et al., 2000). Ultimately, Egypt came to have one of the world's highest rates of hepatitis C (15 to 20 percent of the country's population) in a distribution that appears to reflect the locations of the inoculation activities. It is believed that this case represents the largest iatrogenic transmission of a blood-borne pathogen in biomedical history.

Clinical Trials and Iatrogenic Syndemics

Even though as described the Egyptian case is not technically a syndemic, it raises the question of whether there are actual cases of iatrogenic syndemics. In principle this is possible where medical treatment or medical research is involved in creating conditions that increase the likelihood that two or more diseases come together in a population. An example of this scenario might involve using gene splicing to unite two pathogenic agents and introducing the resulting novel organism into a population.

There is a possibility that this precise event occurred during a randomized, double-blind clinical trial testing the efficacy of the prototype HIV vaccine V520 (HIV Vaccine Trials Network, 2007). The trial had been launched with great expectations and had enrolled 3,000 HIV-negative volunteers from diverse backgrounds and between eighteen and forty-five years of age who were deemed to be at high risk of HIV infection. On November 6, 2007, the pharmaceutical manufacturer Merck & Co. announced that research on the efficacy of V520 had been stopped because interim findings showed an apparent increased risk for HIV infection among participants in the vaccine group of the study compared to those in the placebo group. Specifically, results showed that among vaccine group participants 3.2 percent developed HIV infection, whereas among the placebo group participants only 2.75 percent developed HIV infection. Study investigators also reported a higher risk of HIV infection among participants who had an existing immunity to the common cold virus (known as adenovirus type 5, or Ad5). Each of the V520 vaccine's three components had been made in the laboratory with the aid of a replication-defective version of Ad5. This was the organism selected to serve as the carrier, or delivery vector, for three synthetically produced HIV genes. Researchers suggested one explanation for the higher rate of HIV infection among individuals in the treatment group was that the vaccine actually lowered defenses against the human immunodeficiency virus.

In other words, in the V520 HIV vaccine case, a novel organism created through the splicing of genes from two naturally occurring pathogens may have increased the rate of disease, supporting Donna Haraway's (1991) observation in her book, *Simians, Cyborgs and Women: The Reinvention of Nature,* that "the boundary between science and science fiction is an optical illusion" (p. 149). Although alternative explanations of the results exist, this case suggests the possibility of the emergence of syndemics with an iatrogenic origin. Further, it reveals that the human role in promoting the spread and interaction of diseases is enormous and potentially disastrous.

Returning to the case of the iatrogenic hepatitis C epidemic in Egypt, it is known that that country overall has tended to retain a comparatively low level of HIV infection. Between 2004 and 2005, for example, the estimated number of HIV cases rose from 12,000 to 17,000. Among HIV cases that have been identified, about 6 percent were caused by injection drug use. Among drug users in Egypt about 13 percent report they inject drugs (UNAIDS, 2004). Rates of injection drug use in poor areas of urban centers, however, have been rising, creating the potential for coinfection and interaction between HIV/AIDS and the iatrogenic hepatitis C infections. As noted in Chapter Four, HIV and hepatitis C coinfection, and the resulting end-stage renal disease, is an important cause of death among HIV-infected individuals, affirming the significant risk of an iatrogenic syndemic in Egypt if rates of risky drug use accelerate. Another potential iatrogenic syndemic may be starting up through the impact of highly active antiretroviral therapy (HAART), now the standard treatment for HIV/AIDS, on leprosy. Research by Pereira et al. (2004) in Brazil with a cohort of coinfected individuals suggests that HAART may trigger acute inflammatory episodes among leprosy sufferers.

There are in fact reasons why, as currently conducted, pharmaceutical clinical trials may pose special hazards for syndemic development. Prior to the 1980s, many of the individuals who participated in phase 1 drug trials were prison inmates. This practice ended when ethics panels determined that as a captive group prisoners could not give fully informed and voluntary consent. The pharmaceutical industry was forced to find a new population to test drug safety and turned to the use of paid, market-recruited, clinical trial participants (called *paid volunteers* by the industry). This has led to the emergence of what Abadie (2008), a former pharmaceutical company representative turned critical health social scientist, calls the *professional guinea pig.* This arrangement, as Abadie notes, opens up the potential for synergistic drug interactions, as professional guinea pigs, to make a living, often take part in simultaneous or sequential trials of different drugs. Despite this common practice, Abadie reports that "the pharmaceutical industry does not keep detailed records of a subject's participation in trials and might be unaware of this problem [of participant involvement in multiple or back-to-back trials]. Besides, it might have little or no interest in such a follow-up, which could jeopardize the current development of clinical trials research based on the professionalization of research subjects" (p. 315).

UNINTENDED COUNTERSYNDEMICS

Although iatrogenic syndemics might occur, so might their opposite, namely unintended countersyndemics. A possible example of this has been reported by Hunter et al. (2003) and others for two emerging infectious diseases: cryptosporidiosis, which is an acute human and livestock diarrheal disease caused by the protozoan parasite *Cryptosporidium parvum* (and which in immunocompromised patients and in children can be severe or even fatal), and foot-and-mouth disease (not to be confused with the human disease of hand-foot-and-mouth disease discussed earlier), which is an emergent epizootic (animal disease outbreak) in the sense that in the United Kingdom, at least, it has become a much more common disease in recent years. For example, in 2001 a major outbreak of foot-and-mouth disease erupted in the United Kingdom that produced over 2,000 cases of animal infections. In response, over 6 million animals were slaughtered to control the disease, and various other measures were enacted (such as restrictions on travel to infected areas) that decreased human contact with livestock. Coincident with this culling was a dramatic decline in reports of *Cryptosporidium* infection in the area struck by foot-and-mouth disease. Smerdon et al. (2003) studied laboratory outbreak reports and concluded that "our results suggest that a decrease in genotype 2 *Cryptosporidium* infection in humans was associated with a decrease in human exposure to reservoirs of infection in livestock in England and Wales during the FMD [foot-and-mouth disease] epidemic interval" (p. 26).

In other words, the public health campaign to eliminate foot-and-mouth disease may have led to a significant drop in cases of cryptosporidiosis, owing to an elimination of the animal reservoir of the disease and limitations on human-animal contact. Although this was not the intention of the slaughter and other restrictive measures, it may have been an unanticipated beneficial result. Similarly, World War II soldiers who were treated for malaria with the antiprotozoal medicine quinacrine (better tolerated by patients than quinine) also stopped having diarrhea, which is not a malarial symptom. Examination of their stools revealed that giardia, which unbeknownst to the physicians treating the soldiers had apparently been the cause of their gastrointestinal problems, was no longer present, killed, presumably, by the quinacrine (Gardner & Hill, 2001).

ECOSYNDEMICS AND THE ANTHROPOCENE

It has been said by the Nobel Prize–winning atmospheric chemist Paul Crutzen that we are living in the **Anthropocene Era,** a geological epoch during which human activity is the greatest force shaping the earth's climate and ecosystems. Focusing on the issue of human health in this era, this section examines the growing impact of **global warming** on the creation of **ecosyndemics,** syndemics sparked by changing biospheric conditions (Baer & Singer, 2008). Ecosyndemics are assessed here within the context of the broad biosocial model referred to as *ecohealth*. This concept has emerged in recent years in the field of disease ecology, which itself is part of the growing trend in disciplines like tropical medicine, veterinary medicine, pathology, and immunology toward understanding the interaction of organisms at both the micro- and the macrolevels. Interest in disease ecology has grown significantly in the last twenty-five years in response to the health challenges of emergent diseases, antibiotic resistance, bioterrorism, and global warming. Within this milieu of new ideas, ecohealth researchers have embraced the goal of assessing the multiple interactions that occur among components of the ecosystem, local and global political economies, and cultural beliefs and practices that influence the nature, concentration, and impact of health problems.

Global Warming and Health

Global warming is driving increases in the frequency of intense storms, the length of droughts, the gravity of heat waves, the severity of flooding, the toll of forest fires, the water level of the oceans, the melting of the ice caps, the production of allergens, and the geographical range of climate-sensitive vectors of infectious diseases. Primarily, global warming is anthropogenic, and as we move deeper into the twenty-first century, what we have wrought appears increasingly likely to be a major force shaping many aspects of our future including our health. Along with other forms of environmental degeneration—such as reductions in fish and sea animals, the bleaching of coral reefs, die-offs of sea grass beds and mangroves, plastics pollution, man-made atmospheric radioactivity, and toxic dumping—and the global distribution of toxic commodities sold to the public (Singer & Baer, 2008), global warming is likely to become a worldwide engine of syndemic production.

The considerable potential for an ecosyndemic is illustrated by events in the countries in the Horn of Africa in 1997 and 1998, when ocean current and climate patterns linked to El Niño brought about soaking rains 60 to 100 times heavier than normal. These rains, the heaviest downpours recorded in the area in over thirty years, and the subsequent flooding set off a dramatic epidemic of cholera as well as two mosquito-borne epidemics: malaria and Rift Valley fever (Epstein, 2002), creating the opportunity for interdisease contact and adverse synergistic interaction. During 1997, the World Health Organization (1998) received almost 150,000 reports of cases of cholera worldwide, with over 6,000 deaths and a case fatality rate of 4 percent. Eighty percent of these cholera cases and over 90 percent of the deaths were reported from Africa.

At the same time, malaria struck, producing over 30 percent of all illnesses in the Horn of Africa during this period. The heavy rains also caused Rift Valley fever–infected mosquito eggs to hatch in abundance. First to be attacked by newly hatched adult mosquitoes were livestock, followed closely by humans. Almost 90,000 people in northeastern Kenya and southern Somalia were infected; 200 of them died of Rift Valley fever. Combining infections among both animals and human, it is believed that the Horn of Africa epidemic was the worst Rift Valley fever epidemic in the world to date (World Health Organization, 1998). Unfortunately, from the standpoint of syndemic understanding, the multiple and severe onslaughts of flooding, loss of food sources, damage to infrastructure, forced migration, and epidemics of cholera, malaria, and Rift Valley fever did not allow close examination of disease interactions, although such interactions were likely given available knowledge about these diseases. As Woods et al. (2002) report, in northwest Kenya, in the Garissa District, there were 170 hemorrhagic fever–associated deaths during the flooding in 1997. Laboratory testing identified evidence of acute Rift Valley fever virus infection; however, "many individuals did not undergo thorough clinical and laboratory investigations, and most persons who reported hemorrhaging were not directly observed by a clinician. Laboratory testing also found evidence of infection with other viral agents [including malaria]" (p. 141).

A similar potential for disease interaction related to a climatic event may be seen in Myanmar following Cyclone Nargis in 2008, which wrecked southern coastal areas and offshore islands, destroying at least half of the health care facilities and the majority of residential dwellings in seven townships and leaving over 60,000 people dead or missing. The storm created conditions that could spawn simultaneous outbreaks of malaria, cholera, measles, and dengue fever, among other infectious diseases. According to the World Health Organization (2008a), these conditions were

- Loss of access to safe water

- Population displacement and overcrowding at relief centers and resulting exposure to respiratory and other infections

- Increased exposure to waterborne disease vectors

- Increased numbers of wounds and injuries, with the potential to become infected

- Malnutrition, particularly among children

- Lack of access to health services

- Exposure to snakebites (the affected area has one of the highest rates of snakebite in the world)

- Involvement in the survival sex trade and forced participation in the commercial sex trade and resulting exposure to sexually transmitted diseases including HIV/AIDS

Moreover, international aid was slow in reaching the cyclone's victims because the military rulers of Myanmar are suspicious of foreign influences that could weaken their control. Consequently, assessment of the nature and health consequences of syndemic disease interaction in the aftermath of this cyclone is not likely.

As these examples suggest, global warming opens up the possibility for various kinds of novel interactions among diseases, some of which could develop into ecosyndemics of historic proportion. In addition to creating conditions for the radiation of mosquitoes to new areas, warming of the planet has contributed to the spread of many disease-bearing rodent and vector species—including those responsible for the outbreak of hantavirus in the U.S. Southwest in 1993 and pneumonic plague in India the following year—as well as the spread of the ticks that carry Lyme disease and the sand flies that transmit visceral leishmaniasis. Warmer climates have led to notable jumps in encephalitis rates in Sweden and to cases of dengue in The Netherlands. Since 1987, major outbreaks of encephalitis have been recorded in Florida, Mississippi, Texas, California, and Colorado. Further, as a result of global warming, disease movements are occurring at a quickening pace. Notes Epstein (quoted in Struck, 2006): "Things we projected to occur in 2080 are happening in 2006. . . . Our mistake was underestimation" (p. A16). Beyond rapid migration, global warming has a direct effect on the metabolism of pathogenic organisms, resulting in increased rates of growth and cell division. Syndemic interaction among migrating diseases and endemic diseases raises one more critical flag signaling the grave seriousness of global warming and the multiple threats it presents to human health and well-being, especially among highly vulnerable populations, including the poor, who are likely to feel the effects of these hazards most keenly.

Other human impacts on the environment are also of considerable concern as factors in the development of syndemics. One newly discovered ecosyndemic, for example, is a product of exposure to microscopic diesel fuel particles (pumped into the atmosphere by diesel-powered vehicles). Among people with high levels of low-density lipoprotein (LDL), or "bad cholesterol," the interaction between diesel pollutants and LDL cholesterol increases the risk for both heart attack and stroke significantly above levels found among similar individuals exposed to only one of these health risks. Affirming the "syndemic formula," André Nel, chief of nanomedicine at the David Geffen School of Medicine at UCLA, and a leading researcher of dual exposure, observes: "When you add one plus one, it normally totals two. . . . But we found that adding diesel particles to cholesterol fats equals three. Their combination creates a dangerous synergy that wreaks cardiovascular havoc far beyond what's caused by the diesel or cholesterol alone" (quoted in Schmidt, 2007). Experimentation has shown that these two factors stimulate genes that promote cell inflammation, a primary risk for hardening and blockage of blood vessels (atherosclerosis) and, as narrowed arteries collect cholesterol deposits and trigger blood clots, for heart attacks and strokes as well. Beyond its effects on global warming, in short, pollution of various sorts can be a trigger for syndemic disease.

Storms and Syndemics: Hurricane Katrina

As the prior discussion of climate-related outbreaks in the Horn of Africa and in Myanmar suggests, there are a number of risk factors for disease outbreaks following natural disasters. As noted, many of these stem from the displacement of populations and the subsequent shortages of clean drinking water and sanitation facilities, the exposure to crowding, and the limited access to health care services. Also of importance is the prior health status of the population. All these factors interact to influence the degree of risk for infectious or other diseases and for death after natural disasters. A case in point involves the numerous risk factors delivered by Hurricane Katrina.

More than 1 million people were displaced when Katrina slammed into New Orleans and the surrounding Gulf Coast on August 29, 2005 (Petterson, Stanley, Glazier, & Philipp, 2006). The category 5 hurricane, one of the strongest ever to make landfall in the United States, laid waste to 150 miles of coastline and plunged half a million homes into rising and heavily polluted floodwaters. A sister storm, Hurricane Rita, further battered the area two weeks later. As a result of the massive flooding, extensive infrastructure destruction, and considerable social disruption caused by Hurricane Katrina, the potential for infectious diseases was considerable. Concern about contaminants in the dark, filmy sediment left behind by Katrina's floodwaters was especially high. Environmental Protection Agency tests conducted in the first weeks after the hurricane found high levels of *Escherichia coli* (ten times the federal safety limit) in the flood water (Appel, 2005). Hepatitis was also a significant danger among people exposed to floodwaters containing untreated sewage and to contaminated and unrefrigerated food.

Of special concern was the potential spread of various vector-borne infections, including those caused by the West Nile virus. Hurricane Katrina was the first major hurricane to make landfall in the United States after the flavivirus that causes West Nile–related diseases was introduced into the country in the summer of 1999. Prior to the storm, Louisiana was a major site of West Nile virus infection, with over 170 cases reported for the state out of a total of 2,744 cases reported nationally in 2005. Eight of those pre-Katrina cases resulted in the death of the infected individual (Centers for Disease Control and Prevention, 2005). Stagnant pools of water left behind by the storm (including the swimming pools of abandoned houses) appeared to be ideal and abundant breeding grounds for pathogen-bearing mosquitoes and hence a dangerous origin site for a significant post-Katrina outbreak.

Survey research in Louisiana and Mississippi by Caillouët, Michaels, Xiong, Foppa, and Wesson (2008) in fact confirmed that areas directly damaged by Katrina experienced an increase in West Nile neuroinvasive diseases compared with the pre-storm period. Neuroinvasive diseases, which include West Nile encephalitis, West Nile meningitis, and West Nile meningoencephalitis (involving inflammation of various parts of the nervous system and the brain) are the most dangerous health conditions resulting from West Nile virus infection. Less intense is West Nile fever, which is characterized by high temperature, headache, fatigue, aches, and possibly a skin rash. Because neuroinvasive diseases are seen in only about 1 percent of West Nile infections, even a small jump in the incidence of this set of diseases suggests that a large increase in the transmission of the West Nile virus has occurred. Despite significant loss of population, areas of Louisiana damaged by the storm experienced a jump from an annual case load of thirty patients diagnosed with neuroinvasive diseases in the years from 2002 to 2005, to forty-five patients in 2006. Affected areas of Mississippi saw an even greater increase, from twenty-three cases in the years from 2002 to 2005 to fifty-five cases the year after the hurricane. Overall, the incident rate ratios in 2006 were more than twice those of the prior four years. In contrast, areas in Louisiana and Mississippi that were not directly harmed by the storm exhibited either a decrease (in Louisiana) or no change (in Mississippi) in West Nile infection rates.

The Caribbean and Gulf Coast have witnessed a major leap in the number of devastating storms in recent years—including Hurricanes Katrina and Ike—that have taken a heavy toll in human lives, destroyed communities, and cost billions of dollars. Many climate scientists see the growing frequency of substantial storms as reflecting the heating up of the oceans caused by global warming: the warmer the surface of the ocean the more energy that is available to fuel storm winds and the more water in the atmosphere that can become torrential rainfall. The extent of the damage caused by extreme storms is also a consequence of the population buildup that has been occurring along the U.S. coastline, especially in the states of Texas, Florida, and North Carolina. Between 1980 and 2003, the population living along the Gulf and Southeastern U.S. shores increased to 33 million people, a significant jump in the number of people being put in harm's way by the growing number of violent storms (Crossett, Culliton, Wiley, & Goodspeed, 2004). Moreover, building coastal communities results in the destruction of the protective storm buffer provided by coastal wetlands. Research shows that every mile of wetlands reduces storm surge by three to nine inches and every acre of wetlands reduces the cost of storm damage by over $3,000. The building boom along the coast, along with agricultural expansion elsewhere in the United States, has resulted in a significant drop (about 50 percent) in the U.S. watershed over the last 300 years (Evjen, 2004). The violent storms that are increasing due to global warming, in conjunction with other anthropogenic ecocrises, indeed present a grave threat to human health and well-being.

The hurricane also led to the spread of *Norovirus* infection. This genus of viruses causes at least half of all gastroenteritis cases globally, a disease marked by stomach pain, diarrhea, lethargy, weakness, muscle aches, headache, and vomiting. Named after Norwalk, Ohio, which witnessed an intense outbreak of acute gastroenteritis among elementary school children in 1968, noroviruses have been radiating globally, with a significant increase in infections in 2006. Although they can be spread through various means, including hand-to-hand contact, touching infected surfaces, and eating contaminated food, they also are transmitted by water, and may be present in municipal waterlines, wells, lakes, swimming pools, and even ice machines. Some of the crowded shelters set up in the wake of Katrina became transmission zones for noroviruses (Palacio et al., 2005).

Although the total disease burden of Katrina was not as bad as many feared (in part because of population dispersal), this deadly hurricane suggests the potential for epidemic and ecosyndemic outbreaks if, as has been predicted given the fact of climate change, the frequency of major hurricanes, cyclones, tornados, and other major storms increases.

Syndemics and Instability

There is little doubt any longer among climate, environmental, and health scientists that intensifying climate change is beginning to have significant impacts on human health and well-being. As McMichael et al. (2003) stress, "Populations of all animal species depend on supplies of food and water, freedom from excess infectious disease, and the physical safety and comfort conferred by climatic stability. The world's climate system is fundamental to this life-support" (p. 2). Syndemics are more likely under unstable social and environmental conditions. Social disruption frays personal and communal support networks, increasing individual emotional stress and reducing the capacity to mount an effective immune response to microbial threat. Environmental instability threatens subsistence while also ushering in the damaging effects of malnutrition. Other forms of environmental degradation, including pollution, deforestation, and species extinction, further imperil human health directly and indirectly. Together, these various forces increase the likelihood of ecosyndemics in a world out of balance.

SUMMARY

This chapter has examined the role of human interaction with the environment in the development and character of a set of emergent syndemics. Societal interactions with the physical environment are creating opportunities for the rapid spread of new diseases while various social practices and living conditions are contributing to the reemergence of older diseases that for a time had withdrawn to the backstage of history. Together these emergent and reemergent conditions have brought forth new syndemics, with sometime devastating impacts on human morbidity and mortality.

KEY TERMS

animal reservoirs of disease
Anthropocene Era
ecosyndemics
emergent diseases

emergent syndemics
global warming
reemergent diseases
superinfection

QUESTIONS FOR DISCUSSION

1. Why has there been a sudden jump in recent years in disease emergence? How are emergent diseases becoming a factor in the development of syndemics? Name and describe an emergent syndemic in the contemporary world. How is it affecting human health?

2. What are reemergent diseases, and how are they becoming entwined in syndemics? Name and discuss one example.

3. What role do animal populations play in the development of syndemics in human communities?

4. What are the primary diseases that now threaten the population of Dhaka, Bangladesh? What factors will influence their potential to become part of emergent syndemics in the future?

5. What is superinfection? Discuss the role of multistrain infectious diseases in the development of syndemics.

6. The term *iatrogenic syndemics* has been introduced to label syndemics caused or promoted by the actions of biomedicine. Can you name and describe an example of an iatrogenic syndemic?

7. Discuss the human impact on the natural environment and its role in the development of ecosyndemics. What role might global warming play in the development of syndemics?

8. Discuss the ways in which extreme storms can contribute to the development of syndemics, and describe the role of Hurricane Katrina in syndemic emergence, in 2004.

PART

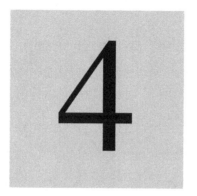

APPLICATIONS
OF THE SYNDEMIC
PERSPECTIVE

Chapter Nine, "Practical Utility: Mobilizing the Syndemic Model in the Promotion of Health and Treatment of Disease," constitutes the final part of this book and addresses a critical public health and health care question: what is the practical utility of the syndemics concept for improving human health and well-being? This final chapter answers this question, demonstrating that an understanding of syndemics can contribute both to health promotion (and disease prevention) and to health care.

CHAPTER

9

PRACTICAL UTILITY

Mobilizing the Syndemic Model
in the Promotion of Health
and Treatment of Disease

After studying this chapter, you should be able to

■ Recognize the value of taking a syndemic perspective in order to respond effectively to disease threats to public health.

■ See the value of developing syndemic treatment protocols, including the mobilization of countersyndemics in the treatment of disease.

■ Understand the importance of syndemics as a factor in health development initiatives and the achievement of public health planning goals.

■ Review emergent efforts in computer modeling of syndemics.

■ Be aware of the importance of public health planning for the syndemics of the future.

WHY STUDY SYNDEMICS?

An initial answer to this question is offered by Mark Nichter in his book, *Global Health* (2008), where he writes: "What is appealing about a syndemic approach to health social science research is both its explicit emphasis on examining connections between health and development and its attention to routes of transmission that affect clusters of interrelated health problems" (p. 159). In other words, addressing syndemics requires public health, biomedical, and health development models that move beyond individual risk, individual diseases, and individual behavior change. This chapter explores this domain of emergent patterns of public health mobilization and biomedical response.

PUBLIC HEALTH AND SYNDEMIC PREVENTION

In 1942, as part of the broader World War II effort, an entity known as the Office of Malaria Control in War Areas was formed by the U.S. government. Its mission was to ensure that the vicinities around U.S. military bases in the southern states remained malaria free, to protect soldiers from this debilitating illness. In 1946, building on this initial antimalarial work, the Communicable Disease Center, a small branch of the U.S. Public Health Service concerned with control of both mosquito-borne diseases and typhus, was established. From these roots, the modern Centers for Disease Control and Prevention (CDC) developed into a large national agency, operating on a global level and charged with the responsibility of improving and protecting public health by assessing epidemiological threats to health, enhancing the health impact of interventions, reducing health disparities, and preparing for emerging threats to health. Before long, the CDC's focus grew to include not only all infectious diseases but also occupational health, toxic chemicals, injury, chronic diseases, health statistics, birth defects, and more.

Among the numerous initiatives undertaken by the CDC to accomplish its increasingly complex mission was the creation of the Syndemics Prevention Network, an online resource for advancing research, discussion, and public health activities in response to the growing impact of interacting epidemics. Milstein (2008) reports that as of January 2008, over 600 individuals representing over 400 organizations in twenty countries had joined the network, which continues to grow at a pace of about 8 percent per month.

It is the perspective of the founders of the Syndemics Prevention Network that even though epidemiological science has produced noteworthy accomplishments in public health, additional progress can be made by integrating a syndemic perspective into the field. With specific reference to the HIV and malaria syndemic, for example, Abu-Raddad (2007) observes: "The synergy between HIV and other diseases such as malaria provides us with more opportunities to combat HIV/AIDS by treating its co-infections with these other diseases. This outcome highlights the fact that global public health challenges require comprehensive and multi-pronged approaches to dealing with them. Current efforts that focus on a single infection at a time may be losing substantial rewards of dealing synergistically and concurrently with multiple infectious diseases."

As described in previous chapters, human populations are facing an increasing number of health threats in a world that is enduring profound and diverse changes, many of which are of human origin and in which social and health disparities have proven to be of great consequence as well as notoriously resistant to change. As a result the Syndemics Prevention Network (2005c) argues on its Web site that "[n]ew ways of thinking and working will be needed to find solutions for today's and tomorrow's challenges." The challenges of achieving these new ways of thinking and working in public health are evident in the following discussion.

Public Health Applied Science: From Silos to Systems

In her book *Hidden Arguments: Political Ideology and Disease Prevention Policy,* Sylvia Tesh (1988) observes that modern public health has moved far beyond simple linear and reductionist understandings of disease causation to a recognition of the need for **multicausal models.** Such models (sometimes displayed as complex interacting nodes connected by a forest of bidirectional lines or as series of overlapping or concentric circles) include many factors believed to *go together* in the production of disease, including contamination of the air, water, soil, and food; psychological stressors; lack of health knowledge and risky personal practices; genetic predisposition; barriers to equitable access to preventive resources; and even certain governmental policies and the activities of political and economic institutions. Although not denying the interaction of diverse domains in the making of public health, Tesh emphasizes that multicausal models offer little direction for what to prioritize and where to begin in building public health responses. Consequently, echoing Michael Terris, Tesh (1988) points out that most epidemiologists mistakenly "spend their time looking for identifiable risk factors, precisely as though they were looking for particular disease agents" (p. 66).

A syndemic approach, in contrast, provides a very different orientation for public health by reinforcing "the idea that the focal mission of public health goes beyond epidemic control to include improvements in the public's health" (Syndemics Prevention Network, 2008b). As emphasized by a holistic but theoretically focused syndemic perspective, this means advancing past narrowly conceived efforts toward an understanding of the epidemiological patterns of a specific disease in order to prevent or control it and, further, moving toward the development of a big-picture awareness of diseases, disease clustering, and disease interactions in biological, ecological, and social contexts and ultimately toward correspondingly broad-based public health initiatives.

State and local departments of public health across the United States, for example, are commonly organized into separate and often somewhat isolated divisions or programs centered around specific diseases and preventive measures (such as diabetes, HIV/AIDS, cancer, lead abatement, and nutrition), related health issues (such as health literacy), or particular populations (such as mothers and children, teens, and seniors). These programs and divisions function as semi-independent silos, with few opportunities to address interactions between syndemically linked diseases or the interconnected health and social problems facing communities. The inherent problem with this arrangement is illustrated by an assessment of state public health programming in Illinois, conducted by the Illinois Public Health Futures Institute (2004), that concluded that "efforts are taking place in Illinois to deliver the 10 essential public health services. However . . . a deeper emphasis needs to be placed on coordinating and integrating the public health services in order to build a true public health system. Developing a sense of the 'system' of public health practice is essential to improve performance" (p. 38).

Consequently, the assessment emphasized the critical need of public health organizations to move "from silos to systems." However, there are problems to be overcome in achieving systemic integration, and they stem in part from a reductionist definition of the health problems to be addressed and the calcification of organizational responses into the well-worn and familiar grooves that constitute public health business-as-usual practices.

Another way of looking at this issue is by way of a review of the challenges that face public health efforts. Margaret Hamburg (2001), a former New York City health commissioner, has identified the following challenges:

- Raising public and policymaker awareness of the importance of public health in troubled times

- Translating this awareness into real and effective programs

- Engaging the public in public health initiatives

- Building integrated public health infrastructure, and training needed personnel at all levels

- Advancing information technology capability, including real-time public health surveillance

- Enhancing integration and communication

In New York City, Hamburg (2001) comments, the will to meet these challenges was elevated by direct confrontation with a health crisis: "the resurgence of TB (including its more frightening form of multiple-drug-resistant TB) helped to change the debate" (p. 60). A syndemic, in short, one that united the emergent syndrome of HIV/AIDS and the resurgent disease of tuberculosis in creating significant adverse consequences, helped to refocus public discourse about the real challenges of public health.

What had been the focus of the debate in New York City prior to the reemergence of TB? As Freudenberg, Fahs, Galea, and Greenberg (2006), building on the work of Deborah Wallace and Rodrick Wallace (1998), have described, beginning in the mid-1970s, public policy decisions in New York City were driven by a cost-cutting mission intended, ostensibly, to save money for the city. Instead, these decisions contributed to deteriorating living conditions, a 20 percent rise in the number of poor people in the city (despite an overall population decrease of 10 percent), and a significant rise in the health burden of the poor. As Freudenberg et al. (2006) point out:

First, city, state, and federal budget cuts diminished the public health, public safety, medical, and social service infrastructures that respond to health emergencies, compromising their ability to respond effectively to emerging threats such as HIV infection and crack addiction. Second, the cuts led to reductions in services such as drug treatment, preventive clinical services, health education, and policing and thus contributed to increases in TB, HIV infection, and homicide. Third, these policy decisions amplified other trends that were pushing vulnerable populations such as the homeless, drug users, the incarcerated, single mothers, and the unemployed into living situations that put them squarely in the path of TB, HIV infection, and violence [p. 431].

In the aftermath of these changes, TB rates began to rise following a previous century of declining TB infection. At the same time, AIDS cases also became more frequent, particularly among drug users. Homicide rates began going up and continued to climb through 1990. In short, neither was public health prioritized as a social good nor were the significant interactions that occur between health and social issues a basis for the making of public policy. The costs of cost cutting, as a result, were enormous (fiscally and in terms of social suffering) and included sparking a costly tripartite syndemic of HIV, TB, and violence.

Recognizing the role social structural factors play both in creating living conditions that promote syndemic formation and in erecting barriers to the adoption of a syndemic orientation in public health, underlines the need for paying close attention to the issue of **environmental justice.** A popular social movement in support of environmental justice emerged as an outgrowth of the coming together, toward the end of the twentieth century, of the civil rights and environmental movements to respond to issues like the disproportionately higher blood lead levels in black children compared to white children. This development reflects as well the longstanding tendency of powerful governmental and industry forces to locate environmentally damaging and frequently health-damaging facilities, like solid waste or toxic chemical landfills and other anthropogenic pollution sources, near poor and ethnic minority communities (a tendency that gave rise to the coining of the term *environmental racism* by Benjamin F. Chavis Jr., director of the United Church of Christ). Two of the earliest environmental justice actions involved members of African American communities who fought the building of landfills near the North Hollywood section of Houston, Texas, and in Warren County, North Carolina, during the late 1970s and early 1980s.

Healthy People Initiatives

As the example in the sidebar suggests, structural influences on policy can lead to the kinds of unhealthy health policies (Castro & Singer, 2004) that promote syndemics. Structural factors can also become unintended barriers to the development of a broadly based syndemic orientation in public health. In 1979, for example, the Office of the Surgeon General issued a report titled *Healthy People: The Surgeon General's Report on Health Promotion and Disease Prevention* (U.S. Department of Health and Human Services, 1979). This report, driven by a commitment to significantly improving public health, was designed to, first, establish national health objectives for the United States that would serve, in effect, as a ten-year prevention agenda for the nation and, second, would provide a model for the development of health activities at the federal, state, and local levels. The targets of the proposed agenda were to reduce mortality among four age groups (infants, children, adolescents and young adults, and adults) and to increase independence among older adults and thus implement a full life course approach to public health. This report was updated with the publication of *Healthy People 2000: National Health Promotion and Disease Prevention Objectives* (U.S. Department of Health and Human Services, 1990), which provided an agenda consisting primarily of individual health issues of central concern in improving the nation's health (for example, malnutrition, use of tobacco, abuse of alcohol and other drugs, mental disorders, violence, heart problems and stroke, HIV/AIDS, diabetes, sexually transmitted diseases, and cancer). As this list suggests, the focus was on specific diseases and not for the most part on their interactions. In this the Healthy People approach wedded an innovative outlook to a narrow and traditional approach to health problems.

Currently, the national health effort is guided by *Healthy People 2010* (U.S. Department of Health and Human Services, 2000), which set out goals intended to reflect life in the twenty-first century. A central theme of *Healthy People 2010* is health choices. The report urges Americans to make better choices for themselves and their families when selecting doctors, health insurance, online health information, and a lifestyle. Of course, with almost 50 million people without health insurance, either public or private, and often as a result forced to delay treatment; with the majority of Americans who declare bankruptcy each year citing medical expenses as a major cause of their fiscal crises; with various restrictions imposed on people with insurance or government health care support when it comes to choosing doctors (as most are covered by a single plan) or receiving routine preventive care (many insurance plans do not cover routine gynecological screening, for example); and with multiple structural barriers to healthy lifestyles (such as lack of access to well-stocked supermarkets in the inner city, pressure to buy food that is affordable and energy-dense in a time of rapidly rising food costs, and an unending barrage of corporate promotion of unhealthy diets, lifestyles, and attitudes), stressing choice might appear to be more ideological than realistic for many people, including those who are least healthy.

Healthy People 2010 lists ten leading health indicators:

- Physical activity

- Overweight and obesity

- Tobacco use

- Substance abuse

- Responsible sexual behavior

- Mental health

- Injury and violence

- Environmental quality

- Immunization

- Access to health care

Here too, the general emphasis is on individual issues and individual choices.

Healthy People 2010 does offer encouragement to make connections across indicators. As explained by the Office of Disease Prevention and Health Promotion (2000), "Thinking 'outside the indicator' means that we can look at how one contributing factor or one important change may affect several indicators. The indicators can also provide the foundation for new partnerships across health issues and new thinking about how to address the many health concerns we face." Some examples of "innovative thinking" and cross-cutting action provided by the Office of Disease Prevention and Health Promotion are

- Arranging collaboration among those who want to increase the amount of physical activity individuals do and promote weight loss to reach a healthy weight

- Combining education for parents into a "healthy home" program that addresses injury prevention, nutrition, and the impact of environmental tobacco smoke on children and other family members

- Designing worksite wellness programs to address several indicators simultaneously, such as physical activity, overweight and obesity, and tobacco use

- Using existing communication and outreach efforts for immunization to promote enrollment of children in health insurance programs

Again, transition to a holistic approach suggested by a syndemic perspective appears limited. As Milstein (2008) notes, the primary focus is "on how to manage each item on a long list of risks and diseases without necessarily joining those questions with ones about creating and assuring the related conditions for health." There is, he stresses, little attention given to "policies for improving adverse conditions, out of which all diseases and risks emerge" (p. 23), or to the interaction among diseases that results from socially adverse conditions like those discussed in Chapter Six, including conditions that have lifelong consequences even if individuals are removed to other settings or the immediate threat is contained.

Work is currently under way to develop the *Healthy People 2020* objectives, a fairly competitive effort for issue-oriented health advocates and promoters because inclusion of a health issue in the Healthy People objectives increases the likelihood that federal funding will be available to address it. Consequently, even though public comment is solicited every ten years before the release of a Healthy People report, the relation of the health issues included in the final report to subsequent government funding for health programs favors a single-issue orientation over a syndemic perspective.

Beyond the public health arena, there is a critical need as well for expanded consideration of syndemic issues in biomedicine, as discussed below.

MEDICAL TREATMENT OF SYNDEMICS

From the perspective of biomedicine, awareness of syndemics raises five critical questions:

1. How does syndemic interaction among diseases complicate diagnosis?

2. What can biomedicine do to address the social causes of syndemics?

3. For patients who are suffering from multiple interacting diseases, what is the best course of medical treatment? Can entwined syndemic diseases be treated simultaneously?

4. How can biomedicine avoid iatrogenic syndemics?

5. Conversely, can countersyndemics play an innovative role in treatment?

Each of these questions is addressed in turn.

Diagnostic Complications

Diagnosis of disease relies on the identification and interpretation of signs and symptoms. A significant complication of syndemics is that they can alter the landmark characteristics of diseases that are commonly used to confirm a diagnosis. Coinfection with herpes simplex virus type 2 and HIV-1, for example, reduces the expression of typical HIV-specific responses in T cells (Sheth et al., 2008). Similarly, detecting hepatitis C virus (HCV) in people who are immunocompromised by HIV infection can be difficult because they may not produce an antibody response sufficient to be detected with the existing HCV blood test. In HIV-positive people with a CD4 T-cell count below 200 cells/μl, an HCV RNA viral load test may be necessary to diagnose hepatitis C.

With reference to the diagnostic complications caused by coinfection with leptospirosis and malaria, Wongsrichanalai et al. (2003) report they have found

Although leptospirosis, a bacterial infection of the kidneys and liver, is not common in humans, it may be relatively prevalent as a human disease in some locations. Although the *Leptospira* pathogen can be cultured, the process takes three weeks to three months, making it difficult to obtain a timely diagnosis. Coinfection that masks leptospirosis complicates the process.

compelling evidence for leptospirosis-malaria co-infection in [the] Thailand-Myanmar border community [that] raises dual issues concerning its diagnosis. First, leptospirosis is difficult to diagnose on the spot and diagnostic tools are usually unavailable in remote settings. Second, it is common practice in a malaria-endemic area that if an acutely febrile patient is found to be malaria-positive, malaria is naturally assumed as the sole cause of the fever. Failure to recognize acute leptospirosis co-infection means a delay in the initiation of its proper therapy and possibly ensuing severe complications such as Weil's syndrome (jaundice and renal failure), pulmonary hemorrhage, and uveitis [inflammation of the inner eye] [p. 585].

Diagnostic complications are not limited to syndemics of infectious diseases, but occur as well with mixed noninfectious and infectious disease syndemics and with syndemics that do not involve an infectious disease. With regard to the former, Shaikh, Singla, Khan, Sharif, and Saigh (2003), in a study of patients at the Sahary Chest Hospital, in Riyadh, Saudi Arabia, have examined how diabetes mellitus alters the radiological image of pulmonary tuberculosis. Radiographic findings of pulmonary TB patients suffering from diabetes were compared with those of TB patients who did not have diabetes. These researchers found that diabetes sufferers had more frequent lung lesions and that these tended to be located in the lower lung field. Logistic regression analysis showed that diabetes was the only significant independent risk factor associated with lung lesions in the lower lung.

With regard to noninfectious disease syndemics, the common co-occurrence of mental health and substance abuse disorders is known to "make diagnosis complicated, and treatment . . . difficult" (Rosack, 2003, p. 30). One factor that burdens diagnostic efforts is that the side effects of some psychiatric medications, including sedation, dry mouth, agitation, and fine motor tremor, mimic symptoms of substance abuse. Similarly, a considerable body of research shows that major depression is significantly more common in patients with medical conditions like cardiovascular disease, diabetes, and cancer than it is in the general population. Although depression is ten times more prevalent in medically ill individuals, it presents significant diagnostic and therapeutic challenges for physicians (Mok & Lin, 2002). Consequently, it is estimated that as many as half of the depressive episodes in patients with medical illness are not accurately diagnosed (Beliles & Stoudemire, 1998). One of the most important barriers to accurate diagnosis in such cases is the problematic but common idea that *reactive depression* (that is, depression that develops in response to a major medical diagnoses) is not pathological. Unwillingness to stigmatize medically ill patients with a psychiatric diagnosis may also be a factor. In addition, there is the difficulty of differentiating the neurovegetative symptoms of depression (for example, poor sleep, impaired concentration, loss of energy, lack of appetite) from various physiological processes associated with organic disease (Cohen-Cole, Brown, & McDaniel, 1993).

As these cases imply, syndemics can obscure the identities of their constituent disease components and confuse the diagnostic process. Awareness of syndemics, of commonly interacting diseases that are locally prevalent, and of the signs and symptoms of syndemic expression becomes all the more important as a constituent of biomedical education and knowledge as new disease interactions become increasingly common.

Biomedicine and the Social Origins of Syndemics

Can biomedicine be broadened to address the social origins of disease? Some physicians believe it can. Farmer, Nizeye, Stulac, and Keshavjee (2006), for example, comment:

> If structural violence is often a major determinant of the distribution and outcome of disease, why is it or a similar concept not in wider circulation in medicine and public health, especially now that our interventions can radically alter clinical outcomes? One reason is that medical professionals are not trained to make structural interventions. Physicians can rightly note that structural interventions are "not our job." Yet, since structural interventions might arguably have a greater impact on disease control than do conventional clinical interventions, we would do well to pay heed to them.

Farmer et al. (2006) consequently urge a resocialization process to promote medical understanding of disease distribution in light of structural inequality. They suggest that as part of this process, health care providers "insist that [their] services be delivered equitably" and that fellow physicians accept this as a basic responsibility of their role in society. Farmer et al. further note that only when physicians and other health care providers link their efforts "to those of others committed to initiating virtuous social cycles can we expect a future in which medicine attains its noblest goals." Finally, they offer as an example of the new approach the model employed by Partners in Health (PIH), an organization cofounded by Farmer with his colleague and fellow physician and anthropologist Jim Yong Kim (Farmer et al., 2001). The PIH model, which is being tested on the front lines of clinical treatment among the poor in Haiti, Peru, Rwanda, Boston, and elsewhere, comprises several components (the selection actually used is conditioned by local factors, resources, and needs):

- Removing clinical and community barriers to care, with diagnosis and treatment being declared a public good and made available free of charge to patients living in poverty.

- Treating patients with respect and sensitivity in light of the structural realities they face.

- Delivering health care not only in the conventional way at the clinic, but also in the community settings in which patients work and live.

- Addressing health-related social conditions (for example, in Rwanda this included launching a potable water project in the clinic's catchment area; distributing kerosene stoves, kerosene, bottles, and infant formula; and providing food aid and housing assistance when possible).

- Modeling the treatment plan to the realities of patients' lives (for example, when highly active antiretroviral therapy is provided for AIDS, each patient is urged to select a partner, often a neighbor, who is trained to deliver drugs and other supportive care in the patient's home).

- Paying for treatment transportation costs and providing other incentives.

- Having a comprehensive approach that addresses comorbid conditions ranging from drug addiction to mental illness.

Advocates of the PIH model recognize that activities like those just described "are not the tasks for which clinicians were trained," but they also recognize that such activities must become "central to the struggle to reduce premature suffering and death" (Farmer et al., 2006). As the last of the activities listed suggests, one approach that needs to be developed more broadly, beyond the specific health conditions mentioned, is the incorporation of a syndemic perspective into the new biomedical gaze.

Social Medicine   An orientation that has parallels to the PIH model can be found in a corner of biomedicine known as **social medicine,** although this approach is actively embraced at present by only a minority of physicians and medical training programs (it is the Department of Social Medicine that Paul Farmer, Jim Kim, and like-minded colleagues are in at Harvard). Another place such an approach finds support is at the Albert Einstein College of Medicine in the Department of Family and Social Medicine. In this program, social medicine is defined as an approach that "looks at . . . interactions in a systematic way and seeks to understand how health, disease and social conditions are interrelated" (Kark & Kark, 2008). Consequently, following the principle articulated in Chapter Two, that reliance on biomedicine alone to address health problems is not likely to have an enduring impact (Gandy & Zumla, 2003), clinicians in this program are taught to be concerned with individual and social change and not just with biological change. In the department's social internal medicine track, for example, medical residents provide care to an indigent urban and immigrant medically underserved community in the South Bronx, a job with both clinical and advocacy components. Another center of social medicine is the Sophie Davis School of Biomedical Education at the City College of New York. This program tailors its curriculum to preparing students to be community-oriented primary care physicians working in medically underserved areas. Medical students receive training in four somewhat different but related roles as

- Clinicians who provide first contact, continuing, integrated health care to individuals and their families in urban communities

- Community health promoters who serve to protect the health of all people in a defined population

■ Agents of change who work with the community to improve its residents' health by altering the social, biological, and physical environments and the distribution of health care resources

■ Researchers engaged in studies in primary clinical care, epidemiology, and social and institutional issues that affect the health of community residents

Although conventional biomedicine "has traditionally been slow to accept the fact that social factors play an important role in disease" (Anderson, Smith, & Sidel, 2005), the theoretical model of social medicine, as reflected in the medical school training programs described previously, offers a set of propositions that are very harmonious with the syndemic perspective (Rosen, 1974), namely:

1. Social and economic conditions profoundly influence health, disease, and the practice of medicine.

2. The health of the population is a matter of social concern.

3. Society should promote health through both individual and social means.

Given these principles, the job of physicians is, in the words of Rudolph Virchow, a noted mid-nineteenth century physician and one of the primary founders of social medicine, "to create institutions to protect the poor, who have no soft bread, no good meat, no warm clothing, and no bed, and who through their work cannot subsist on rice soup and chamomile tea. . . . [And to ensure that] the rich remember during the winter, when they sit in front of their hot stoves and give Christmas apples to their little ones, that the ship hands who brought the coal and the apples died from cholera" (quoted in Waitzkin, 2006, p. 7).

Simultaneous Treatment A recognition of syndemics highlights the need to attend to the clinical consequences of dual infections and to identify best practices for the simultaneous treatment of interlocked conditions. At present, however, the randomized controlled trials that produce much of the evidence on which treatment guidelines for physicians are based do not adjust for comorbidities in trial participants. Furthermore, to enhance the internal validity of the research, comorbidity is commonly used as a criterion for excluding volunteers from research samples (as if each disease existed in a pathological vacuum in the real world). The end result is inadequate knowledge of how to treat such patients. As Fortin et al. (2006) comment, "Excluding a subset of the population from such trials or from the final reports means important information about the proper use of a treatment or intervention for that subset is not available. Numerous pharmacological treatments and interventions dealing with isolated chronic conditions take little account of the multiple morbidities experienced by the majority of patients in general practice. . . . The resulting guidelines may offer a simplified, potentially inadequate approach to the treatment because of inadequate attention to the comorbid illnesses" (p. 105). Exemplary is the exclusion of people with Alzheimer's disease from clinical trials designed to study the treatment of diseases that commonly are comorbid with and appear to interact with this progressive neurodegenerative condition. Hospitalized patients with Alzheimer's disease have an average of eight comorbid conditions, such as diabetes, cardiovascular disease, and musculosketelal and neuropsychiatric conditions (Zamrini, Parrish, Parsons, & Harrell, 2004). As Tschanz et al. (2004) found in their research in Utah, among Alzheimer disease patients, cardiovascular disease and pneumonia are both more common immediate causes of death than dementia itself. If individuals with Alzheimer disease continue to be excluded from research on comorbid conditions, as Wall (2009) stresses, "optimal and safe treatments for these conditions in this population will remain unknown" (pp. 1–2).

Some research has been done further indicating the importance of including individuals with comorbid conditions in clinical trials. Reddy et al. (2007), for example, recognizing that the distributions of many of the neglected tropical diseases (discussed in Chapter Four) overlap and that people in some tropical zones are commonly coinfected with two or more of them, reviewed the available research on simultaneous, multidisease treatment. This team established that twenty-nine randomized clinical trials had been carried out on the treatment of various co-occurring neglected tropical diseases and that three of these trials addressed the concurrent treatment of four diseases, twenty targeted three diseases, and six looked at two diseases. At the same time, the team found that some prominent conditions were not included in any multidisease clinical trials. The studies reviewed had three main findings. First, joining the drugs albendazole (used for worm infestations) with diethylcarbamazine (a synthetic compound used to treat parasites) significantly reduced prevalence of elephantiasis, hookworm, roundworm, and whipworm. Second, combining albendazole with ivermectin (an antiparasite medication) significantly reduced the prevalence of elephantiasis, hookworm, roundworm, and whipworm. Finally, mixing levamisole (an antibiotic) with mebendazole (used to treat worms) significantly reduced the prevalence of hookworm, roundworm, and whipworm. Based on this meta-analysis, Reddy and his coworkers concluded that several of the most prevalent neglected tropical diseases can be treated simultaneously with existing oral medications, facilitating effective and efficient syndemic treatment. This study supports findings by other researchers suggesting that the constituent diseases that make up some syndemics can be treated with combined drug regimes (assuming that treatments exist) or even that a single pharmacological agent may be effective with two or more interacting diseases.

Sometimes, however, syndemic treatment is much more complicated. A case in point is the syndemic produced by dual infection with the hepatitis delta virus (also known as the hepatitis D virus, or HDV) and hepatitis B virus. Patients can become infected with both viruses at the same time through sexual contact, intravenous drug use, or some other route of exposure to infected blood. HDV, first identified in 1977, is an incomplete virus and cannot survive on its own independent of HBV because it needs a component of HBV (its outer cover) to infect cells of the liver. Of the 300 million people worldwide infected with HBV, it is estimated that about 1.5 million (5 percent) also have HDV infection, although rates vary considerably by region and by population. The western sector of the Brazilian Amazon Basin has been reported to be endemic for HBV and HDV, whereas in the United States, infection currently tends to be limited to either injection drug users or hemophiliacs (Viana, Paraná, Moreira, Compri, & Macedo, 2005). Triple hepatitis infection (with HCV as well) is also known in Mongolia (including among some asymptomatic patients), Taiwan, and elsewhere. When HDV and HBV are both present, infection tends to be more severe and the patient is more likely to develop chronic liver disease. In chronically ill patients (those in whom the viruses persist longer than six months), the combined viruses cause inflammation all over the liver and ultimately destroy liver cells, which are then replaced by scar tissue, a condition known as cirrhosis.

Diagnosis of this dual infection is complicated because the available blood test for detecting HDV antibody is not very effective much in advance of symptom onset, necessitating a liver biopsy. Patients with this life-threatening syndemic condition often need at least one year of interferon-alpha (IFN-alpha) therapy. Even with this prolonged therapeutic regimen, many sufferers relapse once interferon treatment is suspended (Koytak, Yurdaydin, & Glenn, 2007). Complications are enhanced further when HIV is copresent.

Another example of the complications of syndemic medical treatment is seen in the case of HIV and HBV coinfection. Research by Soriano et al. (2005) in Madrid, for example, has found that treatment of chronic hepatitis B poses specific challenges in the presence of HIV coinfection, because both infections must be addressed simultaneously. Even though interferon (specifically, IFN-alpha) is valuable in the treatment of HBV infection, its effectiveness is diminished among coinfected individuals, especially those in advanced stages of immunosuppression. Introduction of more potent pegylated forms of IFN-alpha (that is, interferon that has undergone a process that prolongs its circulatory time by reducing clearance by the kidneys) has improved treatment outcomes. Nonetheless, as Dieterich (2007) emphasizes, in treating coinfected individuals multiple decisions must be made about the various effects of the available therapies (for example, whether an antiviral medicine is specific for HBV or acts on both HBV and HIV, whether a drug has potential for producing drug resistance and cross-resistance, and whether a drug produces hepatotoxicity).

As these examples indicate, the complexities of many syndemics magnify the challenges of treatment while illustrating the critical importance of ongoing syndemic research to enhance treatment effectiveness. At the same time, as the case of triple hepatitis suggests, co-infection does not automatically produce symptoms in some individuals, which raises important research questions about differences within populations, biologically and socially, that may contribute to asymptomatic comorbidity.

Bayliss (2006) has introduced a typological system for assessing the relationship between comorbid conditions in order to help establish a treatment plan. The three categories in her typology are (1) pathophysiologically related conditions that require congruent treatment plans, (2) co-occurring conditions that have discordant and potentially competing treatments, and (3) comorbid conditions that do not affect the disease of primary interest. She points out that participants in a random control trial to explore the use of exercise in the management of blood glucose levels may variously suffer from diabetes, hypertension, osteoarthritis, dyspepsia, and asthma, and that (1) the patients suffering from hypertension might have improved chances of achieving the desired outcomes, (2) the patients with the comorbid conditions of arthritis or asthma might have a decreased likelihood of having the same outcomes, and (3) the patients experiencing dyspepsia would have outcomes unaffected by their comorbidity. Bayliss, in short, shows the critical importance of paying close attention to potentially positive, negative, or neutral treatment effects of comorbidity, underlying the significance of a syndemic approach in clinical research.

Avoidance of Iatrogenic Syndemics

Heightened awareness of the nature of syndemic interactions, including both the effects of interaction and of the channels and mechanisms of interaction, is needed to diminish the likelihood of triggering iatrogenic syndemics as well. Similarly, fuller recognition of the complex interactions that occur across disease categories commonly assumed to be separate (as emotional diseases and physical diseases are often thought to be) would enhance assessment of what the potential iatrogenic consequences of treating one disease might be for other comorbid conditions. For example, patients with Parkinson's disease and related conditions often also suffer from daytime sleepiness and sleep disorders such as apnea. The treatment of Parkinson's with dopamino-mimetics—drugs that have been proven to have both immediate and long-term benefits for advanced Parkinson's patients—may at the same time exacerbate sleepiness in some patients (Rye, 2003). Given the health risks of daytime sleepiness, inattention to comorbidity and disease interaction may diminish the effectiveness of disease-specific treatment.

Assessment of Countersyndemics' Medical Value

If the presence of one disease diminishes or eradicates another, might countersyndemic knowledge be of value to biomedicine? This is actually a very old idea. A belief that disease-induced fever, for example, can have a curative effect on emotional and mental disorders dates to antiquity. Galen cited a case of melancholy that was cured following a bout of "quartan fever" (that is, malaria). Similarly, writings attributed to followers of Hippocrates mentioned the beneficial effects of fever caused by malaria on epilepsy.

The potential value of fever in treating a range of emotional problems has been mentioned in the reports of various later physicians into modern times. In the late 1800s, for example, a psychiatrist by the name of Julius Wagner-Jauregg, working at the Asylum of Lower Austria in Vienna, carried out a series of observations on the short- and long-term beneficial effects of fevers caused by typhoid, cholera, or other diseases on psychoses. He became convinced of the value of this line of inquiry after compiling a table of over 160 asylum patient cases and began to put the notion of developing a "fever therapy" into experimental practice (Whitrow, 1990). After testing and reporting various approaches over a number of years, in 1917 he began use of intentionally induced malarial infection as a treatment for neurosyphilis. Of the first nine patients so treated (using the blood of a soldier with confirmed malaria to cause infection and quinine afterward to treat the induced malaria), Wagner-Jauregg reported that six showed considerable improvement, at least in the short run. Many other patients were treated subsequently with malaria or other fever therapies, both by Wagner-Jauregg and by those he influenced in several countries in Europe as well as in the United States, with beneficial results in about half the treated patients (although some others died of malaria, sparking ethical concerns in some quarters). For this work, Wagner-Jauregg received the Nobel Prize in medicine in 1927. While his treatment was subsequently discontinued and has faded into the shadows of medical history, the basis for its effect has now become clear to researchers: *Treponema pallidum,* the bacterium that causes syphilis, cannot tolerate the high body temperatures brought on by malarial infection (Covell & Nicol, 1951). In effect, Wagner-Jauregg had discovered what has since been realized is a bodily defensive strategy, namely that the immune system can trigger a spike in body temperature to kill off invasive bacteria. This immune mechanism works by causing a drop in the availability of iron in the body while stimulating an increased need for iron in the bacteria (Greiger & Kluger, 1978).

A countersyndemic that remains of active interest is based on (at least initially) the relationship of two types of bacteria, *Mycobacterium indicus pranii* (MIP), a benign microbe found in many species including humans, and *Mycobacterium leprae,* the pathogen responsible for leprosy (Hansen's disease), a disease mentioned in the last chapter. *M. leprae* was first identified in 1873 by G. H. Armauer Hansen, earning it the status of the first bacterium to be definitively linked to a human disease. For centuries before this discovery, the distinctive skin and neurological expressions of leprosy were well known in several parts of the world. Moreover, because of the disfigurements that it can cause and the fear that these tend to generate, leprosy became a highly stigmatized condition. Indeed, leprosy has long been the epitome of stigmatizing diseases characterized by forced quarantine and other abuse of sufferers (for example, patients taken by sea to the "leper colony" in the isolated Kalaupapa area of the Hawaiian island of Molokai were sometimes forced to jump ship and swim through rough waters to shore so that sailors would not have to get too close to the quarantined area).

Leprosy has long been the type of disease that medical anthropologist Susan Estroff (1989) has called an "I am" as opposed to an "I have" condition. With an "I am" condition, the person does not merely have a disease, his or her social identity is defined by that disease, and hence a person infected with leprosy was not described as suffering from leprosy but as a "leper." This dehumanization has sparked social protest by both people with leprosy and others. During his motorcycle travels around South America as a young medical student, for example, Ernesto "Che" Guevara was pushed toward a lifelong revolutionary perspective in part by the mistreatment and ostracism accorded to "lepers" that he witnessed in São Paulo, Brazil. Although antibiotic treatments (involving multidrug cocktails) have been developed, the course of treatment is long, and leprosy remains a significant problem in many parts of the developing world, including places that were first exposed to the causative agent as a result of the slave trade. Today approximately 250,000 cases of leprosy are diagnosed annually around the world. It is estimated that over 100 million people are directly or indirectly affected by leprosy as patients and as family members who are also subject to ostracism. Consequently, there has been pressure to identify even more effective treatment options.

It was this concern in India (which had over 3 million cases of leprosy at the time) that led to an invitation being sent in the early 1970s to J. P. Talwar, a promising researcher in biochemistry at the All India Institute of Medical Sciences in New Delhi, to direct a new immunology research and training center and to take up finding a vaccine for leprosy. His first reaction was to turn down the invitation and to stay focused on developing the place of biochemistry in Indian medicine. Then, he reports (Talwar, 2005), he received a message from the inviting committee that changed his mind: "[The] statement [that] floored me squarely [read]: 'India has the world's largest number of leprosy patients. . . . Do we expect Americans to come and work on this disease to find solutions? Scientists in India should take up the problems of India'" (p. 438).

Talwar began his leprosy research by considering why most people exposed do not develop the disease and why even most of those who do express it develop only a single lesion rather than the worst symptoms, involving disseminated lesions all over the body that are filled with proliferating mycobacteria. The reason for this vast difference in disease expression is believed to be that most (but not all) people have effective innate resistance to the disease. Those who develop disseminated lesions, in contrast, suffer from a "maximal immune deficit. Instead of killing the bacteria, their macrophages offer a hospitable territory for them to multiply" (Talwar, 2005, p. 438). These patients, Talwar and his team discovered, did not have a generalized immune problem (they did develop antibodies in response to exposure to cholera or tetanus); rather, their immune systems had either an inherent (that is, a genetic) or a disease-induced inability to recognize *M. leprae*.

Vaccines are commonly made with partial, dead, or attenuated pathogens and are intended to stimulate immune response without causing disease. This approach is not feasible with leprosy because the immune systems of vulnerable individuals fail to identify the invasive microorganism. Instead, the research team looked at other mycobacteria to see if a cross-reaction (an evocation of antibodies for another bacterium that were also effective in controlling *M. leprae*) occurred. *Mycobacterium indicus pranii* proved to have the desired properties, including demonstrating marked improvement in people with leprosy. A phased series of clinical trials followed that demonstrated safety and efficacy and led to the first leprosy vaccine to receive approval for public use from both the drug controller general of India and the U.S. Food and Drug Administration. Subsequently, human clinical trials have begun to assess the efficacy of MIP in interventions against HIV/AIDS, psoriasis, bladder cancer, and tuberculosis (Ahmed et al., 2007).

Another line of broadly related research involves the use of disease-causing bacteria in the treatment of cancer. The basis for this countersyndemic conception is a discovery dating from the nineteenth century that bacteria often colonize cancerous tumors. Although the appeal of tumors for bacterial multiplication is not fully understood, researchers like Siegfried Weiss at the Helmholtz Centre for Infection Research, a component of the Helmholtz Association, Germany's largest biological and medical research organization, believe that "dead tissue inside the tumor provides . . . bacteria with a protective and nutrient-rich environment. . . . Tumor interiors . . . are low in oxygen, conditions under which many types of bacteria thrive" (quoted in Helmholtz Association, 2007). Weiss heads Molecular Immunity, a project group that has successfully planted genetically modified salmonella bacteria in the tumors of cancer-bearing mice. These microbes are programmed (via a simple sugar molecule called L-arabinose) to produce substances on command. The ultimate goal is to have the bacteria migrate to cancerous areas and secrete cell toxins that kill cancerous tissue (Loessner et al., 2007). In a first step in this work, Weiss and his colleagues have implanted genes with encoded light-emitting proteins into *Salmonella typhimurium*, infected cancerous mice with these bacteria, waited for the bacteria to migrate to and infect tumors in the mice, and then fed the mice a dose of L-arabinose. This caused the bacteria to fluoresce, allowing the locations and sizes of tumors to be seen and analyzed. According to Weiss, "Until now, people have viewed salmonella as a threat to their health . . . so there would be a certain charm in using such bacteria for treatment of such a terrible disease as cancer" (quoted in Helmholtz Association, 2007).

One of the countersyndemic solutions currently being proposed as a medical response to the emergence of drug-resistant bacteria and the resulting antibiotic crisis is the use of **bacteriophage therapy.** Bacteriophages (from the Greek word *phagein,* which means "to eat") are viruses that infect bacteria. Discovered early in the twentieth century, bacteriophages are ubiquitous in the environment and have been used therapeutically to a limited degree (primarily in Eastern Europe) almost since their discovery. Interest in them has grown significantly of late because, unlike antibiotics, bacteriophages are living organisms that can mutate and evolve, which allows them to adapt to the antiphage evolution of bacteria (Hausler, 2006). Various companies have begun clinical trials on phage therapies, including investigation of phage cocktails that blend multiple bacteriophages in a single medicine (as phage attacks on bacteria are species-specific) and phage patches for skin and wound infections. Independent researchers, it should be noted, have expressed some enthusiasm over the therapeutic promise of bacteriophages, although caution has also been voiced about the need for safe and controlled use of phage therapy (Skurnik & Strauch, 2006). The latter reaction is propelled in part by the discovery by Broudy and Fischetti (2003) that bacteriophages, such as those that attack the *Streptococcus pyogenes* bacterium that causes scarlet fever, can transfer genes for encoding toxin production from one bacterium group to another, leading to the conversion of bacteria from a nonpathogenic to a pathogenic orientation (a process known as **acquired pathogenicity**). Nonetheless, in 2006 the U.S. Food and Drug Administration approved the use of bacteriophages to kill the bacterium *Listeria monocytogenes* on cheese, and the following year the same bacteriophages, which are isolates from wastewater sources, were approved for use on all food products.

As these various examples suggest, there is considerable potential in harnessing countersyndemic approaches in the treatment of disease, and it is likely that this line of work will expand significantly as antibiotic weapons of mass protection diminish in their capacity to contain pathogenic activity.

MODELING SYNDEMICS

One tool of note in syndemic control and prevention is mathematical modeling (Keeling & Rohani, 2007; Nowak & May, 2000). A mathematical model is a simplified representation using mathematical language to describe patterns of behavior in natural, mechanical, or social systems. An appeal of modeling is that it allows improved understanding in a world marked by enormous complexity and rapid change. Daniel Bernoulli carried out mathematical modeling of smallpox epidemics in the mid-1700s and formally presented his findings to the French Academy of Sciences in 1760 (Daley & Gani, 1999). Beginning early in the twentieth century, and with the aid of ever more powerful technologies, epidemiologists became increasingly interested in the use of modeling procedures to project possible patterns in the spread of infectious diseases, including potential outcomes of an epidemic. To achieve these goals, epidemiological modelers unite several types of information and analytical capacity: (1) mathematical equations and computational algorithms; (2) computer technology; (3) epidemiological knowledge about infectious disease dynamics, including information about specific pathogens and disease vectors; and (4) research data on social conditions and human behavior. Advances in the modeling of disease have been propelled by the HIV/AIDS pandemic (Ghani & Boily, 2003), especially in the understanding of how sexual behavior can drive an epidemic (Anderson & May, 1991). Building on earlier models of STD transmission (Hethcoke & Yorke, 1984), this work has led in turn to improved STD models and greater appreciation of the value of modeling in epidemiology generally (Aral & Roegner, 2000; Donnelly & Cox, 2001). Consequently, modeling has become an influential factor in health policy and planning, as seen in the modeling carried out in preparation for the next major influenza pandemic (Feurguson et al., 2006; Halloran et al., 2008). Beyond individual epidemics, mathematical modeling in epidemiology is also beginning to be applied to syndemics.

Abu-Raddad, Patnaik, and Kublin (2006), for example, used modeling to quantify the syndemic effects of malaria and HIV in sub-Saharan Africa, basing their work on research in Kisumu, Kenya. These researchers point out that infection with HIV facilitates disease progression in individuals exposed to malaria. At the same time, immune reaction to malaria doubles the infectious level of HIV-infected individuals. In short, in typical syndemic fashion, each of these diseases amplifies the effects of the other. Using mathematical modeling, Abu-Raddad and coworkers found that 5 percent of HIV infections (that is, 8,500 cases of HIV since 1980) in Kisumu were the result of the higher HIV infectiousness of malaria-infected HIV patients. Additionally, their model attributed 10 percent of adult malaria episodes (or almost 1 million excess malaria infections since 1980) to the greater susceptibility of HIV-infected individuals to malaria. Their model also suggests that HIV has contributed to the wider geographical spread of malaria in Africa, a process previously thought to be the consequence primarily of global warming.

Other researchers also have begun to apply mathematical models to syndemics. Herring and Sattenspiel (2007), for example, have been interested in understanding the set of factors that influenced the spread of the 1918 influenza epidemic among aboriginal communities in Manitoba; of special concern to this research team have been questions about intercommunity and within-household heterogeneity in patterns of illness. For this purpose they combine demographic and historical analyses with mathematical and computer models. Also factored into their models is information about seasonal and longer term changes in mobility rates, the effects of social structure, and the influence of quarantine policies implemented during the epidemic (Herring & Sattenspiel, 2003; Sattenspiel & Herring, 1998). Initially, these researchers used population-based, deterministic mathematical models that did not allow for random factors. Although easy to implement, this approach has a shortcoming in that it assumes large, homogeneous populations in the three aboriginal communities of concern (the Hudson Bay Company's posts at Norway House, Oxford House, and God's Lake). In fact, not only were each of these communities subdivided into extended family groups but during winter fur trapping, the season when influenza struck, these family groups were dispersed over a wide area tending to their traps. Consequently, a new model was developed that was better suited to the analysis of small population groups. Thus, Herring and Sattenspiel selected an individual-based, fully stochastic (that is, random) modeling approach that was designed to include both settlement structure and family dispersal over a large geographical area.

In the new individual-based models for each community, each person was assumed to be in one of four health states: susceptible to infection, exposed, already infected (and infectious), and recovered. Further, the population was distributed into heterogeneous (by age and gender) family groups that dispersed during the winter and clustered together at the post communities in the summer (where some family members remained as year-round residents). Runs of the new model confirmed a finding of the population model: "epidemic severity is more strongly influenced by within-community factors, such as settlement structure and the nature of within-community contacts than by between-community factors, such as travel from one community to another" (Herring & Sattenspiel, 2007, p. 198).

In the next phase, Herring and Sattenspiel plan to consider the interplay of biological and social factors in an epidemic, including factors such as nutritional status and its impact on health, the social location of the study communities in the political economy of the Hudson's Bay Company at the time of the 1918 epidemic (involving, for example, the economic decline of Norway House owing to the local hunting-out of fur-bearing animals), and the effects of other infections, like tuberculosis, on immune capacity to fight influenza infection. As they note (Herring & Sattenspiel, 2007), tuberculosis "likely exacerbated the effects of influenza in 1918, contributing to the high proportion of deaths" (p. 199). In related historical research on the health of the Mushkegowuk Cree living at the Moose Factory settlement in the Hudson Bay region of the Canadian north during the 1940s, Herring, Abonyi, and Hoppa (2003) found evidence of significant reduction in survivorship. This decline in community health from the nineteenth to the mid-twentieth century was associated with an increased dependence on store-bought food (especially flour, sugar, and lard) and a faltering food security and dietary quality tied to overall economic decline "that, in turn, undermined the ability to resist infectious diseases such as tuberculosis" (p. 299).

Modeling of this sort offers an enormously useful tool not only for explaining disease patterns and effects in the past but also for anticipating future syndemics, including ecosyndemics, based on information about the spread of various diseases across the planet and the coinfections and disease interactions that will likely result.

In this regard, Jeremy Lauer et al. (2003) have developed PopMod, a longitudinal population tool that models distinct and possibly interacting diseases. Unlike other life-table population models, PopMod is specifically designed to not assume the statistical independence of the diseases of interest. PopMod has several intended purposes, including describing the evolution over time of population health for standard demographic purposes (such as estimating healthy life expectancy in a population), and providing a standard measure of effectiveness for health interventions and cost-effectiveness analysis. Typically, PopMod is used to simulate the evolution of morbidity and mortality in a population in which health status, health risk, and mortality risk are all influenced by overall disease state and in which the two primary diseases of concern interact and mutually influence prevalence, incidence, remission, and mortality risk. PopMod is one of the standard tools of the CHOICE (Choosing Interventions that are Cost-Effective) program of the World Health Organization (WHO), an initiative designed to provide national health policymakers in the WHO's fourteen epidemiological subregions around the world with findings on a range of health intervention costs and effects.

Although PopMod is not designed to model infectious diseases, Lauder and his colleagues (Pretorius et al., 2007) are using microsimulation models to examine HIV and TB interactions. For this, they have developed the HIV microsimulation model (HIVMM), a stochastic, agent-based simulation program based on knowledge about interacting HIV and TB epidemics gained from research on Masiphumelele, a small township outside Cape Town, South Africa, in which a significant jump in TB cases was tied to HIV infection. Consequently, HIVMM is designed to allow HIV to affect TB infection. Modeling is based on HIV status and CD4+ T-cell count, with helper cell decline making people more susceptible to contracting TB. Important social variables in risk assessment, like social networks and sexual orientation and practices, are also incorporated into the program. HIVMM, in short, moves the field closer toward the ability to model complex, multidirectional syndemic interactions involving two or more health problems and various social factors that promote mutually enhancing disease effects.

FUTURE SYNDEMICS

Humans always have and always will suffer diseases and disorders, as all living organisms do. Also, there is little doubt that syndemics will be part of the future health of human populations. The tomorrow of syndemics, like its yesterday and today, will be determined in large part by human activities, policies, structural relations, and impacts on the planet. Failure to seriously address issues like global warming, environmental degradation, global health disparities, human rights violations, structural violence, and low- and high-impact wars, all but ensures that syndemics will exact a tremendous human toll in the years and decades ahead. Growing awareness of syndemics, and knowledge about their dynamics, biosocial causes, and consequences, offers part of what is needed to limit the health burden of syndemic disease interactions and provide an improved and safer life for all peoples. Such a global course is certainly possible, as simulation modeling reveals various plausible futures. The will and commitment to find and use this knowledge at local, national, and international levels is what is most sorely needed to ensure a just and healthier future. Although microsolutions such as health education, treating individual cases of disease, and caring for the ill and intermediate solutions such as developing and broadly disseminating new vaccines and other medical interventions are necessary for responding to some syndemics, macrosolutions that address the socioenvironmental conditions and structural relations of inequality that foster syndemics are mandatory. There will certainly be syndemics in our future, but the level of their contribution to human suffering truly is in our own hands.

SUMMARY

The goal of this final chapter has been to demonstrate that an awareness of syndemics contributes to public health prevention, health development, and disease treatment. In short, syndemics knowledge has immediate practical utility. Adding to this knowledge, computer modeling is now being used to gain an understanding of syndemic formation. Syndemics have had dramatic impacts in the past and are having significant consequences for human health currently; given our changing environment, it may well be that syndemics will be even more significant in the future.

KEY TERMS

acquired pathogenicity
bacteriophage therapy
environmental justice

Healthy People initiative
multicausal models
social medicine

QUESTIONS FOR DISCUSSION

1. Summarize the key reasons why it is important to study syndemics.

2. How can understanding syndemics contribute to health promotion? Is this a good investment of scarce resources? How do syndemics challenge the current organization of state departments of health?

3. How can the syndemic perspective contribute to breaking down the silos that separate sectors of public health, and contribute to the integration of health promotion efforts?

4. How can medical treatment contribute to the development of syndemics? What changes will be needed in disease understanding to advance the medical treatment of syndemics?

5. Discuss developments in the computer modeling of syndemics and how this effort can contribute to syndemics prevention.

6. For what reasons can we expect consequent syndemics in the future? How important might such syndemics be in shaping health in the future?

GLOSSARY

Accelerated virulence. A syndemic interaction in which one disease causes another to be more lethal than it would be without comorbidity.

Acquired pathogenicity. The transfer between bacteria of genes for encoding toxin production that results in the conversion of bacteria from nonpathogenic to pathogenic.

Animal reservoirs of disease. Animals that serve as hosts for pathogens that may evolve into human diseases.

Anthropocene. A geological epoch during which human activity is the greatest force shaping the earth's climate and ecosystems.

Antigenic shift. The result of two different viruses attacking the same cell; the genetic material from both recombines to form a new strain of the virus (*see gene assortment*).

Asthma-influenza syndemic. A syndemic in which asthma and influenza interact, causing enhancement of one or both conditions.

Autoimmune disease. A disease characterized by the failure of a person's immune system to recognize cells of the person's own body, resulting in an immune attack on the person's own cells.

Bidirectional disease interaction. A type of syndemic interaction in which comorbid conditions both influence and are influenced by each other.

Biologizing experience. Undergoing biochemical and psychophysiological processes through which the body converts emotions and experiences into biological states, such as converting the experience of enduring stress into disease.

Biomedical individualism. The concept that each individual is different from all others in terms of the particular mix of genetic makeup and life experience factors that influence his or her current health status.

Body mass index. A formula that uses a person's weight and height to determine obesity.

CD4 T cell *or* **CD4+ T cell.** A type of immune cell attacked by HIV.

Comorbidity. The state of having two or more diseases at the same time (a syndemic is a kind of comorbidity in which such interaction leads to adverse outcomes under a given set of social conditions).

Countersyndemic. Comorbid disease interaction that limits the adverse impact of one or more of the diseases that are copresent.

Cytokines. Hormones released by wounded or infected cells; they are critical to immune response because they attract immune cells to infection areas.

Deleterious interaction. Interaction among diseases that produces negative health outcomes.

Diabulimia syndemic. A syndemic involving interaction between diabetes and a food disorder; this interaction is intentionally induced by avoidance of diabetes medication.

Disease carrier. An individual who is infected and spreads infectious disease to others but who is personally asymptomatic.

Disease clustering. A situation in which multiple diseases are active within a vulnerable population.

Disease interaction. The impact comorbid diseases have on each other; it may be biological, chemical, or involve some other mediator.

Drunkorexia. The colloquial name for a syndemic interaction between abusive drinking (or other drug use) and an eating disorder.

Dutch hypothesis. The view that airway obstruction diseases like asthma, chronic bronchitis, and emphysema constitute a single disease.

Ecosocial. Having entwined environmental and social aspects, as in an ecosocial health condition.

Ecosyndemic. A syndemic triggered by changing environmental and climatic conditions (often anthropogenic), such as global warming.

Emergent syndemic. A newly recognized adverse interaction among diseases or other disorders, or a syndemic known from one geographical area that is now appearing in another area where it has not been seen previously.

Enhanced contagiousness. A condition in which a disease is more contagious than it would be ordinarily, typically as a result of a syndemic interaction with another disease.

Environmental justice. A social movement that advocates equal access to natural resources and opposes the exposure of people to the unhealthy and polluting waste products of commercial and industrial production.

Explosive syndemic. A deleterious interaction among comorbidities that develops very rapidly in a population.

Folk syndemic. Local cultural beliefs about a disease interaction that causes enhanced health consequences.

Food choice constraint model. A model showing that a person's ability to purchase healthy foods declines as his or her income falls or as economic constraint increases.

Food insufficiency. A diet with inadequate levels of protein or calories (*macronutrients*) or of vitamins and minerals (*micronutrients*).

Gene assortment. The movement of genes between organisms; such movement involving two or more pathogens can produce a syndemic.

Germ theory. An explanation of disease in terms of pathogenic agents, such as bacteria, viruses, and other parasites.

HAART. Highly active antiretroviral therapy; a combination of three or more drugs that target retroviruses like HIV.

Health and social disparities. Uneven distributions of health status and social status within and across populations; social disparities can lead to health disparities and vice versa.

Health inequality. A higher disease burden in a group or population as a consequence of mistreatment, social injustice, and structural injustice.

Helminths. Parasitic worms of various species.

HIVAN. Human immunodeficiency virus–associated nephropathy.

Host-pathogen interactions. Ways in which the body responds to the detection of a pathogen; these ways include pain and fever, which are efforts by the body to rid itself of infectious agents.

Humors. The body fluids of blood, yellow bile, black bile, and phlegm; most people from ancient Greek to late Renaissance times believed that good health depended on maintaining a balance among the humors. Beliefs about the importance of maintaining balance continue in ethnomedical systems in many parts of the world.

Hyperinfective syndrome. A condition of massive infection in which threadworm (*Strongyloides stercoralis*) larvae multiply and spread rapidly throughout the body.

Iatrogenic syndemic. A syndemic interaction caused by medical treatment.

Interferons. Proteins that are part of the immune system biochemistry and that inhibit viral replication.

Internalized racism. A racist stereotype accepted as valid by a member of the vilified ethnic minority group.

Intimate partner violence. Emotional and physical abuse that occurs in close dyadic relationships; for example, among current and former spouses, dating partners, and sexual partners.

Koch's postulates. A set of sequential conditions; fulfilling these conditions affirms that a particular pathogen causes a particular disease (found to be impracticable with some pathogens and some health conditions).

Life course perspective. An examination of health and influences on health status across the several life stages: infancy, adolescence, adulthood, and old age).

Macronutrients. The proteins and calories in a person's diet; people are vulnerable when macronutrients are inadequate.

Macroparasites. Large entities, usually other humans, particularly elite social strata, that live off of and extract resources from subordinated populations.

Making of disease. A doctor or other health care provider detecting and assembling a set of signs and/or symptoms and constructing from them a disease diagnosis.

Making individual of disease. A doctor or other health care provider conducting an interactive process to help a patient to conceptualize his or her symptoms (or even a lack of symptoms) as a biomedically verified disease.

Making social of disease. Analytically revealing the structure of the social relationships and inequalities that shape the making of disease and making individual of disease processes.

Marginal coping. Adopting behaviors that in the long run may be self-destructive but that offer short-term relief from uncomfortable emotional states (for example, depression).

Miasma. The vapors given off by decomposing organic matter in the environment; until the acceptance of germ theory, miasma was believed to be the cause of many diseases.

Microlevel of disease interaction. The specific pathways and mechanisms of contact and exchange between two or more comorbid conditions clustered within a population that result in enhanced disease morbidity and morality.

Micronutrients. The vitamins and minerals in a person's diet; people are vulnerable when these are inadequate.

Microparasites. Generally microscopic parasites that infect human populations, extracting from them the resources (such as genetic materials) needed for survival and replication.

Motivated behavior. Actions undertaken to fulfill a need or craving or to seek a particular reward.

Multidisciplinarity. The quality of involving two or more scientific disciplines in collaborative knowledge development.

Mutualism. A mutually beneficial symbiotic relationship between species.

Neglected tropical diseases. A group of approximately fifteen infectious diseases, found in often underdeveloped tropical countries, that contribute to as many as half a million deaths annually but that have not attracted adequate global health and pharmacological attention.

Neutrophil. A white blood cell component of the immune system.

Opportunistic infections. Diseases that generally are able to infect only individuals with compromised immune systems.

Oxidative stress. A condition in which oxidants flow through the body's cells (including immune cells), cause damage, and accelerate cell destruction.

Paradigm shift. A change in the dominant explanatory model in a discipline; the shift from using miasma as an explanation of disease to using germ theory was a paradigm shift in biomedicine and the biological sciences.

Pathogenicity. A disease's combined speed of development in the body and degree of lethality.

Pathogens of everyday life. A cluster of persistent, endemic infections that routinely produce significant rates of morbidity and mortality in a population.

Polyparasitism. The condition of suffering from multiple parasitic infestations.

Popular epidemiology. The efforts of local communities to document the social origins of the health problems they are experiencing.

Reemergent disease. An old disease once on the decline that reappears as a threat to human health, usually after a population has developed resistance to available antimicrobial drugs.

Renocardiac syndemic. A disease interaction in which kidney disease accelerates heart disease, including myocardial infarction, heart failure, arrhythmias, and cardiac death.

Reverse zoonosis. Spread of an infectious disease from humans to a nonhuman animal species.

SAVA. A tripartite syndemic that brings together a behavior-linked emotional disease (substance abuse), interpersonally inflicted physical or emotional suffering (violence victimization), and an infectious disease (AIDS) within the context of a particular set of social conditions (structural violence and social suffering).

Self-medication. Use of psychotropic drugs, not prescribed (or not as prescribed) by an authorized health care provider, in order to self-treat a conflicted and upsetting emotional state.

Sexually transmitted disease syndemic. A deleterious interaction among comorbid sexually transmitted diseases.

Shantytown. An unofficial and often illegal and impoverished settlement, often seen in large cities of developing countries and commonly a center of disease clustering.

Simultaneous treatment. Integrated treatment of comorbid and interlocked health conditions that avoids producing an iatrogenic syndemic.

Social epidemiology. An approach to the study of health issues that builds on the classic epidemiological interactive triangle of host, agent, and environment while also emphasizing the social determinants of health at all three points on this triangle.

Social injustice. Discriminatory mistreatment perpetrated on a group by others with greater social power; it is one expression of structural violence and a contributor to disease.

Social suffering. The widespread and shared human misery produced by discrimination, stigmatization, war, famine, poverty, and torture; in short, the assemblage of human problems that result from the exercise of political, economic, and institutional power.

Spectral disease. A disease whose symptoms may vary considerably from person to person.

Structural violence. Social inequality that is embedded in social structures and that increases human suffering to a level that merits its being seen as a form of socially sanctioned brutality; an important source of human injury and ill health.

Superinfection. Coinfection by and interaction between two or more genetically different strains of the same or related pathogens, especially after immune response to the first infection has begun.

Supersyndemic. A synergistic interaction among two or more previously independent syndemics.

Symptomatology. The set of symptoms characteristic of a disease.

Syndemic. A concentration and deleterious interaction of two or more diseases or other health conditions in a population, especially as a consequence of social inequity and the unjust exercise of power.

Syndemic theory. An explanatory framework for the analysis of disease interactions, including their origins in disease clustering, dynamics of interaction, stages of disease enhancement, and the social conditions that facilitate these processes.

Syndemics of history. Syndemics that have played a role in shaping historical events and directions.

Syndemics of war Syndemics arising from and spread by the social disruptions caused by war.

Syndemogenic. Having a tendency to become involved in syndemic interaction; for example, HIV/AIDS tends to be syndemogenic.

Synergistic enlightenment. Recognition of the value of taking interdisciplinary approaches and overcoming barriers erected by discipline-centric attitudes.

Third epidemic. The stigma that is socially inflicted on those with HIV infection and AIDS, referred to as an epidemic because it not only acts as a barrier to seeking testing and treatment and hampers the ability of a society to respond effectively to the epidemics of HIV and AIDS but also inflicts extensive health-degrading suffering in its own right.

Unculturable. Used to describe a pathogen that cannot be grown (cultured) in an artificial environment outside the body.

Unidirectional disease interaction. A syndemic interaction in which only one of the co-occurring diseases or disorders influences the impact of the other.

VL/HIV syndemic. An interaction between a very damaging form of the infectious disease leishmaniasis (visceral leishmaniasis) and HIV/AIDS.

Wasting syndrome. Severe weight loss accompanied by fever or diarrhea (commonly associated with HIV infection).

World Health Organization (WHO). The coordinating authority for public health within the United Nations; WHO is responsible for providing guidance to member countries on global health issues, shaping the global health research agenda, setting norms and standards for public health internationally, providing technical support to countries, and monitoring and assessing health trends.

Zoonotic transmission. Spread of a disease from a nonhuman animal species to humans.

REFERENCES

Abadie, R. (2008). A guinea pig's wage: Risk and commoditization in pharmaceutical research in America. In M. Singer & H. Baer (Eds.), *Killer commodities: Public health and the corporate production of harm* (pp. 311–334). Lanham, MD: AltaMira Press.

Abrams, K., Teplin, L., McClelland, G., & Dulcan, M. (2003). Comorbid psychiatric disorders in youth in juvenile detention. *Archives of General Psychiatry, 60*, 1097–1108.

Abu-Raddad, L. (2007, January 11). HIV and malaria: A vicious cycle. *Scitizen.* Retrieved February 10, 2009, from http://www.scitizen.com/stories/AIDS/2007/01/HIV-and-Malaria—A-Vicious-Cycle.

Abu-Raddad, L., Patnaik, P., & Kublin, J. (2006). Dual infection with HIV and malaria fuels the spread of both diseases in sub-Saharan Africa. *Science, 314*, 1603–1606.

Action on Smoking and Health. (2006). *Secondhand smoke: The impact on children.* London: Author.

Acuna-Soto, R., Romero, L. C., & Maguire, J. (2000). Large epidemics of hemorrhagic fever in Mexico 1545–1845. *American Journal of Tropical Medicine and Hygiene, 62*, 733–739.

Adams, J. (1999). Victorian sexualities. In H. Tucker (Ed.), *A companion to Victorian literature and culture* (pp. 125–139). Boston, MA: Wiley-Blackwell.

Adewuya, A., Afolabi, M., Ola, B., Ogundele, O., Ajibare, A., & Oladipo, B. (2008). Psychiatric disorders among the HIV-positive population in Nigeria: A control study. *Journal of Psychosomatic Research, 63*(2), 203–206.

Agar, M. (2006). *Dope double agent: The naked emperor on drugs.* Morrisville, NC: Lulu.

Agerberth, B., & Gudmundsson, G. (2006). Host antimicrobial defense peptides in human disease. *Current Topics in Microbiology and Immunology, 306*, 67–90.

Aguirre, P. (2000). Socioanthropological aspects of obesity and poverty. In M. Peña and J. Bacallao (Eds.), *Obesity and poverty: A new public health challenge* (pp. 11–22). Washington, DC: Pan American Health Organization.

Ahmed, N., Saini, V., Raghuvanshi, S., Khurana, J., Tyagi, A., Tyagi, A., et al. (2007). Molecular analysis of a leprosy immunotherapeutic bacillus provides insights into Mycobacterium evolution. *PLoS ONE, 2*(10), e968.

Ahuja, T., Grady, J., & Khan, S. (2002). Changing trends in the survival of dialysis patients with human immuno-deficiency virus in the United States. *Journal of the American Society of Nephrology, 13*, 1889–1893.

Akinbami, L., Rhodes, J., & Lara, M. (2005). Racial and ethnic differences in asthma diagnosis among children who wheeze. *Pediatrics, 115*, 1254–1260.

Akolo, C., Ukoli, C., Ladep, G., & Idoko, J. (2008). The clinical features of HIV/AIDS presentation at the Jos University Teaching Hospital. *Nigerian Journal of Medicine, 17*(1), 83–87.

Alan, M., Hauser, S., Lavori, P., Wolfsdorf, J., Herskowitz, R., Milley, J., et al. (1990). Adherence among children and adolescents with insulin-dependent diabetes mellitus over a four-year longitudinal follow-up: I. The influence of patient coping and adjustment. *Journal of Pediatric Psychology, 15*, 511–526.

Albert, M., Ostheimer, K., Liewehr, D., Steinberg, S., & Breman, J. (2002). Smallpox manifestations and survival during the Boston epidemic of 1901 to 1903. *Annals of Internal Medicine, 13*, 993–1000.

Alcott, L. M. (1872). *Little women, or Meg, Jo, Beth and Amy.* London: Sampson Low, Marston Low, and Searle.

Amaro, H., Fried, L., Cabral, H., & Zuckerman, B. (1990). Violence during pregnancy and substance use. *American Journal of Public Health, 80*, 575–579.

American Association of Public Health Physicians. (2006). *Preventive Services ToolKit Project: Instructor's manual and supplemental materials.* Rolling Meadows, IL: Author.

American Lung Association. (2003). *Trends in asthma morbidity and mortality.* New York: Author.

Ami, Y., Nagata, N., Shirato, K., Watanabe, R., Iwata, N., Nakagaki, K., et al. (2008). Co-infection of respiratory bacterium with severe acute respiratory syndrome coronavirus induces an exacerbated pneumonia in mice. *Microbiology and Immunology, 52*(2), 118–127.

Amici, R. (2001). The history of Italian parasitology. *Veterinary Parasitology, 98*(1–3), 3–30.

Amos, A., McCarty, D., & Zimmet, P. (1997). The rising global burden of diabetes and its complications: Estimates and projections to the year 2010. *Diabetic Medicine, 14*(Suppl. 5), S7–S84.

Anabwani, G. (2003, February). *Nutritional disorders among children with HIV*. Paper presented at the Nestlé Nutrition Institute Africa Workshop, Gaborone, Botswana.

Anabwani, G., & Navario, P. (2005). Nutrition and HIV/AIDS in sub-Saharan Africa: An overview. *Nutrition, 21*, 96–99.

Anderson, M., Smith, L., & Sidel, V. (2005). What is social medicine? *Monthly Review.* Retrieved January 3, 2008, from http://www.monthlyreview.org/0105anderson.htm.

Anderson, R., & May, R. (1991). *Infectious diseases of humans: Dynamics and control.* New York: Oxford University Press.

Annan, K. (2004). *Report on the global AIDS epidemic.* Geneva: UNAIDS.

Annie E. Casey Foundation. (2008). *Kids Count data book.* Baltimore, MD: Author.

Appel, A. (2005, September 30). Gulf wracked by Katrina's latest legacy—Disease, poisons, mold. *National Geographic News.* Retrieved June 3, 2007, from http://news.nationalgeographic.com/news/2005/09/0930_050930_katrina_health.html.

Aral, S., & Roegner, R. (2000). Mathematical modeling as a tool in STD prevention and control: A decade of progress, a millennium of opportunities. *Sexually Transmitted Diseases, 27*, 556–557.

Arias, E., Anderson, R., Kung, H., Murphy, S., & Kochanek, K. (2003). Deaths: Final data for 2001. *National Vital Statistics Reports, 52*(3), 1–115.

Arnott, D. (2006). *Poverty and smoking strongly linked, new maps show clearly.* Retrieved June 16, 2008, from http://www.ash.org.uk/ash_5355qukf.htm.

Auyang, S. (2003). *Reality and politics in the war on infectious diseases.* Retrieved April 22, 2008, from http://www.creatingtechnology.org/biomed/germs.pdf.

Bachar, J., Lefler, L., Reed, L., McCoy, T., Bailey, R., & Bell, R. (2006). Cherokee choices: A diabetes prevention program for American Indians. *Preventing Chronic Disease.* Retrieved March 15, 2008, from http://www.cdc.gov/pcd/issues/2006/ jul/05_0221.htm.

Baer, H., & Singer, M. (2008). *Global warming and the political ecology of health: Emerging crises and systemic solutions.* Walnut Creek, CA: Left Coast Press.

Baer, H., Singer, M., & Susser, I. (2003). *Medical anthropology and the world system* (2nd ed.). Westport, CT: Praeger.

Baillargeon, J., Paar, D., Wu, H., Giordano, T., Murray, O., Raimer, B., et al. (2008). Psychiatric disorders, HIV infection and HIV/hepatitis co-infection in the correctional setting. *AIDS Care, 20*(1), 124–129.

Baingana, F., Thomas, R., & Comblain, C. (2005). *HIV/AIDS and mental health* (Health, Nutrition, and Population Discussion Paper). Washington, DC: World Bank.

Bair-Merritt, M., Crowne, S., Burrell, L., Caldera, D., Cheng, T., & Duggan, A. (2008). Impact of intimate partner violence on children's well-child care and medical home. *Pediatrics, 121*, e473–e480.

Baker, S. (2002). Illness and mortality in nineteenth-century Mormon immigration. *Mormon Historical Studies.* Retrieved April 19, 2008. from http://parentfrost.netfirms.com/MormonImmigrationIllness.pdf.

Bangladesh capital hosts at least 50,000 beggars. (1999, March 19). Reuters. Retrieved June 17, 2008, from http://hpn.asu.edu/archives/Mar99/0156.html.

Bangladesh Institute of Development Studies. (2001). *Fighting human poverty: Bangladesh human development report 2000.* Dhaka: Author.

Barclay, R. (2002). *Melal: A novel of the Pacific.* Honolulu: University of Hawai'i Press.

Barnes, E. (2005). *Disease and human evolution.* Albuquerque: University of New Mexico Press.

Bartholow, B., Doll, L., Joy, D., Douglas, J., Bolan, G., Harrison, J., et al. (1994). Emotional behavior and HIV risks associated with sexual abuse among adult homosexual and bisexual men. *Child Abuse & Neglect, 18*, 747–761.

Baum, M., Shor-Posner, G., & Lai, S. (1997). High risk of mortality in HIV infection is associated with selenium deficiency. *Journal of AIDS and Human Retrovirology, 15*, 370–374.

Bayliss, E. (2006). *A methodological suggestion for the management of comorbidities in randomized controlled trials* [E-Letter]. Retrieved April 4, 2008, from http://www.annfammed.org/cgi/eletters/4/2/104#3914.

BBC. (2004). *UN Darfur mission 'within days.'* Retrieved June 3, 2008, from http://news.bbc.co.uk/1/hi/world/africa/3641457.stm.

BBC. (2008). *A short history of Ireland: 1741 "The year of slaughter."* Retrieved April 24, 2008, from http://www.bbc.co.uk/northernireland/ashorthistory/archive/intro123.shtml.

Beliles, K., & Stoudemire, A. (1998). Psychopharmacologic treatment of depression in the medically ill. *Psychosomatics, 39*(Suppl. 1), S2–S19.

Bennett, L., & Larson, M. (1994). Barriers to cooperation between domestic violence and substance abuse programs. *Families in Society, 75,* 277–286.

Ben-Shlomo, Y., & Kuh, D. (2002). A life course approach to chronic disease epidemiology: Conceptual models, empirical challenges and interdisciplinary perspectives. *International Journal of Epidemiology, 31,* 285–293.

Bensley, L., Van Eenwyk, J., & Simmons, K. (2000). Self-reported childhood sexual and physical abuse and adult HIV-risk behaviors and heavy drinking. *American Journal of Preventive Medicine, 18,* 151–158.

Bensley, L., Van Eenwyk, J., & Simmons, K. (2003). Childhood family violence history and women's risk for intimate partner violence and poor health. *American Journal of Preventive Medicine, 25,* 38–44.

Bentivoglio, M., & Pacini, P. (1995). Flippo Pacini: A determined observer. *Brain Research Bulletin, 38,* 161–165.

Bentwich, Z., Maartens, G., Torten, D., Lal, A., & Lal, R. (2000). Concurrent infections and HIV pathogenesis. *AIDS, 14,* 2071–2081.

Berenson, A., Wiemann, C., & McCombs, C. (2001). Exposure to violence and associated health-risk behaviors among adolescent girls. *Archives of Pediatric Adolescent Medicine, 155,* 1238–1242.

Berger, J. (2000). *Beating the heat: Why and how we must combat global warming.* Berkeley, CA: Berkeley Hills Books.

Berger-Greenstein, J., Cuevas, C., Brady, S., Trezza, G., Richardson, M., & Keane, T. (2007). Major depression in patients with HIV/AIDS and substance abuse. *AIDS Patient Care and STDS, 21,* 942–955.

Bernal, E., Masiá, M., Padilla, S., Hernández, I., & Gutiérrez, F. (2008). Low prevalence of peripheral arterial disease in HIV-infected patients with multiple cardiovascular risk factors. *Journal of Acquired Immune Deficiency Syndromes, 47,* 126–127.

Bernstein, K., Tulloch, R., Montes, J., Golan, G., Dyer, I., Lawrence, M., et al. (2000). Outbreak of syphilis among men who have sex with men—Southern California. *Morbidity and Mortality Weekly Report, 50,* 117–120.

Birch, L. (1999). Development of food preferences. *Annual Review of Nutrition, 19,* 41–62.

Björntorp, P. (1988). The associations between obesity, adipose tissue distribution and disease. *Acta Medica Scandinavica, 723*(Suppl.), 121–134.

Black, S., Bashore, M., Bennett, R., Carter, L., Conder, M., Hartley, W., et al. (1998). Do we know how many Latter-day Saints died between 1846–1869 in the migration to the Salt Lake valley? *The Ensign, 28*(7), 40–44.

Bogden, J., Kemp, F., Han, S., Li, W., Bruening, K., Denny, T., et al. (2000). Status of selected nutrients and progression of human immunodeficiency virus type 1 infection. *American Journal of Clinical Nutrition, 72,* 809–815.

Bollet, A. (2004). The major infectious epidemic diseases of Civil War soldiers. *Infectious Disease Clinics of North America, 18,* 293–309.

Bonomi, A., Thompson, R., Anderson, M., Reid, R., Carrell, D., Dimer, J., et al. (2006). Intimate partner violence and women's physical, mental, and social functioning. *American Journal of Preventive Medicine, 30,* 458–466.

Borgundvaag, B., Ovens, H., Goldman, B., Schull, M., Rutledge, T., Boutis, K., et al. (2004). SARS outbreak in the Greater Toronto Area: The emergency department experience. *Canadian Medical Association Journal, 171,* 1342–1344.

Bornovalova, M., Gwadz, M., Kahler, C., Aklin, W., & Lejuez, C. (2008). Sensation seeking and risk-taking propensity as mediators in the relationship between childhood abuse and HIV-related risk behavior. *Child Abuse & Neglect, 32,* 99–109.

Boschi-Pinto, C., Stuver, S., Okayama, A., Trichopoulos, D., Orav, E., Tsubouchi, H., et al. (2000). A follow-up study of morbidity and mortality associated with hepatitis C virus infection and its interaction with human T lymphotropic virus type I in Miyazaki, Japan. *Journal of Infectious Diseases, 181*, 35–41.

Bourgois, P. (2003). *In search of respect: Selling crack in El Barrio* (2nd ed.). New York: Cambridge University Press.

Bourgois, P., Lettiere, M., & Quesada, J. (1997). Social misery and the sanctions of substance abuse: Confronting HIV risk among homeless heroin addicts in San Francisco. *Social Problems, 44*, 155–173.

Braitstein, P., Li, K., Tyndall, M., Spittal, P., O'Shaughnessy, M., Schilder, A., et al. (2003). Sexual violence among a cohort of injection drug users. *Social Science & Medicine, 57*, 561–569.

Brewer, D., Fleming, C., Haggerty, K., & Calalano, R. (1998). Drug use predictors of partner violence in opiate dependent women. *Violence and Victims, 13*, 107–115.

Brodie, T., Holmes, P., & Urquhart, G. (1987). Some aspects of tick-borne diseases of British sheep. *Veterinary Record, 118*, 415–418.

Brooke, J. (1991a, April 19). Cholera kills 1,100 in Peru and marches on, reaching the Brazilian border. *New York Times*, p. 1.

Brooke, J. (1991b, April 19). Feeding on 19th century conditions, cholera spreads in Latin America. *New York Times*, p. 4.

Broudy, T., & Fischetti, V. (2003). In vivo lysogenic conversion of Tox– *Streptococcus pyogenes* to Tox+ with Lysogenic Streptococci or free phage. *Infection and Immunity, 71*, 3782–3786.

Brown, B., & Beschner, G. (Eds.). (1993). *Handbook on risk of AIDS: Injection drug users and sexual partners.* Westport, CT: Greenwood Press.

Brown, G., & Anderson, B. (1991). Psychiatric morbidity in adult inpatients with childhood histories of sexual and physical abuse. *American Journal of Psychiatry, 148*, 55–61.

Brown, H. (1999). *The rape of 100,000 girls.* Retrieved September 20, 2008, from http://freespirit.members.gn.apc.org/100-000.htm.

Brown, L. (2000). *Helicobacter pylori:* Epidemiology and routes of transmission. *Epidemiology Review, 22*, 283–297.

Brown, M., Mawa, P., Kaleebu, P., & Elliot, M. (2006). Helminths and HIV infection: Epidemiological observations on immunological hypotheses. *Parasite Immunology, 28*, 613–623.

Brown, P. (1992). Popular epidemiology and toxic waste contamination: Lay and professional ways of knowing. *Journal of Health and Social Behavior, 33*, 267–281.

Brown, P. (1998). Cultural adaptations to endemic malaria in Sardinia. In P. Brown & M. Inhorn (Eds.), *Understanding and applying medical anthropology* (pp. 119–141). London: Mayfield.

Bryden, K., Neil, A., Mayou, R., Peveler, R., Fairburn, C., & Dunger, D. (1999). Eating habits, body weight, and insulin misuse: A longitudinal study of teenagers and young adults with type 1 diabetes. *Diabetes Care, 22*, 1956–1960.

Buchacz, K., Klausner, J., Kerndt, P., Shouse, R., Onorato, I., McElroy, P., et al. (2008). HIV incidence among men diagnosed with early syphilis in Atlanta, San Francisco, and Los Angeles, 2004 to 2005. *Journal of Acquired Immune Deficiency Syndrome, 47*, 234–240.

Budrys, G. (2003). *Unequal health: How inequality contributes to health or illness.* Lanham, MD: Rowman & Littlefield.

Bundy, D., Sher, A., & Michael, E. (2000). Good worms or bad worms: Do worm infections affect the epidemiological patterns of other diseases? *Parasitology Today, 16*, 273–274.

Burnam, M., Stein, J., Golding, I., Siegel, J., Sorenson, S., Forsythe, A., et al. (1988). Sexual assault and mental disorders in a community population. *Journal of Consulting Clinical Psychology, 56*, 843–850.

Burney, J., & Haughton, B. (2002). EFNEP: A nutrition education program that demonstrates cost-benefit. *Journal of the American Dietetic Association, 102*, 39–45.

Buss, T., Abdu, R., & Walker, J. (1995). Alcohol, drugs, and urban violence in a small city trauma center. *Journal of Substance Abuse Treatment, 12*, 75–83.

Caillouët, K., Michaels, S., Xiong, X., Foppa, I., & Wesson, D. (2008). Increase in West Nile neuroinvasive disease after Hurricane Katrina. *Emerging Infectious Diseases, 14*, 804–807.

Calder, P., & Kew, S. (2002). The immune system: A target for functional foods? *British Journal of Nutrition, 88*(Suppl. 2), S165–S177.

Cameron, D., & Jones, I. (1985). An epidemiological and sociological analysis of the use of alcohol, tobacco, and other drugs of solace. *Community Medicine, 7*, 18–29.

Cameron, S. (2002). *Kidney failure: The facts.* New York: Oxford University Press.

Campa, A., Yang, Z., Lai, S., Xue, L., Phillips, J., Sales, S., et al. (2005). HIV-related wasting in HIV-infected drug users in the era of highly active antiretroviral therapy. *Clinical Infectious Diseases, 41*, 1179–1185.

Canducci, F., Uberti Foppa, C., Boeri, E., Racca, S., Gallotta, G., Grasso, M., et al. (2003). Characterization of GBV-C infection in HIV-1 infected patients. *Journal of Biological Regulators and Homeostatic Agents, 17*, 191–194.

Cantor, K., Weiss, S., Goedert, J., & Battjes, R. (1991). HTLV-I/II seroprevalence and HIV/HTLV coinfection among U.S. intravenous drug users. *Acquired Immune Deficiency Syndrome, 4*, 460–467.

Cantor, N. (2002). *In the wake of the plague: The Black Death and the world it made.* New York: Harper Perennial.

Carballo-Dieguez, A., & Dolezal, C. (1995). Association between history of childhood sexual abuse and adult HIV-risk sexual behavior in Puerto Rican men who have sex with men. *Child Abuse & Neglect, 19*, 595–605.

Carter, L., Weithorn, L., & Behrman, R. (1999). Domestic violence and children: Analysis and recommendations. *The Future of Children, 9*(3), 4–20.

Carvalho, E., & Porto, A. (2004). Epidemiological and clinical interaction between HTLV-1 and *Strongyloides stercoralis. Parasite Immunology, 26*, 487–497.

Castro, A., & Farmer, P. (2005). Understanding and addressing AIDS-related stigma: From anthropological theory to clinical practice in Haiti. *American Journal of Public Health, 95*, 53–59.

Castro, A., & Singer M. (Eds.). (2004). *Unhealthy health policy: A critical anthropological examination.* Lanham, MD: AltaMira Press.

Center for Social and Behavioral Research, University of Northern Iowa. (2007). *Iowa 2006 adult tobacco use survey.* Des Moines: Iowa Department of Public Health, Division of Tobacco Use Prevention and Control.

Centers for Disease Control and Prevention. (2001). *Behavioral risk factor surveillance system, 1991–2000.* Atlanta: Author.

Centers for Disease Control and Prevention. (2005). *2005 West Nile virus activity in the United States.* Retrieved December 2, 2008, from http://www.cdc.gov/ncidod/dvbid/westnile/surv&controlCaseCount05_detailed.htm.

Centers for Disease Control and Prevention. (2006a). *Dengue fever.* Retrieved November 22, 2007, from http://www.cdc.gov/ncidod/dvbid/dengue.

Centers for Disease Control and Prevention. (2006b). *Reported cases of Lyme disease by year, United States, 1991–2005.* Atlanta: Centers for Disease Control and Prevention, Division of Vector-Borne Diseases.

Centers for Disease Control and Prevention. (2007). Reported HIV status of tuberculosis patients—United States, 1993–2005. *Morbidity and Mortality Weekly Report, 56*, 1103–1106.

Centers for Disease Control and Prevention. (2008a). *2007–2008 influenza season week 18, ending May 3, 2008* (FluView). Retrieved May 10, 2008, from http://www.cdc.gov/flu/weekly.

Centers for Disease Control and Prevention. (2008b). *HIV/AIDS surveillance in injection drug users (through 2006).* Retrieved January 12, 2009, from http://www.cdc.gov/hiv/idu/resources/slides/index.htm.

Centre for Health and Population Research. (2005). *Little Sweden in a life saving effort of great importance.* Retrieved May 1, 2008, from http://www.sasnet.lu.se/cont05icd.html.

Chadee, D., Rawlins, S., & Tiwari, T. (2003). Short communication: Concomitant malaria and filariasis infections in Georgetown, Guyana. *Tropical Medicine and International Health, 8*, 140–143.

Chadwick, D. (2003). Pacific suite. *National Geographic, 203*(2), 104–127.

Chan, J., Ng, Y., Chan, T., Mok, W., Who, S., Lee, S., et al. (2003). Short term outcome and risk factors for adverse clinical outcomes in adults with severe acute respiratory syndrome. *Thorax, 58*, 686–689.

Chandra, R. (1997). Nutrition and the immune system: An introduction. *American Journal of Clinical Nutrition, 66*, 460–463.

Chandra, S., & Chandra, R. (1986). Nutrition, immune response, and outcome. *Progress in Food and Nutrition Science, 10*, 1–65.

Charlson, M., Pompei, P., Ales, K., & McKenzie, C. (1987). A new method of classifying prognostic comorbidity in longitudinal studies: Development and validation. *Journal of Chronic Diseases, 40*, 373–383.

Chen, C., Lee, C., Liu, C., Wang, J., Wang, L., & Perng, R. (2005). Clinical features and outcomes of severe acute respiratory syndrome and predictive factors for acute respiratory distress syndrome. *Journal of the Chinese Medical Association, 68*, 4–10.

Chen, J., Dunne, M., & Han, P. (2004). Child sexual abuse in China: A study of adolescents in four provinces. *Child Abuse & Neglect, 28*, 1171–1186.

Child Abuse Prevention and Treatment Act, 42 U.S.C. Annotated §5106g(2) (1998).

Choi, A., Rodriquez, R., Bacchetti, P., Berenthal., D., Volberding, P., & O'Hare, A. (2007). Racial differences in end-stage renal disease in HIV infection versus diabetes. *Journal of the American Society of Nephrology, 18*, 2968–2974.

Church of Jesus Christ of Latter-day Saints. (1996). *Our heritage.* Salt Lake City, UT: Author.

Civil War Society. (2002). *Medical care, battle wounds and disease.* Retrieved May 14, 2008, from http://www.civilwarhome.com/civilwarmedicine.htm.

Clair, S., & Singer, M. (2009). *HIV status, risk, and prevention needs among Latino and non-Latino MSM in Connecticut.* In D. Feldman (Ed.), *AIDS, culture, and gay men.* Westport, CT: Greenwood Press.

Clarkson, L., & Crawford, E. (2001). *Feast and famine: Food and nutrition in Ireland, 1500–1920.* New York: Oxford University Press.

Clements-Nolle, K., Guzman, R., & Harris, S. (2008). Sex trade in a male-to-female transgender population: Psychosocial correlates of inconsistent condom use. *Sex Health, 5*, 49–54.

Cochran, G., Ewald, P., & Cochran, K. (2000). Infectious causation of disease: An evolutionary perspective. *Perspectives in Biology and Medicine, 43*, 406–448.

Cohen, C., Karstaedt, A., Frean, J., Thomas, J., Govender, N., Prentice, E., et al. (2005). Increased prevalence of severe malaria in HIV-infected adults in South Africa. *Clinical Infectious Diseases, 41*, 1631–1637.

Cohen, F., & Densen-Gerber, J. (1982). A study of the relationship between child abuse and drug addiction in patients: Preliminary results. *Child Abuse & Neglect, 6*, 383–387.

Cohen-Cole, S., Brown, F., & McDaniel, J. (1993). *Assessment of depression and grief reactions in the medically ill.* In A. Stoudemire & B. Fogel (Eds.), *Psychiatric care of the medical patient* (pp. 53–59). New York: Oxford University Press.

Coleman, J., LeVine, D., Thill, C., Kuhlow, C., & Benach, J. (2005). Babesia microti and Borrelia burgdorferi follow independent courses of infection in mice. *Journal of Infectious Diseases, 192*, 1634–1641.

Collins, P., von Unger, H., & Armbrister, A. (2008). Church ladies, good girls, and locas: Stigma and the intersection of gender, ethnicity, mental illness, and sexuality in relation to HIV risk. *Social Science & Medicine, 67*(3), 389–397.

Committee on Psychosocial Aspects of Child and Family Health. (2001). The new morbidity revisited: A renewed commitment to the psychosocial aspects of pediatric care. *Pediatrics, 108*, 1227–1230.

Cone, R., & Martin, E. (2003). Corporal flows: The immune system, global economies of food, and new implications for health. In J. Wilce Jr. (Ed.), *Social and cultural lives of immune systems* (pp. 232–266). New York: Routledge.

Conference Board of Canada. (2003). *The economic impact of SARS.* Retrieved September 20, 2008, from http://www.conferenceboard.ca/documents.asp?rnext=539.

Cooper, J. (2008, January 29). Diabetes and bulimia: Skipping insulin shots can result in a thinner body—and a shortened life span. *Hartford Courant*, p. A1.

Cordier, M., Gillet, P., Boucherat, M., Capdeville, J., Rouzioux, J., & François, R. (1981). Lead poisoning revealed by severe encephalopathy: Pica does exist in France. *Archives Françaises de Pédiatrie, 38*, 609–611.

Coreil, J., Mayard, G., Louis-Charles, J., & Addiss, D. (1998). Filarial elephantiasis in Haitian women: Social context and behavioural factors in treatment. *Tropical Medicine and International Health, 3*, 467–473.

Corey, L., Wald, A., Celum, C., & Quinn, T. (2004). The effects of herpes simplex virus-2 on HIV-1 acquisition and transmission: A review of two overlapping epidemics. *Journal of Acquired Immune Deficiency Syndromes, 35*, 435–445.

Covell, G., & Nicol, W. (1951). Clinical, chemotherapeutic and immunological studies on induced malaria. *British Medical Bulletin, 8*, 51–55.

Crosby, A. (2003). *America's forgotten pandemic: The influenza of 1918.* New York: Cambridge University Press.

Crossett, K., Culliton, T., Wiley, P., & Goodspeed, T. (2004). *Population trends along the coastal United States: 1980–2008.* National Oceanic and Atmospheric Administration. Retrieved November 3, 2008, from http://oceanservice.noaa.gov/programs/ mb/supp_cstl_population.html.

Culhane, J., Rauh, V., McCollum, K., Elo, I., & Hogan, V. (2002). Exposure to chronic stress and ethnic differences in rates of bacterial vaginosis among pregnant women. *American Journal of Obstetrics and Gynecology, 187*, 1272–1276.

Cunningham-Rundles, S., McNeeley, D., & Moon, A. (2005). Mechanisms of nutrient modulation of the immune response. *Journal of Allergy and Clinical Immunology, 115*, 1119–1128.

Currie, C., Gabhainn, S., Godeaum E., Roberts, C., Smith, R., Currie, D., et al. (2008). *Inequalities in young people's health: HBSC international report from the 2005/2006 survey.* Copenhagen: WHO Regional Office for Europe.

Dahl, M., Dabbagh, K., Liggitt, D., Kim, S., & Lewis, D. (2004). Viral-induced T helper type 1 responses enhance allergic disease by effects on lung dendritic cells. *Nature Immunology, 5*, 337–343.

Daley, D., & Gani, J. (1999). *Epidemic modelling: An introduction* (Cambridge University Studies in Mathematical Biology). New York: Cambridge University Press.

Dao, C., Blanton, L., Epperson, S., Brammer, L., Finelli, L., Wallis, T., et al. (2008). Update: Influenza activity—United States, September 30, 2007–April 5, 2008, and composition of the 2008–09 influenza vaccine. *Morbidity and Mortality Weekly Report, 57*, 404–409.

Davis-Floyd, R. (1994). The technocratic body: American childbirth as cultural expression. *Social Science & Medicine, 38*, 1125–1140.

Davis-Floyd, R., & St. John, G. (1998). *From doctor to healer: The transformative journey.* New Brunswick, NJ: Rutgers University Press.

Day, A., Thurlow, K., & Woolliscroft, J. (2003). Working with childhood sexual abuse: A survey of mental health professionals. *Child Abuse & Neglect, 27*, 191–198.

Dean, D., Kandel, R., Adhikari, H., & Hessel, T. (2008). Multiple chlamydiaceae species in trachoma: Implications for disease pathogenesis and control. *PloS Medicine, 5*, e14.

del Mar Pujades Rodriguez, M., Obasi, A., Mosha, F., Todd, J., Brown, D., Changalucha, J., et al. (2002). Herpes simplex virus type 2 infection increases HIV incidence: A prospective study in rural Tanzania. *AIDS, 16*, 451–462.

deMause, L. (1998). The history of child abuse. *Journal of Psychohistory, 25*(3), 2–18.

Deo, R., Fyr, C., Fried, L., Newman, A., Harris, T., Angleman, S., et al., & the Health ABC Study. (2008). Kidney dysfunction and fatal cardiovascular disease—an association independent of atherosclerotic events: Results from the Health, Aging, and Body Composition (Health ABC) study. *American Heart Journal, 155*, 62–68.

DevNews Media Center. (2002). *SAR puts HIV/AIDS at top of agenda.* Washington, DC: World Bank Group.

DeWitte, S., & Wood, J. (2008). Selectivity of Black Death mortality with respect to preexisting health. *Proceedings of the National Academy of Sciences of the United States of America, 105*, 1436–1441.

Diaz, R. (1997). *Latino gay men and HIV: Culture, sexuality, and risk behavior.* New York: Routledge.

Dieterich, D. (2007). Special considerations and treatment of patients with HBV-HIV coinfection. *Antiviral Therapy, 12*(Suppl. 3), H43–H51.

Dietrich, A. (2008). Corrosion in the system: The community health by-products of pharmaceutical production in northern Puerto Rico. In M. Singer & H. Baer (Eds.), *Killer commodities: Public health and the corporate production of harm* (pp. 335–366). Lanham, MD: AltaMira Press.

Doherty, M., Garfein, R., Monterroso, E., Brown, D., & Vlahov, D. (2000). Correlates of HIV infection among young adult short-term injection drug users. *AIDS 14*, 717–726.

Dolman, C. (1969). Theobald Smith, 1859–1934, Life and work. *New York State Journal of Medicine, 69*, 2801–2816.

Dominguez, T., Dunkel-Schetter, C., Glynn, L., Hobel, C., & Sandman, C. (2008). Racial differences in birth outcomes: The role of general, pregnancy, and racism stress. *Health Psychology, 27*, 194–203.

Donnelly, C., & Cox, D. (2001). Mathematical biology and medical statistics: Contributions to the understanding of AIDS epidemiology. *Statistical Methods in Medical Research, 10*, 141–154.

Donner, H., Rau, H., Walfish, P., Braun, J., Siegmund, T., Finke, R., et al. (1997). CTLA4 alanine-17 confers genetic susceptibility to Graves' disease and to type 1 diabetes mellitus. *Journal of Clinical Endocrinology and Metabolism, 82*, 143–146.

Draus, P. (2004). *Consumed in the city: Observing tuberculosis at century's end.* Philadelphia: Temple University Press.

Dressler, W. (2004). Culture, stress, and cardiovascular disease. In C. Ember and M. Ember (Eds.), *Encyclopedia of medical anthropology: Health and illness in the world's cultures* (Vol. 1, pp. 328–335). New York: Kluwer Academic/Plenum.

Drewnowski, A., & Specter, S. (2004). Poverty and obesity: The role of energy density and energy costs. *American Journal of Clinical Nutrition, 79*, 6–16.

Drexler, M. (2006). The people's epidemiologists. *Harvard Magazine, 108*(4). Retrieved July 22, 2007, from http://www.harvardmagazine.com/on-line/030636.html.

Duke, M., Singer, M., Li, J., & Pelia, P. (2003). A community-based organization builds an international initiative. *Anthropology News, 44*, 15.

Duke, M., Teng, W., Clair, S., Saleheen, H., Choice, P., & Singer, M. (2006). Patterns of intimate partner violence among drug using women. *Free Inquiry in Creative Sociology, 34*, 29–38.

Duke, M., Teng, W., Simmons, J., & Singer, M. (2003). Structural and interpersonal violence among Puerto Rican drug users. *Practicing Anthropology, 25*(3), 28–31.

Dumler, J., Choi, K.-.S., Carolos, J., Barat, N., Scorpio, D., Garyu, J., et al. (2005). Human granulocytic anaplasmosis and *Anaplasma phagocytophilum. Emerging Infectious Diseases, 11.* Retrieved April 20, 2008, from http://www.cdc.gov/ncidod/EiD/vol11no12/05-0898.htm.

Dushay, R., Singer, M., Weeks, M., Rohena, L., & Gruber, R. (2001). Lowering HIV risk among ethnic minority drug users: Comparing culturally targeted intervention to a standard intervention. *American Journal of Drug and Alcohol Abuse, 27*, 504–524.

Dushoff, J., Plotkin, J., Viboud, C., Earn, D., & Simonsen, L. (2006). Mortality due to influenza in the United States— An annualized regression approach using multiple-cause mortality data. *American Journal of Epidemiology, 163*, 181–187.

Dyer, J., & McGuiness, T. (2008). Reducing HIV risk among people with serious mental illness. *Journal of Psychosocial Nursing and Mental Health Services, 46*(4), 26–34.

Eastman, C. (1977). *From the deep woods to civilization: Chapters in the autobiography of an Indian.* Lincoln: University of Nebraska Press. (Original work published 1936)

Easton, D. (2004). The urban poor: Health issues. In C. Ember and M. Ember (Eds.), *Encyclopedia of medical anthropology: Health and illness in the world's cultures* (Vol. 1, pp. 207–213). New York: Kluwer Academic/Plenum.

Edgardh, K., & Ormstad, K. (2000). Prevalence and characteristics of sexual abuse in a national sample of Swedish seventeen-year-old boys and girls. *Acta Paediatrica, 89*, 310–319.

Edlich, R., Arnette, J., & Williams, F. (2000). Global epidemic of human T-cell lymphotropic virus type-I (HTLV-I). *Journal of Emergency Medicine, 18*, 109–119.

Egwunyenga, A., Ajayi, J., Nmorsi, O., & Duhlinska-Popova, D. (2001). *Plasmodium*/intestinal helminth co-infections among pregnant Nigerian women. *Memórias do Instituto Oswaldo Cruz, 96*, 1055–1059.

Eickhoff, T. (2008). Looking back on the 2008 influenza season and vaccine. *Infectious Disease News.* Retrieved May 10, 2008, from http://www.infectiousdiseasenews.com/200804/teded.asp.

El-Bassel, N., Gilbert, L., & Wasde, T. (2000). Drug abuse and partner violence among women in methadone treatment. *Journal of Family Violence, 15,* 209–225.

El-Bassel, N., Witte, S., Wada, T., Gilbert, L., & Wallace, J. (2001). Correlates of partner violence among female street-based sex workers: Substance abuse, history of childhood abuse, and HIV risks. *AIDS Patient Care and STDS, 15,* 41–51.

Elsayed, E., Tighiouart, H., Griffith, J., Kurth, T., Levey, A., Salem, D., et al. (2007). Cardiovascular disease and subsequent kidney disease. *Archives of Internal Medicine, 167,* 1130–1136.

Engel, G. (1977, April 8). The need for a new medical model: A challenge for biomedicine. *Science, 196,* 129–136.

Epstein, P. (2002, August 4). Choking on climate change. *Boston Globe.*

Erickson, P. (2008). *Ethnomedicine.* Long Grove, IL: Waveland Press.

Erstad, I. (2006). *The resurgence of tuberculosis in South Africa: An investigation into socio-economic aspects of the disease in a context of structural violence in Grahamstown, Eastern Cape.* Unpublished master's thesis, Rhodes University, Grahamstown, South Africa.

Estroff, S. (1989). Self, identity, and subjective experiences of schizophrenia. *Schizophrenia Bulletin, 15,* 189–196.

Evans-Pritchard, A. (2008, July 22). Global warming rage lets global hunger grow. *Daily Telegraph.* Retrieved January 25, 2009, from http://www.telegraph.co.uk/finance/comment/ambroseevans_pritchard/2788092/Global-warming-rage-lets-global-hunger-grow.html.

Evjen, J. (2004). *Wetlands restoration.* Retrieved September 20, 2008, from http://www.ngs.noaa.gov/PROJECTS/Wetlands.

Eyler, J. (1979). *Victorian social medicine: The ideals and methods of William Farr.* Baltimore, MD: Johns Hopkins University Press.

Eyler, J. (2001). The changing assessments of John Snow's and William Farr's cholera studies. *Sozial- und Präventivmedizin, 46,* 225–232.

Fadiman, A. (1997). *The spirit catches you and you fall down: A Hmong child, her American doctors, and the collision of two cultures.* New York: Farrar, Straus & Giroux.

Farley, M., & Barkan, H. (1998). Prostitution, violence against women, and posttraumatic stress disorder. *Women & Health, 27*(3), 37–49.

Farmer, P. (1996). Social inequalities and emerging infectious diseases. *Emerging Infectious Diseases, 2,* 259–269.

Farmer, P. (2003). Pathologies of power: Health, human rights and the new war on the poor. *North American Dialogue, 6*(1), 1–4.

Farmer, P. (2004). An anthropology of structural violence. *Current Anthropology, 45,* 305–325.

Farmer, P., Léandre, F., Mukherjee, J., Claude, M., Nevil, P., Smith-Fawzi, M., et al. (2001). Community-based approaches to HIV treatment in resource-poor settings. *Lancet, 358,* 404–409.

Farmer, P., Nizeye, B., Stulac, S., & Keshavjee, S. (2006). Structural violence and clinical medicine. *PLoS Medicine, 3,* e449.

Fassin, D. (2004). Public health as culture. The social construction of the childhood lead poisoning epidemic in France. *British Medical Bulletin, 69,* 167–177.

Fassin, D., & Naudé, A. (2004). Plumbism reinvented: Childhood lead poisoning in France, 1985–1990. *American Journal of Public Health, 94,* 1854–1863.

Fauci, A. (2005). Emerging and reemerging infectious diseases: The perpetual challenge. *Academic Medicine, 80,* 1079–1085.

Fawzi, W., Msamanga, G., Spiegelman, D., Urassa, E., McGrath, M., Mwakagile, D., et al. (1998). Randomised trial of effects of vitamin supplements on pregnancy outcomes and T cell counts in HIV-1-infected women in Tanzania. *Lancet, 351,* 1477–1482.

Fee, E., & Krieger, N. (1993). Understanding AIDS: Historical interpretations and the limits of biomedical individualism. *American Journal of Public Health, 83,* 1477–1486.

Feinstein, A. (1970). The pre-therapeutic classification of co-morbidity in chronic disease. *Journal of Chronic Diseases, 23,* 455–468.

Feitosa, G., Bandeira, A., Sampaio, D., Badaró, R., & Brites, C. (2001). High prevalence of giardiasis and strongyloidiasis among HIV-infected patients in Bahia, Brazil. *Brazilian Journal of Infectious Diseases, 5*, 339–344.

Fenton, K., & Valdiserri, R. (2006). Twenty-five years of HIV/AIDS—United States, 1981–2006. *Morbidity and Mortality Weekly Report, 55*, 585–589.

Ferencík, M., & Ebringer, L. (2002). Modulatory effects of selenium and zinc on the immune system. *Folia Microbiologica, 48*, 417–426.

Feurguson, N., Cummings, D., Fraser, C., Cajka, J., Cooley, P., & Burke, D. (2006). Strategies for mitigating an influenza pandemic. *Nature, 442*, 488–452.

Field, C., Johnson, I., & Schley, P. (2002). Nutrients and their role in host resistance to infection. *Journal of Leukocyte Biology, 71*, 16–32.

Fiers, W., Beyaert, R., Declercq, W., & Vandenabeele, P. (1999). More than one way to die: Apoptosis, necrosis and reactive oxygen damage. *Oncogene, 18*, 7717–7730.

Fine, D., & Atta, M. (2007). Kidney disease in the HIV-infected patient. *AIDS Patient Care and STDS, 21*, 813–824.

Finkel, M. (2007). Bedlam in the blood: Malaria. *National Geographic, 212*(1), 32–67.

Fisher, J., & Misovich, S. (1990). Social influence and AIDS-prevention behavior. In J. Edwards, R. Tindale, L. Heath, & E. Posavac (Eds.), *Social influence processes and prevention* (pp. 39–70). New York: Plenum.

Fleck, L. (1979). *Genesis and development of a scientific fact.* Chicago: University of Chicago Press. (Original work published 1935)

Fogel, C., & Belyea, M. (1999). The lives of incarcerated women: Violence, substance abuse, and at risk for HIV. *Journal of the Association of Nurses in AIDS Care, 10*(6), 66–74.

Food and Agriculture Organization of the United Nations. (2008, April). Countries in crisis requiring external assistance. *Crop Prospects and Food Situation,* No. 2, p. 2.

Forero, J., & Weiner, T. (2002, June 8). Latin American poppy fields undermine U.S. drug battle. *New York Times,* p. 1.

Fortin, M., Dionne, J., Pinho, G., Gignac, J., Almirall, J., & Lapointe, L. (2006). Randomized controlled trials: Do they have external validity for patients with multiple comorbidities? *Annals of Family Medicine, 4*(4), 104–108.

Foster, G., & Anderson, B. (1978). *Medical anthropology.* New York: Wiley.

Frank, C., Mohamed, M., Strickland, G., Lavanchy, D., Arthur, R., Magder, L., et al. (2000). The role of parenteral antischistosomal therapy in the spread of hepatitis C virus in Egypt. *Lancet, 355*, 887–891.

Frankenberg, R. (1980). Medical anthropology and development: A theoretical perspective. *Social Science & Medicine. Part B, Medical Anthropology. 14B*(4), 197–202.

Franks, P., Muennig, P., Lubetkin, E., & Jia, H. (2006). The burden of disease associated with being African-American in the United States and the contribution of socio-economic status. *Social Science & Medicine, 62*, 2469–2478.

French, N., Nakiyingi, J., Lugada, E., Watera, C., Whitworth, J., & Gilks, C. (2001). Increasing rates of malarial fever with deteriorating immune status in HIV-1-infected Ugandan adults. *AIDS, 15*, 899–906.

Frerichs, R. (2001). *Competing theories of cholera.* Retrieved January 9, 2009, from http://www.ph.ucla.edu/epi/snow/choleratheories.html.

Freudenberg, N., Fahs, M., Galea, S., & Greenberg, A. (2006). The impact of New York City's 1975 fiscal crisis on the tuberculosis, HIV, and homicide syndemic. *American Journal of Public Health, 96*, 424–434.

Frias-Armenta, M., & McCloskey, L. (1998). Determinants of harsh parenting in Mexico. *Journal of Abnormal Child Psychology, 26*, 129–139.

Friedman, M., Marshal, M., Stall, R., Cheong, J., & Wright, E. (2007). Gay-related development, early abuse and adult health outcomes among gay males. *AIDS and Behavior.* Retrieved March 22, 2008, from http://www.ncbi.nlm.nih.gov/pubmed/17990094.

Friis-Møller, N., Reiss, P., El-Sadr, W., D'Arminio Monforte, A., Thiébaut, R., De Wit, S., et al., & the D:A:D Study Group. (2006, February 5–8). Exposure to PI and NNRTI and risk of myocardial infarction: Results from the D:A:D study. In *Program and Abstracts of the 13th Conference on Retroviruses and Opportunistic Infections* (Abstract 144), Denver, CO.

Fuchs, J. (2007). *The cholera outbreak in Peru: A study of then and now* [Independent study case study]. Richmond, VA: University of Richmond.

Fuller, C., Vlahov, D., Ompad, D., Shah, N., Arria, A., & Strathdee, S. (2002). High-risk behaviors associated with transition from illicit non-injection to injection drug use among adolescent and young adult drug users: A case-control study. *Drug and Alcohol Dependence, 66*(2), 189–198.

Gaines, A., & Davis-Floyd, R. (2004). Biomedicine. In C. Ember and M. Ember (Eds.), *Encyclopedia of medical anthropology: Health and illness in the world's cultures* (Vol. 1, pp. 95–109). New York: Kluwer Academic/ Plenum.

Gall, N. (1993). *The death threat*. Fernand Braudel Institute of World Economics. Retrieved June 3, 2008, from http://www.normangall.com/arquivosdoc/dtr.rtf.

Gallagher, M., Malhotra, I., Mungai, P., Wamachi, A., Kioko, J., Ouma, J., et al. (2005). The effects of maternal helminth and malaria infections on mother-to-child HIV transmission. *AIDS, 19*, 1849–1855.

Gallego, L., Gordillo, V., & Catalán, J. (2000). Psychiatric and psychological disorders associated to HIV infection. *AIDS Reviews, 2*(1), 48–60.

Galtung, J. (1969). Violence, peace, and peace research. *Journal of Peace Research, 6*(3), 167–191.

Gandhi, N., Moll, A., Sturm, A., Pawinski, R., Govender, T., Lalloo, U., et al. (2006). Extensively drug-resistant tuberculosis as a cause of death in patients co-infected with tuberculosis and HIV in a rural area of South Africa. *Lancet, 368*, 1575–1580.

Gandy, M., & Zumla, A. (Eds.). (2003). *Return of the white plague: Global poverty and the "new" tuberculosis*. New York: Verso.

García, M., Yu, X., Griffin, D., & Moss, W. (2008). Measles virus inhibits human immunodeficiency virus type 1 reverse transcription and replication by blocking cell-cycle progression of CD4+ T lymphocytes. *Journal of General Virology, 89*, 984–993.

García Márquez, G. (1989). *Love in the time of cholera*. New York: Penguin Books.

Garcia-Moreno, C., Jansen, H., Ellsberg, M., Heise, L., Watts, C., & the WHO Multi-Country Study on Women's Health and Domestic Violence Against Women Study Team. (2006). Prevalence of intimate partner violence: Findings from the WHO Multi-Country Study on Women's Health and Domestic Violence. *Lancet, 368*, 1260–1269.

Gardner, T., & Hill, D. (2001). Treatment of giardiasis. *Clinical Microbiology Reviews, 14*, 114–128.

Garrett, L. (1994). *The coming plague: Newly emerging diseases in a world out of balance*. New York: Farrar, Straus & Giroux.

Gaynes, B., Pence, B., Eron, J., & Miller, W. (2008). Prevalence and comorbidity of psychiatric diagnoses based on reference standard in an HIV+ patient population. *Psychosomatic medicine, 70,* 505–511. Retrieved May 9, 2008, from http://www.ncbi.nlm.nih.gov/pubmed/18378865?ordinalpos=2&itool=EntrezSystem2.PEntrez. Pubmed.Pubmed_ResultsPanel.Pubmed_RVDocSum.

Gehlert, S., Sohmer, D., Sacks, T., Mininger, C., McClintock, M., & Olopade, O. (2008). Targeting health disparities: A model linking upstream determinants to downstream interventions. *Health Affairs, 27*, 339–349.

Geijtenbeek, T., van Vliet, S., Koppel, E., Sanchez-Hernandez, M., Vandenbroucke-Grauls, C., Appelmelk, B., et al. (2003). Mycobacteria target DC-SIGN to suppress dendritic cell function. *Journal of Experimental Medicine, 197*, 7–17.

Gelpi, A. (1987). Alexander Russell and the Aleppo ulcer. *International Journal of Dermatology, 26*(2), 131–134.

Gerberding, J. (2005). Protecting health: The new research imperative. *JAMA, 294*, 1403–1406.

Ghafur, S. (2004). Bangladesh. In D. Levinson (Ed.), *Encyclopedia of homelessness* (pp. 27–29). Thousand Oaks, CA: Sage.

Ghani, A., & Boily, M.-C. (2003). The epidemiology of HIV/AIDS: Contributions to infectious disease epidemiology. In G. Elison, M. Parker, & C. Campbell (Eds.), *Learning from HIV and AIDS* (pp. 59–87). New York: Cambridge University Press.

Gielen, A., Ghandour, R., Burke, J., Mahoney, P., McDonnell, K., & O'Campo, P. (2007). HIV/AIDS and intimate partner violence: Intersecting women's health issues in the United States. *Trauma, Violence and Abuse, 8*, 178–198.

Gilbert, L., El-Bassel, N., Rajah, V., Foleno, A., Fontdevila, J., Frye, V., et al. (2000). The converging epidemics of mood-altering-drug use, HIV, HCV, and partner violence. *Mount Sinai Journal of Medicine, 67*, 452–464.

Global Infectious Diseases and Epidemiology Online Network. (2008). *Emergence of infectious diseases in the 21st century*. Retrieved May 9, 2008, from http://www.gideononline.com/blog/2008/03/05/ emergence-of-infectious-diseases-in-the-21st-century.

Global Network for Neglected Tropical Diseases. (2006). *About neglected tropical diseases (NTDs)*. Retrieved April 13, 2008, from http://gnntdc.sabin.org/what/aboutntds.html.

Glynn, M., & Rhodes, P. (2005, June). *Estimated HIV prevalence in the United States at the end of 2003*. National HIV Prevention Conference, Atlanta (Abstract T1-B1101).

Goebel-Fabbri, A., Fikkan, J., Connell, A., Vangsness, L., & Anderson, B. (2002). Identification and treatment of eating disorders in women with type 1 diabetes mellitus. *Treatments in Endocrinology, 1*(3), 155–162.

Goebel-Fabbri, A., Fikkan, J., Franko, D., Pearson, K., Anderson, B., & Weinger, K. (2008). Insulin restriction and associated morbidity and mortality in women with type 1 diabetes. *Diabetes Care, 31*, 415–419.

Goldberg, R. (2003). The plausibility of micronutrient deficiency in relationship to perinatal infection. *Journal of Nutrition, 133*, 1645–1648.

Goldstein, D. (2003). *Laughter out of place: Race, class, violence, and sexuality in a Rio shantytown*. Berkeley: University of California Press.

Gomez, A., Atzori, C., Ludovisi, A., Rossi, P., Scaglia, M., & Pozio, E. (1995). Opportunistic and non-opportunistic parasites in HIV-positive and negative patients with diarrhoea in Tanzania. *Tropical Medicine and Parasitology, 46*, 109–114.

Gomez, M., Fernandez, D., Otero, J., Miranda, S., & Hunter, R. (2000). The shape of the HIV/AIDS epidemic in Puerto Rico. *Pan American Journal of Public Health, 7*, 377–383.

Good, R., & Lorenz, E. (1992). Nutrition and cellular immunity. *International Journal of Immunopharmacology, 14*, 361–366.

Goodwin, J., Cheeves, K., & Connell, V. (1990). Borderline and other severe symptoms in adult survivors of incestuous abuse. *Psychiatric Annals, 20*, 22–32.

Gordis, L. (1996). *Epidemiology*. Philadelphia: Saunders.

Gorman, M., & Carroll, R. (2000). Substance abuse and HIV: Considerations with regard to methamphetamines and other recreational drugs for nursing practice and research. *Journal of the Association of Nurses in AIDS Care, 11*(2), 51–62.

Gostin, L. (2000). *Public health law: Power, duty, restraint*. Berkeley: University of California Press.

Gould, S. (2000, October). Syphilis and the shepherd of Atlantis: Renaissance poem about syphilis attempts to explain its origin; genetic map revealed in 1998. *Natural History*. Retrieved March 16, 2008, from http://findarticles.com/p/articles/mi_m1134/is_8_109/ai_65913170/pg_1.

Graham, A., Lamb, T., Read, A., & Allen, J. (2005). Malaria-filaria coinfection in mice makes malarial disease more severe unless filarial infection achieves patency. *Journal of Infectious Diseases, 191*, 410–421.

Graham, D., Malaty, H., Evans, D., Evans, D., Jr., Klein, P., & Adam, E. (1991). Epidemiology of *Helicobacter pylori* in an asymptomatic population in the United States: Effect of age, race, and socioeconomic status. *Gastroenterology, 100*, 1495–1501.

Grandin, T. (1997). The design and construction of facilities for handling cattle. *Livestock Production Science, 49*, 103–119.

Grandin, T. (1998). Review: Reducing handling stress improves both productivity and welfare. *The Professional Animal Scientist, 14*, 1–10.

Grandominico, J., & Fichtenbaum, C. (2008). Short-term effect of HAART on blood pressure in HIV-infected individuals. *HIV Clinical Trials, 9*, 52–60.

Gravlee, C., Dressler, W., & Bernard, H. (2005). Skin color, social classification, and blood pressure in southeastern Puerto Rico. *American Journal of Public Health, 95*, 2191–2197.

Gray, R., Wawer, M., Brookmeyer, R., Sewankambo, N., Serwadda, D., Wabwire-Mangen, F., et al., & Rakai Project Team. (2001). Probability of HIV-1 transmission per coital act in monogamous, heterosexual, HIV-1-discordant couples in Rakai, Uganda. *Lancet, 357*, 1149–1153.

Greenberg, D., Givon-Lavi, N., Briodes, A., Blancovich, I., Peled, N., & Dagan, R. (2006). The contribution of smoking and exposure to tobacco smoke to *Streptococcus pneumoniae* and *Haemophilus influenzae* carriage in children and their mothers. *Clinical Infectious Diseases, 42*, 904–906.

Greene, C., & Thornton, R. (2007). *The year the stars fell: Lakota winter counts at the Smithsonian.* Washington, DC: Smithsonian Institution.

Greene, L., & Danubio, M. (Eds.). (1997). *Adaptation to malaria: The interaction of biology and culture.* Amsterdam: Gordon and Breach.

Greenwood, M. (1953). Miasma and contagion. In E. Underwood (Ed.), *Science, medicine and history* (Vol. 2, pp. 501–507). New York: Oxford University Press.

Greiger, T., & Kluger, M. (1978). Fever and survival: The role of serum iron. *Journal of Physiology, 279,* 187–196.

Grimwade, K., French, N., Mbatha, D., Zungu, D., Dedicoat, M., & Gilks, C. (2003). Childhood malaria in a region of unstable transmission and high human immunodeficiency virus prevalence. *Pediatric Infectious Disease Journal, 22,* 1057–1063.

Grimwade, K., French, N., Mbatha, D., Zungu, D., Dedicoat, M., & Gilks, C. (2004). HIV infection as a cofactor for severe falciparum malaria in adults living in a region of unstable malaria transmission in South Africa. *AIDS, 18,* 547–554.

Grinsztejn, B., Bastos, F., Veloso, V., Friedman, R., Pilotto, J., Schechter, M., et al. (2006). Assessing sexually transmitted infections in a cohort of women living with HIV/AIDS, in Rio de Janeiro, Brazil. *International Journal of STD & AIDS, 17,* 473–478.

Gross, J. (2008, May 9). AIDS patients face downside of living longer. *New York Times,* p. A1.

Grundy, S. (2008). Metabolic syndrome pandemic. *Arteriosclerosis, Thrombosis, and Vascular Biology, 28,* 629–636.

Gu, J., & Korteweg, C. (2007). Pathology and pathogenesis of severe acute respiratory syndrome. *American Journal of Pathology, 170,* 1136–1147.

Gupta, E., Dar, L., Kapoor, G., & Broor, S. (2006). The changing epidemiology of dengue in Delhi, India. *Virology Journal, 3.* Retrieved November 22, 2007, from http://www.pubmedcentral.nih.gov/articlerender.fcgi?artid=1636631.

Gupta, S., Eustace, J., Winston, J., Boydstun, I., Ahuja, T., Rodriguez, R., et al. (2005). Guidelines for the management of chronic kidney disease in HIV-infected patients: Recommendations of the HIV Medicine Association of the Infectious Diseases Society of America. *Clinical Infectious Diseases, 40,* 1559–1585.

Ha, L., Bloom, S., Hien, N., Maloney, S., Mai, L., Leitmeyer, K., et al. (2004). Lack of SARS transmission among public hospital workers, Vietnam. *Emerging Infectious Diseases, 12.* Retrieved April 7, 2008, from http://www.cdc.gov/ncidod/EID/vol10no2/03-0707.htm.

Hackett, L. (1937). *Malaria in Europe: An ecological study.* New York: Oxford University Press.

Haley, B. (1978). *The healthy body and Victorian culture.* Cambridge, MA: Harvard University Press.

Halloran, M., Ferguson, N., Eubank, S., Longini, I., Jr., Cummings, D., Lewis, B., et al. (2008). Modeling targeted layered containment of an influenza pandemic in the United States. *Proceedings of the National Academy of Sciences of the United States of America, 105,* 4639–4644.

Hamburg, M. (2001). Challenges confronting public health agencies. *Public Health Reports, 116*(Suppl. 2), 59–63.

Hamburger, M., Leeb, R., & Swahn, M. (2008). Childhood maltreatment and early alcohol use among high-risk adolescents. *Journal of Studies on Alcohol and Drugs, 69,* 291–295.

Handt, L., Fox, J., Dewhirst, F., Fraser, G., Paster, B., Yan, L., et al. (1994). *Helicobacter pylori* isolated from the domestic cat: Public health implications. *Infection and Immunity, 62,* 2367–2374.

Hansen, D., Sedlar, G., & Warner-Rogers, J. (1999). Child physical abuse. In R. Ammerman & M. Hersen (Eds.), *Assessment of family violence: A clinical and legal sourcebook* (pp. 127–156). San Francisco: Jossey-Bass.

Haraway, D. (1991). *Simians, cyborgs and women: The reinvention of nature.* New York: Routledge.

Harcourt-Webster, J., Scaravilli, F., & Darwish, A. (1991). *Strongyloides stercoralis* hyperinfection in an HIV positive patient. *Journal of Clinical Pathology, 44,* 346–348.

Harms, G., & Feldmeier, H. (2002). HIV infection and tropical parasitic diseases: Deleterious interactions in both directions? *Tropical Medicine and International Health, 7*, 479–488.

Hauser, S., Jacobson, A., Lavori, P., Wolfsdorf, J., Herskowitz, R., Milley, J., et al. (1990). Adherence among children and adolescents with insulin-dependent diabetes mellitus over a four-year longitudinal follow-up: II. Immediate and long-term linkages with the family milieu. *Journal of Pediatric Psychology, 15*, 527–542.

Hausler, T. (2006). *Viruses vs. superbugs: A solution to the antibiotics crisis?* New York: Macmillan.

Hays, J. (2000). *The burdens of disease: Epidemics and human response in western history.* New Brunswick, NJ: Rutgers University Press.

Hein, C., & Small, D. (2007). *Combating diabetes, obesity, periodontal disease and interrelated inflammatory conditions with a syndemic approach.* Retrieved August 12, 2007, from http://www.healthdecisions.org/Dental/News/default.aspx?doc_id=109688.

Helfand, R., Moss, W., Harpaz, R., Scott, S., & Cutts, F. (2005). Evaluating the impact of the HIV pandemic on measles control and elimination. *Bulletin of the World Health Organization, 83*, 329–337.

Helmholtz Association. (2007). *Fighting cancer with salmonella: How the medical profession can use bacteria.* Retrieved May 11. 2008, from http://www.helmholtz-hzi.de/en/news_public_relation/press_releases/view/article/complete/fighting_cancer_with_salmonella-1.

Hendricks, M., Eley, B., & Bourne, L. (2007). Nutrition and HIV/AIDS in infants and children in South Africa: Implications for food-based dietary guidelines. *Maternal and Child Nutrition, 3*, 322–333.

Hennen, J. (1830). *Sketches of the medical topography of the Mediterranean comprising an account of Gibraltar, the Ionian Islands, and Malta; to which is prefixed, a sketch of a plan for memoires on medical typology.* London: Thomas and George Underwood.

Henry, K., Melroe, H., Huebsch, J., Hermundson, J., Levine, C., Swensen, L., et al. (1998). Severe premature coronary artery disease with protease inhibitors. *Lancet, 351*, 1328.

Herring, D., Abonyi, S., & Hoppa, R. (2003). Malnutrition among northern peoples of Canada in the 1940s: An ecological and economic disaster. In D. Herring & A. Swedlund (Eds.), *Human biologists in the archives* (pp. 289–310). New York: Cambridge University Press.

Herring, D., & Sattenspiel, L. (2003). Death in winter: Spanish flu in the Canadian subarctic. In H. Phillips & D. Killingray (Eds.), *The Spanish influenza pandemic of 1918–19: New perspectives* (pp. 156–172). New York: Routledge.

Herring, D., & Sattenspiel, L. (2007). Social contexts, syndemics, and infectious disease in northern aboriginal populations. *American Journal of Human Biology, 19*, 190–202.

Hethcoke, H., & Yorke, J. (1984). *Gonorrhea: Transmission dynamics and control.* New York: Springer-Verlag.

Heymann, D. (2004). From smallpox to polio and beyond: Disease surveillance in India. *Indian Journal of Medical Research, 120*(2), 70–72.

Highleyman, L. (2003). HIV and hepatitis coinfection. *Bulletin of Experimental Treatments for AIDS.* Retrieved May 6, 2008, from http://www.thebody.com/content/art2542.html#growing.

Hirshfield, S., Remien, R., Walavalkar, I., & Chiasson, M. (2004). Crystal methamphetamine use predicts incident STD infection among men who have sex with men recruited online: A nested case-control study. *Journal of Medical Internet Research, 6*(4), e41.

Hisada, M., Chatterjee, N., Zhang, M., Battjes, R., & Goedert, J. (2003). Increased hepatitis C virus load among injection drug users infected with human immunodeficiency virus and human T lymphotropic virus type II. *Journal of Infectious Diseases, 188*, 891–897.

HIV Vaccine Trials Network. (2007). Data from STEP study presented at open scientific session confirm Merck's investigational HIV vaccine was not effective. Retrieved May 2, 2008, from http://www.hvtn.org/media/pr/step.html.

Ho, M., Chen, E., Hsu, K., Twu, S., Chen, K., Tsai, S., et al. (1999). An epidemic of enterovirus 71 infection in Taiwan. *New England Journal of Medicine, 341*, 929–935.

Hoehling, A. (1961). *The great epidemic.* Boston: Little, Brown.

Hoerauf, A., Mand, S., Fischer, K., Kruppa, T., Marfo-Debrekyei, Y., Debrah, A., et al. (2003). Doxycycline as a novel strategy against bancroftian filariasis–depletion of *Wolbachia* endosymbionts from *Wuchereria bancrofti* and stop of microfilaria production. *Medical Microbiology and Immunology, 192*(4), 211–216.

Hoffman, R. (2001). Eating disorders in adolescents with type 1 diabetes: A closer look at a complicated condition. *Postgraduate Medicine, 109*(4), 67–69, 73–74.

Hopkins, W., & Frank, B. (1991). Street studies that work and what they show in New York City. *Journal of Addictive Diseases, 11*(1), 89–97.

Hotez, P. (2006, Winter/Spring). The "biblical diseases" and U.S. vaccine diplomacy. *Brown World Affairs Journal, 12*, 247–358.

Hotez, P., Bethony, J., Bottazzi, M., Brooker, S., & Buss, P. (2005). Hookworm: "The great infection of mankind." *PLoS Medicine, 2*, e67.

Hotez, P., Molyneux, D., Fenwick, A., Ottesen, E., Sachs, S., & Sachs, J. (2006). Incorporating a rapid-impact package for neglected tropical diseases with programs for HIV/AIDS, tuberculosis, and malaria. *PLoS Medicine, 3*, e102.

Humphreys, J. (1997). Nursing care of children of battered women. *Pediatric Nursing, 23*, 122–128.

Hunter, P., Chalmers, R., Syed, Q., Hughes, L., Woodhouse, S., & Swift, L. (2003). Foot and mouth disease and cryptosporidiosis: Possible interaction between two emerging infectious diseases. *Emerging Infectious Diseases, 9*, 109–112.

Hunter, S. (1993). Prostitution is cruelty and abuse to women and children. *Michigan Journal of Gender and Law, 1*, 1–14.

Hunter, W., Jain, D., Sadowski, L., & Sanhueza, A. (2000). Risk factors for severe child discipline practices in rural India. *Journal of Pediatric Psychology, 25*, 435–447.

Hyman, S., Paliwal, P., Chaplin, T., Mazure, C., Rounsaville, B., & Sinha, R. (2008). Severity of childhood trauma is predictive of cocaine relapse outcomes in women but not men. *Drug and Alcohol Dependence, 92*(1–3), 208–216.

Igra-Siegman, Y., Kapila, R., Sen, P., Kaminski, Z., & Louria, D. (1981). Syndrome of hyperinfection with *Strongyloides stercoralis*. *Review of Infectious Diseases, 3*, 397–407.

Illinois Public Health Futures Institute. (2004). *From silos to systems: Assessing Illinois' public health system.* Retrieved May 3, 2008, from http://app.idph.state.il.us/phfi/Home%20page/NPHPSP%20Final%20Report%2012-01-04.pdf.

Interuniversity Institute of Research and Development. (2008). *Cité Soleil Project midway report of research findings.* Port-au-Prince: Author.

Ip, M., Lam, B., Ng, M., Lam, W., Tsang, K., & Lam, K. (2002). Obstructive sleep apnea is independently associated with insulin resistance. *American Journal of Respiratory and Critical Care Medicine, 165*, 670–676.

Isaac, R., Jacobson, D., Wanke, C., Hendricks, K., Knox, T., & Wilson, I. (2008). Declines in dietary macronutrient intake in persons with HIV infection who develop depression. *Public Health Nutrition, 11*(2), 124–131.

Jacob, F. (1988). *The statue within: An autobiography.* New York: Basic Books.

Jacobsen, K. (2008). *Introduction to global health.* Sudbury, MA: Jones and Bartlett.

Jadotte, E. (2006). *Income distribution and poverty in the republic of Haiti.* Quebec: Poverty and Economic Policy Research Network—Poverty Monitoring, Measurement, and Analysis (PEP-PMMA).

Jeon, C., & Murray, M. (2008). Diabetes mellitus increases the risk of active tuberculosis: A systematic review of 13 observational studies. *PLoS Medicine, 5*, e152.

Jinich, S., Paul, J., Stall, R., Acree, M., Kegeles, S., Hoff, C., et al. (1998). Childhood sexual abuse and HIV risk-taking behavior among gay and bisexual men. *AIDS and Behavior, 2*, 41–51.

Johnson, J., Windsor, J., & Clark, C. (2004). Emerging from obscurity: Biological, clinical, and diagnostic aspects of *Dientamoeba fragilis*. *Clinical Microbiology Review, 17*, 553–570.

Johnson, S. (2006). *The ghost map: The story of London's most terrifying epidemic—and how it changed science, cities, and the modern world.* New York: Riverhead Books.

Johnston, B. (2007). "More like us than mice": Radiation experiments with indigenous peoples. In B. Johnston (Ed.), *Half lives and half truths: Confronting the radioactive legacies of the Cold War* (pp. 25–54). Santa Fe, NM: School for Advanced Research Press.

Jolles, A., & Ezenwa, V. (2006, August 8). *Macroparasite-microparasite interactions: Worms and TB in African buffalo*. Paper presented at the meeting of the Ecological Society of America, Memphis, TN.

Jolly, C., & Fernandes, G. (2000). Protein-energy malnutrition and infectious disease. In M. Gershwin, J. German, & C. Keen (Eds.), *Nutrition and immunology: Principles and practice* (pp. 195–202). Totowa, NJ: Humana Press.

Jones, C., & Williams, H. (2004). The social burden of malaria: What are we measuring? *American Journal of Tropical Diseases and Hygiene, 71*(Suppl. 2), 156–161.

Jones, M. (2000). The Ceylon malaria epidemic of 1934–35: A case study in colonial medicine. *Social History of Medicine, 13*, 87–109.

Joralemon, D. (1999). *Exploring medical anthropology*. Needham Heights, MA: Allyn & Bacon.

Kalichman, S., Rompa, D., & Cage, M. (2000). Sexually transmitted infections among HIV seropositive men and women. *Sexually Transmitted Infections, 76*, 350–354.

Kamali, A., Nunn, A., Mulder, D., Van Dyck, E., Dobbins, J., & Whitworth, J. (1999). Seroprevalence and incidence of genital ulcer infections in a rural Ugandan population. *Sexually Transmitted Infection, 75*, 98–102.

Kant, L. (2003). Diabetes mellitus-tuberculosis: The brewing double trouble. *Indian Journal of Tuberculosis, 50*(4), 83–84.

Karanja, D., Hightower, A., Colley, D., Mwinzi, P., Galil, K., Andove, J., et al. (2002). Resistance to reinfection with *Schistosoma mansoni* in occupationally exposed adults and effect of HIV-1 co-infection on susceptibility to schistosomiasis: A longitudinal study. *Lancet, 360*, 592–596.

Kark, S., & Kark, E. (2008). *What is social medicine?* Retrieved May 4, 2008, from http://www.socialmedicine .org/2008/03/23/about/what-is-social-medicine.

Keeling, M., & Rohani, P. (2007). *Modeling infectious diseases in humans and animals*. Princeton, NJ: Princeton University Press.

Keller, T., Hader, C., De Zeeuw, J., & Rasche, K. (2007). Obstructive sleep apnea syndrome: The effect of diabetes and autonomic neuropathy. *Journal of Physiology and Pharmacology, 58*(Suppl. 5, Pt. 1), 313–318.

Kellerhals, M. (2008). *Rising global food prices likely to continue, say experts: Higher food costs have led to increasing civil unrest*. Retrieved May 20, 2008, from http://www.america.gov/st/peacesec-english/2008/April/20080411130214dmslahrellek0.9818994.html.

Khantzian, E. (1985). The self-medication hypothesis of addictive disorders: Focus on heroin and cocaine dependence. *American Journal of Psychiatry, 142*, 1259–1264.

Khantzian, E. (1990). Self-regulation and self-medication factors in alcoholism and the addictions: Similarities and differences. In M. Galanter (Ed.), *Combined alcohol and other drug dependence* (Recent Developments in Alcoholism, Vol. 8, pp. 255–271). New York: Springer.

Kijak, G., & McCutchan, F. (2005). HIV diversity, molecular epidemiology, and the role of recombination. *Current Infectious Disease Report, 7*, 480–488.

Kilpatrick, D., O'Neill, H., Beak, S., Resnick, H., Stugis, E., Best, C., et al. (1990). *Parental substance abuse, personal victimization, and women's risks for substance abuse: Results from a national probability sample*. Paper presented at a meeting of the Association for Advancement of Behavior Therapy, San Francisco.

Kilpatrick, D., & Saunders, B. (1997). *The prevalence and consequences of child victimization*. National Institute of Justice Research Preview. Retrieved September 12, 2008, from http://www.casane.org/library/abuse/prevalence.htm.

Kim, A., Schulze zur Wiesch, J., Kuntzen, T., Timm, J., Kaufmann, D., Duncan, J., et al. (2006). Impaired hepatitis C virus-specific T cell responses and recurrent hepatitis C virus in HIV coinfection. *PLoS Medicine, 3*, e492.

Kim, J., Shakow, A., Bayona, J., Rhatigan, J., & de Celis, E. (2000). Sickness amidst recovery: Public debt and private suffering in Peru. In J. Kim, J. Millen, A. Irwin, & J. Gershman (Eds.), *Dying for growth: Global inequality and the health of the poor* (pp. 127–153). Monroe, ME: Common Courage Press.

Kimball, S. (1995). Sail and rail pioneers before 1869. *BYU Studies, 35*(2), 6–42.

Kirmayer, L. (2003). Reflections on embodiment. In J. Wilce Jr. (Ed.), *Social and cultural lives of immune systems* (pp. 282–302). New York: Routledge.

Kjetland, E., Ndhlovu, P., Gomo, E., Mduluza, T., Midzi, N., Gwanzura, L., et al. (2006). Association between genital schistosomiasis and HIV in rural Zimbabwean women. *AIDS, 20*, 593–600.

Kleinman, A. (1978). Culture, illness and cure: Clinical lessons from anthropologic and cross-cultural research. *Annals of Internal Medicine, 88*, 251–258.

Knobler, S., O'Connor, S., Lemon, S., & Najafi, M. (Eds.). (2002). *The infectious etiology of chronic diseases: Defining the relationship, enhancing the research, and mitigating the effects.* Washington, DC: National Academies Press.

Koch, R. (1987). *Essays of Robert Koch* (K. Codell Carter, Trans.). Westport, CT: Greenwood Press. (Original work published 1890)

Konomi, N., Lebwohl, E., Mowbray, K., Tattersall, I., & Zhang, D. (2002). Detection of mycobacterial DNA in Andean mummies. *Journal of Clinical Microbiology, 40*, 4738–4740.

Korppi, M., Leinonen, M., Koskela, M., Mäkelä, P., & Launiala, K. (1989). Bacterial coinfection in children hospitalized with respiratory syncytial virus infections. *Pediatric Infectious Disease Journal, 8*, 6878–6892.

Koutsilieri, E., Scheller, C., Sopper, S., ter Meulen, V., & Riederer, P. (2002). Psychiatric complications in human immunodeficiency virus infection. *Journal of NeuroVirology, 8*, 129–133.

Kovach, J. (1983). *The relationship between treatment failures of alcoholic women and incestuous histories with possible implications for post traumatic stress disorder symptomatology.* Unpublished doctoral dissertation, Wayne State University Graduate School.

Koytak, E., Yurdaydin, C., & Glenn, J. (2007). Hepatitis D. *Current Treatment Options in Gastroenterology, 10*, 456–463.

Kraft, M. (2006). Asthma and chronic obstructive pulmonary disease exhibit common origins in any country! *American Journal of Respiratory and Critical Care Medicine, 174*, 238–240.

Krause, P., Telford, S., Spielman, A., Sikand, V., Ryan, R., Christianson, D., et al. (1996). Concurrent Lyme disease and babesiosis: Evidence for increased severity and duration of illness. *JAMA, 275*, 1657–1660.

Krause, R. (2001). Microbes and emerging infections: The compulsion to become something. *American Society for Microbiology News, 67*(1), 15–20.

Kravitz, R., Hays, R., Sherbourne, C., DiMatteo, M., Rogers, W., Ordway, L., et al. (1993). Recall of recommendations and adherence to advice among patients with chronic medical conditions. *Archives of Internal Medicine, 153*, 1863–1868.

Krieger, N. (2005). *Health disparities and the body.* Boston: Harvard School of Public Health.

Krieger, N., Jarvis, T., Chen, J., Waterman, P., Rehkopf, D., & Subramanian, S. (2003). Race/ethnicity, gender, and monitoring socioeconomic gradients in health: A comparison of area-based socioeconomic measures— the public health disparities geocoding project. *American Journal of Public Health, 93*, 1655–1671.

Kuhn, K. (1999). Global warming and leishmaniasis in Italy. *Bulletin of Tropical Medicine and International Health, 7*(2), 1–2.

Kuhn, T. (1970). *The structure of scientific revolutions* (2nd ed.). Chicago: University of Chicago Press.

Kumwenda, N., Miotti, P., Taha, T., Broadhead, R., Biggar, R., Jackson, J., et al. (2002). Antenatal vitamin A supplementation increases birth weight and decreases anemia among infants born to human immunodeficiency virus–infected women in Malawi. *Clinical Infectious Diseases, 35*, 618–624.

Kwena, A., Terlouw, D., De Vlas, S., Phillips-Howard, P., Hawley, W., Friedman, J., et al. (2003). Prevalence and severity of malnutrition in pre-school children in a rural area of Western Kenya. *American Journal of Tropical Medicine and Hygiene, 68*(Suppl. 4), 94–99.

Lagacé-Wiens, P., VanCaeseele, P., & Koschik, C. (2006). *Dientamoeba fragilis:* An emerging role in intestinal disease. *Canadian Medical Association Journal, 175*(5), 48–49.

Lane, S., Keefe, R., Rubinstein, R., Webster, N., Rosenthal, A., Cibula, D., et al. (2004). Structural violence and racial disparity in heterosexual HIV infection. *Journal of Health Care for the Poor and Underserved, 15*, 319–335.

Lane, W., Rubin, D., Monteith, R., & Christian, C. (2002). Racial differences in the evaluation of pediatric fractures for physical abuse. *JAMA, 288*, 1603–1609.

Laserson, K., & Wells, C. (2007). Reaching the targets for tuberculosis control: The impact of HIV. *Bulletin of the World Health Organization, 85*(5). Retrieved November 24, 2008, from http://www.who.int/bulletin/volumes/85/5/06.035329/en/index.html.

Latour, B. (1979). *Laboratory life: The social construction of scientific facts.* Thousand Oaks, CA: Sage.

Lauer, J., Röhrich, K., Wirth, H., Charette, C., Gribble, S., & Murray, C. (2003). PopMod: A longitudinal population model with two interacting disease states. *Cost Effectiveness and Resource Allocation, 1*(6). Retrieved April 20, 2008, from http://www.pubmedcentral.nih.gov/articlerender.fcgi?artid=156025.

Layseca, C., Parodi, C., & Carrasco, L. (1991). Cholera—Peru, 1991. *Morbidity and Mortality Weekly Report, 40*, 108–110.

le Carré, J. (2005). *The constant gardener.* New York: Simon & Schuster.

Lee, C.-H., & Liu, J.-W. (2007). Coinfection with leptospirosis and scrub typhus in Taiwanese patients. *American Journal of Tropical Medicine and Hygiene, 77*, 525–527.

Lee, J. (1989). *The modernization of Irish society, 1848–1910.* Dublin: Gill and Macmillan.

Lee, N., Hui, D., Wu, A., Chan, P., Cameron, P., Joynt, G., et al. (2003). A major outbreak of severe acute respiratory syndrome in Hong Kong. *New England Journal of Medicine, 348*, 1986–1994.

Leischow, S., & Milstein, B. (2006). Systems thinking and modeling for public health practice. *American Journal of Public Health, 96*, 403–405.

Leo, Y., Chen, M., Lee, M., Paton, N., Ang, B., Choo, P., et al. (2003). Severe acute respiratory syndrome—Singapore. *Morbidity and Mortal Weekly Report, 52*, 405–411.

Leontiev, V., Maury, W., & Hadany, L. (2008). Drug induced superinfection in HIV and the evolution of drug resistance. *Infection, Genetics and Evolution, 8*, 40–50.

Lessnau, K., Can, S., & Talvera, W. (1993). Disseminated *Strongyloides stercoralis* in human immunodeficiency virus-infected patients: Treatment failure and a review of the literature. *Chest, 4*, 119–122.

Leung, G., Hedley, A., Ho, L.-M., Chau, P., Wong, I., Thach, T., et al. (2004). The epidemiology of severe acute respiratory syndrome in the 2003 Hong Kong epidemic: An analysis of all 1755 patients. *Annals of Internal Medicine, 141*, 662–673.

Levine, A., Kotz, C., & Gosnell, B. (2003). Sugars and fats: The neurobiology of preference. *Journal of Nutrition, 133*(Suppl.), 831S–834S.

Levins, R., & Lewontin, R. (1985). *The dialectical biologist.* Cambridge, MA: Harvard University Press.

Lin, E., Katon, W., Von Korff, M., Rutter, C., Simon, G., Oliver, M., et al. (2004). Relationship of depression and diabetes self-care, medication adherence, and preventive care. *Diabetes Care, 27*, 2154–2160.

Lindblom, C., & Cohen, D. (1979). *Usable knowledge: Social science and social problem solving.* New Haven, CT: Yale University Press.

Lindqvist, P. (2007). Mental disorder, substance misuse and violent behaviour: The Swedish experience of caring for the triply troubled. *Criminal Behaviour and Mental Health, 17*(4), 242–249.

Livingston, F. (1958). Anthropological implications of sickle-cell gene distribution in West Africa. *American Anthropologist, 60*, 533–562.

Lockman, S., Hone, N., Kenyon, T., Mwasekaga, M., Villauthapillai, M., Creek, T., et al. (2003). Etiology of pulmonary infections in predominantly HIV-infected adults with suspected tuberculosis, Botswana. *International Journal of Tuberculosis and Lung Disease, 7*, 714–723.

Loessner, H., Endmann, A., Leschner, S., Westphal, K., Rohde, M., Miloud, T., et al. (2007). Remote control of tumour-targeted *Salmonellen enterica* serovar Typhimurium by the use of L-arabinose as inducer of bacterial gene expression in vivo. *Cellular Microbiology, 9*, 1529–1537.

Louisiana State Museum. (2007). *Antebellum Louisiana: Disease, death, and mourning.* Retrieved April 20, 2008, from http://lsm.crt.state.la.us/cabildo/cab8a.htm.

Loureiro, S., Spinola, A., Martins, F., and Barreto, M. (1983). Lead poisoning and hookworm infection as multiple factors in anaemia. *Tropical Medicine and Hygiene, 7*(3), 321–322.

Lucas, G., Mehta, S., Atta, M., Kirk, G., Galai, N., Vlahov, D., et al. (2007). End-stage renal disease and chronic kidney disease in a cohort of African-American HIV-infected and at-risk HIV-seronegative participants followed between 1988 and 2004. *AIDS, 21,* 2435–2443.

Lyon, M. (2003). "Immune" to emotion: The relative absence of emotion in PNI, and its centrality to everything else. In J. Wilce Jr. (Ed.), *Social and cultural lives of immune systems* (pp. 82–102). New York: Routledge.

Maas, C., Herrenkohl, T., & Sousa, C. (2008). Review of research on child maltreatment and violence in youth. *Trauma, Violence & Abuse, 9,* 56–67.

Machel, G. (1996). *Promotion and protection of the rights of children: Impact of armed conflict on children.* United Nations, UNICEF. Retrieved January 15, 2009, from http://www.unicef.org/graca/a51-306_en.pdf.

MacQueen, K. (2002). Anthropology and public health. In L. Breslow (Ed.), *Encyclopedia of Public Health.* New York: Macmillan Reference.

Madu, S., & Peltzer, K. (2000). Risk factors and child sexual abuse among secondary students in the Northern Province (South Africa). *Child Abuse & Neglect, 24,* 259–268.

Magner, L. (2002). *A history of the life sciences* (3rd ed.). New York: Decker.

Malaty, H., Kim, J., Kim, S., & Graham, D. (1996). Prevalence of *Helicobacter pylori* infection in Korean children: Inverse relation to socioeconomic status despite a uniformly high prevalence in adults. *American Journal of Epidemiology, 143,* 257–262.

Mamidi, A., DeSimone, J., & Pomerantz, R. (2002). Central nervous system infections in individuals with HIV-1 infection. *Journal of NeuroVirology, 8,* 158–159.

Manfredi, C. (1999). Can the resurgence of malaria be partially attributed to structural adjustment programmes? *Parasitologia, 41,* 389–390.

Mankodi, K. (1996). Political and economic roots of disease: Malaria in Rajasthan. *Economic and Political Weekly, 31*(4), 42–48.

Mann, J., Gostin, L., Gruskin, S., Brennan, T., Lazzarini, Z., & Fineberg, H. (1999). Health and human rights. In J. Mann, S. Gruskin, M. Grodin, & G. Annas (Eds.), *Health and human rights: A reader* (pp. 7–20). New York: Routledge.

Marcos, L., Terashima, A., Dupont, H., & Gotuzzo, E. (2008). Strongyloides hyperinfection syndrome: An emerging global infectious disease. *Transactions of the Royal Society of Tropical Medicine and Hygiene, 102,* 314–318.

Marmot, M., & Bell, R. (2006). The socioeconomically disadvantaged. In B. Levy & V. Sidel (Eds.), *Social injustice and public health* (pp. 25–44). New York: Oxford University Press.

Marr, A., & Dasqupta, N. (2008, July 22–25). *Strategies for water pollution control in Dhaka, Bangladesh: An institutional and economic analysis.* Paper presented at the Third International Conference on Interdisciplinary Social Sciences, Monash University Centre, Prato, Tuscany, Italy.

Marshal, M., Friedman, M., Stall, R., King, K., Miles, J., Gold, M., et al. (2008). Sexual orientation and adolescent substance use: A meta-analysis and methodological review. *Addiction, 103,* 546–556.

Marshall, B., Armstrong, J., McGechie, D., & Glancy, R. (1985). Attempt to fulfill Koch's postulates for pyloric campylobacter. *Medical Journal of Australia, 142,* 436–439.

Marshall, B., & Warren, J. (1984). Unidentified curved bacilli in the stomach of patients with gastritis and peptic ulceration. *Lancet, 1,* 1311–1315.

Marshall, M. (2005). Carolina in the Carolines: A survey of patterns and meanings of smoking on a Micronesian island. *Medical Anthropology Quarterly, 19,* 354–382.

Marshall, P., Singer, M., & Clatts, M. (Eds.). (1999). *Integrating cultural, observational, and epidemiological approaches in the prevention of drug abuse and HIV/AIDS.* Rockville, MD: National Institute on Drug Abuse.

Marston, W. (1998, December 8). In Peru's shantytowns, cholera comes by the bucket. *New York Times,* p. 1.

Martin, P., & Leibovich, S. (2005). Inflammatory cells during wound repair: The good, the bad and the ugly. *Trends in Cell Biology, 15,* 599–607.

Martin, P., & Martin-Granel, E. (2006). 2,500-year evolution of the term epidemic. *Emerging Infectious Diseases.* Retrieved March 12, 2008, from http://www.cdc.gov/ncidod/EID/vol12no06/05-1263.htm.

Martín-Carbonero, L., Soriano, V., Valencia, E., García-Samaniego, J., López, M., & González-Lahoz, J. (2001). Increasing impact of chronic viral hepatitis on hospital admissions and mortality among HIV-infected patients. *AIDS Research and Human Retroviruses, 17,* 1467–1471.

Martinez, J. (1999). *Peru: Country health briefing paper.* London: Department for International Development, Health Systems Resource Centre.

Mata, L. (1994). Cholera El Tor in Latin America, 1991–1993. In M. Wilson, R. Levins, & A. Spielman (Eds.), *Disease in evolution: Global changes and emergence of infectious diseases* (pp. 55–68). New York: New York Academy of Sciences.

Matteelli, A., Beltrame, A., Carvalho, A., Casalini, C., Forleo, M., Gulletta, M., et al. (2003). *Chlamydia trachomatis* genital infection in migrant female sex workers in Italy. *International Journal of STD & AIDS, 14,* 591–595.

Mazzeo, S., Trace, S., Mitchell, K., & Gow, R. (2007). Effects of a reality TV cosmetic surgery makeover program on eating disordered attitudes and behaviors. *Eating Behaviors, 8,* 390–397.

McArthur, J. (2004). HIV dementia: An evolving disease. *Journal of Neuroimmunology, 157*(1–2), 3–10.

McCombie, S. (1987). Folk flu and viral syndrome: An epidemiological perspective. *Social Science & Medicine, 25,* 987–993.

McCullers, J., & Rehg, J. (2002). Lethal synergism between influenza virus and *Streptococcus pneumoniae:* Characterization of a mouse model and the role of platelet-activating factor receptor. *Journal of Infectious Diseases, 186,* 341–350.

McCullogh, D. (2005). *Knowing history and knowing who we are.* Retrieved March 23, 2008, from http://www.freerepublic.com/focus/f-news/1380518/posts.

McCullough, P., Jurkovitz, C., Pergola, P., McGill, J., Brown, W., Collins, A., & the KEEP Investigators. (2007). Independent components of chronic kidney disease as a cardiovascular risk state: Results from the Kidney Early Evaluation Program (KEEP). *Archives of Internal Medicine, 167,* 1122–1129.

McCullough, P., Nowak, R., Foreback, C., Tokarski, G., Tomlanovich, M., Khoury, N., et al. (2002). Emergency evaluation of chest pain in patients with advanced kidney disease. *Archives of Internal Medicine, 162,* 2464–2468.

McFarland, W., Gwanzura, L., Bassett, M., Machekano, R., Latif, A., Ley, C., et al. (1999). Prevalence and incidence of herpes simplex virus type 2 infection among male Zimbabwean factory workers. *Journal of Infectious Diseases, 180,* 1459–1465.

McFarlane, J., Groff, J., O'Brien, J., & Watson, K. (2003). Behaviors of children who are exposed and not exposed to intimate partner violence: An analysis of 330 black, white, and Hispanic children. *Pediatrics, 111,* e202–e207.

McMichael, A., Cambell-Lendrum, H., Corvalan, C., Ebi, K., Githeko, A., Schwraga, J. et al. (2003). *Climate change and human health: Risks and responses.* Geneva: World Health Organization.

McNeal, C., & Amato, P. (1998). Parents' marital violence: Long-term consequences for children. *Journal of Family Issues, 19,* 123–139.

McNeil, W. (1976). *Plagues and peoples.* Garden City, NY: Anchor Books.

McNeil, W. (1980). *The human condition: An ecological and historical view.* Princeton, NJ: Princeton University Press.

Meade, C., & Sikkema, K. (2005). HIV risk behavior among adults with severe mental illness: A systematic review. *Clinical Psychology Review, 25,* 433–457.

Medco Health Solutions. (2008, May 14). *Chronic medication nation: Research finds chronic health problems now afflict more than half of all Americans* (Press Release). Retrieved May 14, 2008, from http://money.aol.com/news/articles/qp/pr/_a/chronic-medication-nation-research-finds/rfid103100799.

Medical Information Group. (1998). *Dhaka air pollution.* Retrieved May 2, 2008, from http://www.angelfire.com/ak/medinet/dhakutp.html.

Melia, M. (2007). *Dengue fever surges in Latin America.* Associated Press. Retrieved November 24, 2008, from http://news.aol.com/story/ar/_a/dengue-fever-surges-in-latin-america/20070930122409990001?ncid=NWS00010000000001.

Mendelsohn, N. (2008). *A different face of eating disorders: Diabulimia.* Retrieved March 6, 2008, from http://www.savvyhealth.com/disp.asp?doc_id=25.

Merican, I., Guan, R., Amarapuka, D., Alexander, M., Chutaputti, A., Chien, R., et al. (2000). Chronic hepatitis B virus infection in Asian countries. *Journal of Gastroenterology and Hepatology, 15,* 1356–1361.

Mermin, J., Lule, J., Ekwaru, J., Downing, R., Hughes, P., Bunnell, R., et al. (2005). Cotrimoxazole prophylaxis by HIV-infected persons in Uganda reduces morbidity and mortality among HIV-uninfected family members. *AIDS, 19,* 1035–1042.

Miller, B., Downs, W., Gondoli, D., & Keil, A. (1987). The role of childhood sexual abuse in the development of alcoholism in women. *Violence and Victims, 2,* 157–171.

Miller, B., Downs, W., & Testa, M. (1993). Interrelationships between victimization experiences and women's alcohol use. *Journal of Studies on Alcohol, 11,* 109–117.

Miller, J. (2000). The effects of race/ethnicity and income on early childhood asthma prevalence and health care use. *American Journal of Public Health, 90,* 428–430.

Miller, M., Liao, Y., Wagner, M., & Korves, C. (2008). HIV, the clustering of sexually transmitted infections, and sex risk among African American women who use drugs. *Sexually Transmitted Disease.* Retrieved April 17, 2008, from http://www.ncbi.nlm.nih.gov/pubmed/18418289?ordinalpos=1&itool=EntrezSystem2.PEntrez.Pubmed.Pubmed_ResultsPanel.Pubmed_RVDocSum.

Milstein, B. (2005). Syndemics. In S. Mathison (Ed.), *Encyclopedia of evaluation* (pp. 404–405). Thousand Oaks, CA: Sage.

Milstein, B. (2008). *Hygeia's constellation: Navigating health futures in a dynamic and democratic world.* Atlanta: Centers for Disease Control and Prevention.

Minnes, S., Singer, L., Humphrey-Wall, R., & Satayathum, S. (2008). Psychosocial and behavioral factors related to the post-partum placements of infants born to cocaine-using women. *Child Abuse & Neglect, 32,* 353–366.

Moerman, D. (2003). Reflections on embodiment. In J. Wilce (Ed.), *Social and cultural lives of immune systems* (pp. 206–231). New York: Routledge.

Mok, H., & Lin, D. (2002, December). Major depression and medical comorbidity. *Canadian Psychiatry Association Bulletin,* pp. 25–28.

Molina, R., Gradoni, L., & Alvar, J. (2003). HIV and the transmission of leishmania. *Annals of Tropical Medicine and Parasitology, 97*(Suppl. 1), S29–S45.

Mooney, J. (2006). *The ghost dance religion and the Sioux outbreak of 1890.* Whitefish, MT: Kessinger.

Moorman, J., Rudd, R., Johnson, C., King, M., Minor, P., Bailey, C., et al. (2007). National surveillance for asthma—United States, 1980–2004. *Morbidity and Mortality Weekly Report Surveillance Summaries, 56*(8), 18–54.

Morens, D., & Fauci, A. (2007). The 1918 influenza pandemic: Insights for the 21st century. *Journal of Infectious Diseases, 195,* 1018–1028.

Mosack, K., Abbott, M., Singer, M., Weeks, M., & Rohena, L. (2005). If I didn't have HIV I'd be dead now: Illness narratives of drug users living with HIV/AIDS. *Qualitative Health Research, 15,* 586–605.

Moss, W., Ryon, J., Monze, M., Cutts, F., Quinn, T., & Griffin, D. (2002). Suppression of human immunodeficiency virus replication during acute measles. *Journal of Infectious Diseases, 185,* 1035–1042.

Muela, S., Ribera, J., & Tanner, M. (1998). Fake malaria and hidden parasites: The ambiguity of malaria. *Anthropology & Medicine, 5,* 43–61.

Mujawar, Z., Rose, H., Morrow, M., Pushkarsky, T., Dubrovsky, L., Mukhamedova, T., et al. (2006). Human immunodeficiency virus impairs reverse cholesterol transport from macrophages. *PLoS Biology, 4,* e365.

Mullings, J., Marquart, J., & Brewer, V. (2000). Assessing the relationship between child sexual abuse and marginal living conditions on HIV/AIDS-related risk behavior among women prisoners. *Child Abuse & Neglect, 24,* 677–688.

Mustanski, B., Garofalo, R., Herrick, A., & Donenberg, G. (2007). Psychosocial health problems increase risk for HIV among urban young men who have sex with men: Preliminary evidence of a syndemic in need of attention. *Annals of Behavioral Medicine, 34,* 37–45.

Muturi, E., Mbogo, C., Mwangangi, J., Ng'ang'a, Z., Kabiru, E., Mwandawiro, C., et al. (2006). Concomitant infections of *Plasmodium falciparum* and *Wuchereria bancrofti* on the Kenyan coast. *Filaria Journal, 5.* Retrieved April 16, 2008, from http://www.filariajournal.com/content/pdf/1475-2883-5-8.pdf.

Narain, J., Raviglione, M., & Kochi, A. (1992). HIV-associated tuberculosis in developing countries: Epidemiology and strategies for prevention. *Tubercle and Lung Disease, 73,* 311–321.

Nash, N. (1991, February 17). Spread of cholera brings frenzy and improvisation to model Lima hospital. *New York Times,* p. 1.

National Center on Addiction and Substance Abuse. (2003). *Individuals with eating disorders up to five times likelier to abuse alcohol and illicit drugs* (Press Release). Retrieved November 21, 2008, from http://www .casacolumbia.org/absolutenm/templates/PressReleases.aspx?articleid=350&zoneid=46.

National Department of Health [South Africa]. (2006). *HIV & AIDS and STI strategic plan for South Africa, 2007–2011.* Retrieved November 12, 2007, from http://data.unaids.org/pub/ExternalDocument/2007/ 20070604_sa_nsp_final_en.pdf.

National Foundation for Infectious Diseases. (2004). *Influenza and children with asthma.* Chicago: Author.

National Institutes of Health, Office of AIDS Research. (2006). *Research on AIDS benefits efforts against other diseases.* Retrieved March 1, 2008, from http://www.25yearsofaids.oar.nih.gov/crossovers.htm.

National Research Council. (1993). *Understanding child abuse and neglect.* Washington, DC: National Academies Press.

Neale, M., & Kendler, K. (1995). Models of comorbidity for multifactorial disorders. *American Journal of Human Genetics, 57,* 935–953.

Neergaard, L. (2007). Kidney, heart disease spur each other. *USA Today.* Retrieved April 9, 2008, from http:// www.usatoday.com/news/health/2007-06-25-3480578305_x.htm.

Neihardt, J. (2004). *Black Elk speaks: Being the life story of a holy man of the Oglala Sioux.* Lincoln: University of Nebraska Press, Bison Books.

Nichter, M. (2008). *Global health: Why cultural perceptions, social representations, and biopolitics matter.* Tucson: University of Arizona Press.

Nielsen, N., Friis, H., Magnussen, P., Krarup, H., Magesa, S., & Simonsen, P. (2007). Co-infection with subclinical HIV and *Wuchereria bancrofti,* and the role of malaria and hookworms, in adult Tanzanians: Infection intensities, CD4/CD8 counts and cytokine responses. *Transactions of the Royal Society of Tropical Medicine and Hygiene, 101,* 602–612.

Nowak, M., & May, R. (2000). *Virus dynamics: Mathematical principles of immunology and virology.* New York: Oxford University Press.

Noymer, A., & Garenne, M. (2000). The 1918 influenza epidemic's effects on sex differentials in mortality in the United States. *Population and Development Review, 26,* 565–581.

Obel, N., Thomsen, H., Kronborg, G., Larsen, C., Hildebrandt, P., Sørensen, H., et al. (2007). Ischemic heart disease in HIV-infected and HIV-uninfected individuals: A population-based cohort study. *Clinical Infectious Diseases, 44,* 1625–1631.

O'Connell, J., Lampinen, T., Weber, A., Chan, K., Miller, M., Schechter, M., et al. (2004). Sexual risk profile of young men in Vancouver, British Columbia, who have sex with men and inject drugs. *AIDS and Behavior, 8,* 17–23.

O'Connor, S., Taylor, C., & Hughes, J. (2006). Emerging infectious determinants of chronic diseases. *Emerging Infectious Diseases, 21*(Suppl. 1), 15–24.

Office of Disease Prevention and Health Promotion. (2000). *Leading health indicators: Priorities for action.* U.S. Department of Health and Human Services. Retrieved May 4, 2008, from http://www.healthypeople.gov/ LHI/Priorities.htm.

Ogden, C., Carroll, M., Curtin, L., McDowell, M., Tabak, C., & Flegal, K. (2006). Prevalence of overweight and obesity in the United States, 1999–2004. *JAMA, 295,* 1549–1555.

Oleckno, W. (2008). Remembering Dr. John Snow on the sesquicentennial of his death. *Canadian Medical Association Journal, 178,* 1691–1692.

Oliver, M., Bararo, R., Medrano, F., & Moreno, J. (2003). The pathogenesis of leishmania/HIV co-infection: Cellular and immunological mechanisms. *Parasitology, 97*(Suppl. 1), S79–S98.

Olsen, S., Chang, Y., Moore, P., Biggar, R., & Melbye, M. (1998). Increasing Kaposi's sarcoma–associated herpesvirus seroprevalence with age in a highly Kaposi's sarcoma endemic region, Zambia in 1985. *AIDS, 12,* 1921–1925.

Orlic, D., Kajstura, J., Chimenti, S., Limana, F., Jakoniuk, I., Quaini, F., et al. (2001). Mobilized bone marrow cells repair the infarcted heart, improving function and survival. *Proceedings of the National Academy of Sciences of the United States of America, 98,* 10344–10349.

Pace, G., & Leaf, C. (1995). The role of oxidative stress in HIV disease. *Free Radical Biology & Medicine, 19,* 523–528.

Page, B., Lai, S., Chitwood, D., Klimas, N., Smith, P., & Fletcher, M. A. (1990). HTLV-I/II seropositivity and death from AIDS among HIV-1 seropositive intravenous drug users. *Lancet, 335,* 1439–1441.

Palacio, H., Shah, U., Kilborn, C., Martinez, D., Page, V., Gavagan, T., et al. (2005). Norovirus outbreak among evacuees from Hurricane Katrina—Houston, Texas, September 2005. *Morbidity and Mortality Weekly Report, 54,* 1016–1018.

Pan American Health Organization. (2004). Situation of severe growth retardation in first-grade schoolchildren in countries of Central America around 2000. *Epidemiological Bulletin, 25*(1), 9–13.

Panchanadeswaran, S., Johnson, S., Sivaram, S., Srikrishnan, A., Latkin, C., Bentley, M., et al. (2008). Intimate partner violence is as important as client violence in increasing street-based female sex workers' vulnerability to HIV in India. *International Journal of Drug Policy, 19*(2), 106–112.

Parker, S., Nuara, A., Buller, R., & Schultz, D. (2007). Human monkeypox: An emerging zoonotic disease. *Future Microbiology, 2,* 17–34.

Parriott, R. (1994). *Health experiences of Twin Cities women used in prostitution: Survey findings and recommendations.* St. Paul, MN: Breaking Free.

Pearl, R. (1919). Preliminary note on the incidence of epidemic influenza among the actively tuberculous. *Publications of the American Statistical Association, 16*(128), 536–540.

Pearl, R. (1928). On the pathological relations between cancer and tuberculosis. *Proceedings of the Society for Experimental Biology and Medicine, 26,* 73–75.

Penner, L. (2004). Florence Nightingale's sensational narrative of contagion and contamination. In P. Twohig & V. Kalitzkus (Eds.), *Making sense of: Health, illness and disease* (pp. 87–102). Amsterdam: Rodolpi.

Pereira, G., Stefani, M., Araújo Filho, J., Souza, L., Stefani, G., & Martelli, C. (2004). Human immunodeficiency virus type 1 (HIV-1) and *Mycobacterium leprae* co-infection: HIV-1 subtypes and clinical, immunologic, and histopathologic profiles in a Brazilian cohort. *American Journal of Tropical Medicine and Hygiene, 71,* 679–684.

Personal histories: Stories of the flu, passed from generation to generation. (2006). *Baltimore Sun.* Retrieved February 19, 2008, from http://www.baltimoresun.com/news/health/bal-flurewrite,0,3959916.story?coll=bal-health-utility.

Petaschnick, J. (2004). *The asthma-influenza connection.* Medical College of Wisconsin HealthLink. Retrieved April 2, 2008, from http://healthlink.mcw.edu/article/1031002437.html.

Petterson, J., Stanley, L., Glazier, E., & Philipp, J. (2006). A preliminary assessment of the social and economic impacts associated with Hurricane Katrina. *American Anthropologist, 108,* 643–670.

Pettit, D., & Bailie, J. (2008). *A cruel wind: Pandemic flu in America, 1918–1920.* Murfreesboro, TN: Timberlane Books.

Pingali, P., Stamoulis, K., & Stringer, R. (2006). *Eradicating extreme poverty and hunger: Towards a coherent policy agenda* (ESA Working Paper No. 06-01). Rome: Food and Agriculture Organization of the United Nations.

Pinlaor, S., Mootsikapun, P., Pinlaor, P., Pipitgool, V., & Tuangnadee, R. (2005). Detection of opportunistic and non-opportunistic intestinal parasites and liver flukes in HIV-positive and HIV-negative subjects. *Southeast Asian Journal of Tropical Medicine and Public Health, 36,* 841–845.

Plankey, M., Ostrow, D., Stall, R., Cox, C., Li, X., Peck, J., et al. (2007). The relationship between methamphetamine and popper use and risk of HIV seroconversion in the Multicenter AIDS Cohort Study. *Journal of Acquired Immune Deficiency Syndromes, 45,* 85–92.

Playfair, J. (2004). *Living with germs in health and disease.* New York: Oxford University Press.

Polgreen, L. (2006, May 24). As Darfur war rages on, disease and hunger kill. *New York Times.* Retrieved October 2, 2008, from http://www.nytimes.com/2006/05/31/world/africa/31darfur.html?pagewanted=1&_r=1.

Porter, C. (2006). *HIV/AIDS and malnutrition locked in "vicious cycle": International community working to address hunger among people with HIV/AIDS.* Retrieved May 12, 2008, from http://www.america.gov/st/washfile-english/2006/October/20061016151256cmretrop0.9265253.html.

Porto, A., Neva, F., Bittencourt, H., Lisboa, W., Thompson, R., Alcântara, L., et al. (2001). HTLV-1 decreases Th2 type of immune response in patients with strongyloidiasis. *Parasite Immunology, 23*, 503–507.

Porto, A., Santos, S., Alcântara, L., Guerreiro, J., Passos, J., Gonzalez, T., et al. (2004). HTLV-1 modifies the clinical and immunological response to schistosomiasis. *Clinical and Experimental Immunology, 137*, 424–429.

Post, J. (1977). *The last great subsistence crisis in the Western World.* Baltimore, MD: Johns Hopkins University Press.

Poundstone, K., Strathdee, S., & Celentano, S. (2004). The social epidemiology of human immunodeficiency virus/acquired immunodeficiency syndrome. *Epidemiologic Reviews, 26*, 22–35.

Prentice, A., & Jebb, S. (2006). TV and inactivity are separate contributors to metabolic risk factors in children. *PLoS Medicine, 3*, 2197–2198.

Preti, A., Usai, A., Miotto, P., Petretto, D., & Masala, C. (2008). Eating disorders among professional fashion models. *Psychiatry Research, 159.* Retrieved April 6, 2008, from http://www.ncbi.nlm.nih.gov/pubmed/18355925?ordinalpos=1&itool=EntrezSystem.

Pretorius, C., Borgdorf, J., Mateer, R., Lauer, J., Welte, A., & Ouifki, R. (2007). *HIVMM model* (Technical Report). SACEMA (South African Centre of Excellence for Epidemiological Modelling and Analysis). Retrieved August 2, 2008, from http://www0.sun.ac.za/sacema/projects/index.html.

Prevention Institute. (2002). *Eliminating health disparities: The role of primary prevention* (Briefing Paper for the California Endowment Board of Directors). San Francisco: Author.

Pribor, E., & Dinwiddie, S. (1992). Psychiatric correlates of incest in childhood. *American Journal of Psychiatry, 149*, 52–56.

Pugliese, A., Andronico, L., Gennero, L., Pagliano, G., Gallo, G., & Torre, D. (2002). Cervico-vaginal dysplasia-papillomavirus-induced and HIV-1 infection: Role of correlated markers for prognostic evaluation. *Cell Biochemistry and Function, 20*(3), 233–236.

Pugliese, A., Torre, D., Saini, A., Pagliano, G., Gallo, G., Pietro, G., et al. (2002). Cytokine detection in HTV-1/HHV-8 co-infected subjects. *Cell Biochemistry and Function, 20*(3), 191–194.

Punjabi, N., Sorkin, J., Katzel, L., Goldberg, A., Schwartz, A., & Smith, P. (2002). Sleep-disordered breathing and insulin resistance in middle-aged and overweight men. *American Journal of Respiratory and Critical Care Medicine, 165*, 677–682.

Ragsdale, K. (2008). Intervention studies. In S. Boslaugh (Ed.), *Encyclopedia of epidemiology* (Vol. 1, pp. 561–564). Thousand Oaks, CA: Sage.

Raso, G., Vounatsou, P., Singer, B., N'Goran, E., Tanner, M., & Utzinger, J. (2006). An integrated approach for risk profiling and spatial prediction of *Schistosoma mansoni*–hookworm coinfection. *Proceedings of the National Academy of Sciences of the United States of America, 103*, 6934–6939.

Ravindran, B., Sahoo, P., & Dash, A. (1998). Lymphatic filariasis and malaria: Concomitant parasitism in Orissa, India. *Transactions of the Royal Society of Tropical Medicine and Hygiene, 92*, 21–23.

Raymond, J., D'Cunha, J., Ruhaini, S., Hynes, H., Rodriguez, Z., & Santos, A. (2002). *Comparative study of women trafficked in the migration process: Patterns, profiles and health consequences of sexual exploitation in five countries (Indonesia, the Philippines, Thailand, Venezuela and the United States).* Washington, DC: Coalition Against Trafficking in Women.

Reback, C., & Grella, C. (1999). HIV risk behaviors of gay and bisexual male methamphetamine users contacted through street outreach. *Journal of Drug Issues, 29*, 155–166.

Reddy, M., Gill, S., Kalkar, S., Wu, W., Anderson, P., & Rochon, P. (2007). Oral drug therapy for multiple neglected tropical diseases: A systematic review. *JAMA, 298*, 1911–1924.

Reiter, P. (2000). From Shakespeare to Defoe: Malaria in England in the Little Ice Age. *Emerging Infectious Diseases, 6*, 1–11.

Relf, M., Huang, B., Campbell, J., & Catania, J. (2004). Gay identity, interpersonal violence, and HIV risk behaviors: An empirical test of theoretical relationships among a probability-based sample of urban men who have sex with men. *Journal of the Association of Nurses in AIDS Care, 15*, (2), 14–26.

Renia, L., & Potter, S. (2006). Co-infection of malaria with HIV: An immunological perspective. *Parasite Immunology, 28*, 589–595.

Renzi, C., Douglas, J., Jr., Foster, M., Zenilman, J., Brookmeyer, R., Paranjape, R., et al. (2003). Herpes simplex virus type 2 infection as a risk factor for human immunodeficiency virus acquisition in men who have sex with men. *Journal of Infectious Diseases, 187*, 19–25.

Restifo, N. (2000). Review of flu: The story of the great influenza pandemic of 1918 and the search for the virus that caused it. *Nature Medicine, 6*, 12–13.

Reynolds, S., Risbud, A., Shepherd, M., Zenilman, J., Brookmeyer, R., Paranjape, R., et al. (2003). Recent herpes simplex virus type 2 infection and the risk of human immunodeficiency virus type 1 acquisition in India. *Journal of Infectious Diseases, 187*, 1513–1521.

Rhodes, T., Singer, M., Bourgois, P., Friedman, S., & Strathdee, S. (2005). The social structural production of HIV risk among injecting drug users. *Social Science & Medicine, 61*, 1026–1044.

Richardson, G. (1991). *Feedback thought in social science and systems theory.* Philadelphia: University of Pennsylvania Press.

Riches, D. (1986). *The anthropology of violence.* Boston, MA: Wiley-Blackwell.

Ridgell, R. (1995). *Pacific nations and territories: The islands of Micronesia, Melanesia, and Polynesia.* Honolulu: Pacific Resources for Education and Learning.

Riese, R., Finn, P., & Shapiro, S. (2004). Influenza and asthma: Adding to the respiratory burden. *Nature Immunology, 5*, 243–244.

Rijken, M., van Kerkhof, M., Dekker, M., & Schellevis, F. (2005). Comorbidity of chronic diseases: Effects of disease pairs on physical and mental functioning. *Quality of Life Research, 14*, 45–55.

Riley, S., Fraser, C., Donnelly, C., Ghani, A., Abu-Raddad, L., Hedley, A., et al. (2003). Transmission dynamics of the etiological agent of SARS in Hong Kong: Impact of public health interventions. *Science, 300*, 1961–1966.

Robinson, K., Kenefeck, R., Pidgeon, E., Shakib, S., Patel, S., Polson, R., et al. (2008). Helicobacter pylori-induced peptic ulcer disease is associated with inadequate regulatory T-cell responses. *Gut, 57*. Retrieved June 16, 2008, from http://www.ncbi.nlm.nih.gov/pubmed/18467372?ordinalpos=25&itool=EntrezSystem2.PEntrez.Pubmed.Pubmed_ResultsPanel.Pubmed_RVDocSum.

Rock, M., Buntain, B., Hatfield, J., & Hallgrímsson, B. (2009). Animal-human connections, "one health," and the syndemic approach to prevention. *Social Science & Medicine,68*, 991–995.

Rodriguez, R., Mendelson, M., O'Hare, A., Hsu, L., & Schoenfeld, P. (2003). Determinants of survival among HIV-infected chronic dialysis patients. *Journal of the American Society of Nephrology, 14*, 1307–1313.

Rohsenow, D., Corbett, R., & Devine, D. (1988). Molested as children: A hidden contribution to substance abuse? *Journal of Substance Abuse Treatment, 5*, 13–18.

Rolph, H., Lennon, A., Riggio, M., Saunders, W., MacKenzie, D., Coldero, L., et al. (2001). Molecular identification of microorganisms from endodontic infections. *Journal of Clinical Microbiology, 39*, 3282–3289.

Romero-Alvira, D., & Roche, E. (1998). The keys of oxidative stress in acquired immune deficiency syndrome apoptosis. *Medical Hypotheses, 51*, 169–173.

Romero-Daza, N., Weeks, M., & Singer, M. (1998). Much more than HIV! The reality of life on the streets for drug-using sex workers in inner city Hartford. *International Quarterly of Community Health Education, 18*(1), 107–119.

Romero-Daza, N., Weeks, M., & Singer, M. (2003). "Nobody gives a damn if I live or die": Violence, drugs, and street-level prostitution in inner-city Hartford, CT. *Medical Anthropology, 22*, 233–259.

Ronco, C., House, A., & Haapio, M. (2008). Cardiorenal syndrome: Refining the definition of a complex symbiosis gone wrong. *Intensive Care Medicine, 34*. Retrieved March 23, 2008, from http://www.springerlink.com/content/n5706561547k177r.

Rosack, J. (2003). Comorbidity common in addicts, but integrated treatment rare. *Psychiatric News, 38*(2), 30.

Rosen, G. (1974). *From medical police to social medicine: Essays on the history of health care.* New York: Science History.

Rosenberg, L., Palmer, J., Wise, L., Horton, N., & Corwin, M. (2002). Perceptions of racial discrimination and the risk of preterm birth. *Epidemiology, 13*, 646–652.

Rosenberg, Z., & Fauci, A. (1990). Immunopathogenic mechanisms of HIV infection: Cytokine induction of HIV expression. *Immunology Today, 11*(5), 176–180.

Rothschild, B., Martin, L., Lev, G., Bercovier, H., Bar-Gal, G., Greenblatt, C., et al. (2001). *Mycobacterium tuberculosis* complex DNA from an extinct bison dated 17,000 years before the present. *Clinical Infectious Diseases, 33*, 305–311.

Rousseau, C., Learn, G., Bhattacharya, T., Nickle, D., Heckerman, D., Chetty, S., et al. (2007). Extensive intra-subtype recombination in South African human immunodeficiency virus type 1 subtype C infections. *Journal of Virology, 81*, 4492–4500.

Ruhräh, J. (1920). Infectious diseases, including acute rheumatism, croupous pneumonia and influenza. *Progressive Medicine, 1*, 117–224.

Ruskin, J. (1877). *Unto this last: Four essays on the principles of political economy.* Sunnyside, Orpington, Kent, UK: George Allen.

Rye, D. (2003). Sleepiness and unintended sleep in Parkinson's disease. *Current Treatment Options in Neurology, 5*, 231–239.

Sallares, R. (2002). *Malaria and Rome: A history of malaria in ancient Italy.* New York: Oxford University Press.

Sampson, R., & Wilson, W. (1998). Toward a theory of race, crime and urban inequality. In D. Karp (Ed.), *Community justice: An emerging field* (pp. 119–136). Lanham, MD: Rowman and Littlefield.

Sapolsky, R. (2004). Social status and health in humans and other animals. *Annual Reviews in Anthropology, 33*, 393–418.

Sapolsky, R. (2005). The influence of social hierarchy on primate health. *Science, 308*, 648–652.

Sattenspiel, L., & Herring, D. (1998). Structured epidemic models and the spread of influenza in the Norway house district of Manitoba, Canada. *Human Biology, 70*, 91–115.

Sawchuk, L. (2001). *Deadly visitations in dark times: A social history of Gibraltar.* Gibraltar: Gibraltar Government Heritage Publications.

Sawchuk, L., & Burke, S. (2003). The ecology of a health crisis: Gibraltar and the 1865 cholera epidemic. In D. Herring & A. Swedlund (Eds.), *Human biologists in the archives* (pp. 178–215). New York: Cambridge University Press.

Sawchuk, L., Herring, D., & Waks, L. (1985). Evidence of a Jewish advantage: A study of infant mortality in Gibraltar, 1870–1959. *American Anthropologist, 87*, 616–625.

Schacker, T. (2001). The role of HSV in the transmission and progression of HIV. *Herpes, 8*(2), 46–49.

Scheper-Hughes, N., & Lock, M. (1987). The mindful body: A prolegomenon to future work in medical anthropology. *Medical Anthropology Quarterly, 1*, 6–41.

Schmidt, E. (2007). *UCLA study links air pollution to clogged arteries.* Retrieved November 3, 2008, from http://newsroom.ucla.edu/portal/ucla/UCLA-Study-Links-Air-Pollution-8104.aspx?RelNum=8104.

Schrier, R. (2007). Cardiorenal versus renocardiac syndrome: Is there a difference? Nature Clinical Practice. *Nephrology, 3*, 637.

Schuller, M. (2008). *Haitian food riots unnerving but not surprising.* Retrieved June 16, 2008, from http://www.worldpress.org/Americas/3131.cfm.

Schwab, N., Cullen, M., & Schwartz, J. (2000). *A survey of prevalence of asthma among school-age children in Connecticut.* New Haven, CT: Environment and Human Health.

Scott, K. (1992). Childhood sexual abuse: Impact on a community's mental health status. *Child Abuse & Neglect, 16*, 285–295.

Scrimshaw, N., & SanGiovanni, J. (1997). Synergism of nutrition, infection, and immunity: An overview. *American Journal of Clinical Nutrition, 66*, 464–477.

Secor, W., Karanja, D., & Colley, D. (2004). Interactions between schistosomiasis and human immunodeficiency virus in Western Kenya. *Memórias do Instituto Oswaldo Cruz, 99*(Suppl. 1), 93–95.

Secor, W., & Sundstrom, J. (2007). Below the belt: New insights into potential complications of HIV-1/schistosome coinfections. *Current Opinion in Infectious Diseases, 20*, 519–523.

Segurado, A., Braga, P., Etzel, A., & Cardoso, M. (2004). Hepatitis C virus coinfection in a cohort of HIV-infected individuals from Santos, Brazil: Seroprevalence and associated factors. *AIDS Patient Care and STDS, 18*(3), 135–143.

Sejvar, J., Chowdary, Y., Schomogyi, M., Stevens, J., Patel, J., Karem, K., et al. (2004). Human monkeypox infection: A family cluster in the Midwestern United States. *Journal of Infectious Diseases, 190*, 1833–1840.

Seth, M. (2005, Fall). From poverty to obesity: Exploration of the food choice constraint model and the impact of an energy-dense food tax. *American Economist.* Retrieved June 18, 2008, from http://www.allbusiness. com/accounting/1086324-1.html.

Shahinian, V., Rajaraman, S., Borucki, M., Grady, J., Hollander, W., & Ahuja, T. (2000). Prevalence of HIV-associated nephropathy in autopsies of HIV-infected patients. *American Journal of Kidney Disease, 35*, 884–888.

Shaikh, M., Singla, R., Khan, N., Sharif, N., & Saigh, M. (2003). Does diabetes alter the radiological presentation of pulmonary tuberculosis. *Saudi Medical Journal, 24*, 278–281.

Sheth, P., Sunderji, S., Shin, L., Rebbaprgada, A., Huibner, S., Kimani, J., et al. (2008). Coinfection with herpes simplex virus type 2 is associated with reduced, HIV-specific T cell responses and systemic immune activation. *Journal of Infectious Diseases, 197*, 1394–1401.

Shoptaw, S., Reback, C., & Freese, T. (2002). Patient characteristics, HIV serostatus, and risk behaviors among gay and bisexual males seeking treatment for methamphetamine abuse and dependence in Los Angeles. *Journal of Addictive Diseases, 21*(1), 91–105.

Shrewsbury, J. (1970). *A history of bubonic plague in the British Isles.* New York: Cambridge University Press.

Sidat, M., Mijch, A., Lewin, S., Hoy, J., Hocking, J., & Fairley, C. (2008). Incidence of putative HIV superinfection and sexual practices among HIV-infected men who have sex with men. *Sexual Health, 5*, 61–68.

Silliman, J., & Bhattacharjee, A. (2002). *Policing the national body: Sex, race, and criminalization.* Cambridge, MA: South End Press.

Silverman, J., Decker, M., Gupta, J., Dharmadhikari, A., Seage, G., & Raj, A. (2008). Syphilis and hepatitis B co-infection among HIV-infected, sex-trafficked women and girls in Nepal. *Emerging Infectious Diseases.* Retrieved September 18, 2008, from http://www.cdc.gov/EID/content/14/6/932.htm.

Singer, M. (1986). The emergence of a critical medical anthropology. *Medical Anthropology Quarterly, 17*(5), 128–129.

Singer, M. (1994). AIDS and the health crisis of the U.S. urban poor: The perspective of critical medical anthropology. *Social Science & Medicine, 39*, 931–948.

Singer, M. (1996). A dose of drugs, a touch of violence, a case of AIDS: Conceptualizing the SAVA syndemic. *Free Inquiry in Creative Sociology, 24*, 99–110.

Singer, M. (1999). Why do Puerto Rican injection drug users inject so often? *Anthropology & Medicine, 6*, 31–58.

Singer, M. (2004a). Critical medical anthropology. In C. Ember and M. Ember (Eds.), *Encyclopedia of medical anthropology: Health and illness in the world's cultures* (Vol. 1, pp. 23–30). New York: Kluwer Academic/Plenum.

Singer, M. (2004b). The social origins and expressions of illness. In G. Smith & M. Shaw (Eds.), *Cultures of health, cultures of illness* (pp. 9–20). New York: Oxford University Press.

Singer, M. (2005). New drugs on the street: An introduction. *Journal of Ethnicity and Substance Abuse, 4*(2), 1–8.

Singer, M. (2006a). A dose of drugs, a touch of violence, a case of AIDS: Part 2. Further conceptualizing the SAVA syndemic. *Free Inquiry in Creative Sociology, 34*, 39–51.

Singer, M. (2006b). *The face of social suffering: Life history of a street drug addict.* Prospect Heights, IL: Waveland Press.

Singer, M. (2006c). *Something dangerous: Emergent and changing illicit drug use and community health.* Prospect Heights, IL: Waveland Press.

Singer, M. (2007). *Drugging the poor: Legal and illegal drug industries and the structuring of social inequality.* Prospect Heights, IL: Waveland Press.

Singer, M. (2008). *Syndemics.* In S. Boslaugh (Ed.), *Encyclopedia of epidemiology* (Vol. 1, pp. 1024–1026). Thousand Oaks, CA: Sage.

Singer, M. (2009). Desperate measures: A syndemic approach to the anthropology of health in a violent city. In B. Rylko-Bauer, L. Whiteford, & P. Farmer (Eds.), *Global health in the time of violence*. Santa Fe, NM: SAR Press.

Singer, M., & Baer, H. (Eds.). (2008). *Killer commodities: Public health and the corporate production of harm*. Lanham, MD: AltaMira Press.

Singer, M., & Clair, S. (2003). Syndemics and public health: Reconceptualizing disease in bio-social context. *Medical Anthropology Quarterly, 17*, 423–441.

Singer, M., Erickson, P., Badiane, L., Diaz, R., Ortiz, D., Abraham, T., et al. (2006). Syndemics, sex and the city: Understanding sexually transmitted disease in social and cultural context. *Social Science & Medicine, 63*, 2010–2021.

Singer, M., & Marxuach-Rodriquez, L. (1996). Applying anthropology to the prevention of AIDS: The Latino Gay Men's Health Project. *Human Organization, 55*, 141–148.

Singer, M., Salaheen, H., & He, Z. (2004). *The special HIV and related health vulnerabilities of sex workers caught in the international sex trade industry*. Paper presented at the meeting of the Society for Applied Anthropology, Dallas, Texas.

Singer, M., & Singer, E. (2008). Eating disorders. In S. Boslaugh (Ed.), *Encyclopedia of epidemiology* (Vol. 1, pp. 293–295). Thousand Oaks, CA: Sage.

Singer, M., & Snipes, C. (1992). Generations of suffering: Experiences of a pregnancy and substance abuse treatment program. *Journal of Health Care for the Poor and Underserved, 3*, 325–239.

Singer, M., Stopka, T., Siano, C., Springer, K., Barton, G., Khoshnood, K., et al. (2000). The social geography of AIDS and hepatitis risk: Qualitative approaches for assessing local differences in sterile syringe access among injection drug users. *American Journal of Public Health, 90*, 1049–1056.

Singer, M., & Weeks, M. (n.d.). [Intertwined epidemics among Puerto Rican drug users.] Unpublished data.

Skelly, P. (2008). Fighting worm killers. *Scientific American, 298*(5), 94–99.

Skurnik, M., & Strauch, E. (2006). Phage therapy: Facts and fiction. *International Journal of Medical Microbiology, 296*(1), 5–14.

Smallman-Raynor, M., & Cliff, A. (2004). *War epidemics: An historical geography of infectious diseases in military conflict and civil strife*. New York: Oxford University Press.

Smerdon, W., Nichols, T., Chalmers, R., Heine, H., & Reacher, M. (2003). Foot and mouth disease in livestock and reduced cryptosporidiosis in humans, England and Wales. *Emerging Infectious Diseases, 9*, 22–28.

Smith, G. (Ed.). (2003). *Health inequalities: Lifecourse approaches*. Bristol, U.K.: Policy Press.

Smith, G., Wentworth, D., Neaton, J., Stamler, R., & Stamler, J. (2003). Socioeconomic differentials in mortality risk among men screened for the Multiple Risk Factor Intervention Trial: Part II. Results for 20,224 black men. In G. Smith (Ed.), *Health inequalities: Lifecourse approaches* (pp. 47–63). Bristol, U.K.: Policy Press.

Snow, J. (1855). *On the mode of communication of cholera*. London: John Churchill.

Sobo, E. (1995). Finance, romance, social support, and condom use among impoverished inner-city women. *Human Organization, 63*, 115–128.

Soriano, V., Nuñez, M., Sheldon. J., Ramos, B., Garcia-Samaniego, J., Martín-Carbonero, L., et al. (2005). Complications in treating chronic hepatitis B in patients with HIV. *Expert Opinion on Pharmacotherapy, 6*, 2831–2842.

Sousa, N. (1983). *Becoming black*. Rio de Janeiro: Graal.

Speak, S. (2004). Degrees of destitution: A typology of homelessness in developing countries. *Housing Studies, 19*, 465–482.

Spector, M. (2005, May 23). Higher risk: Crystal meth, the Internet, and dangerous choices about AIDS. *New Yorker*, pp. 38–45.

Stall, R., Friedman, M., & Catania, J. (2007). Interacting epidemics and gay men's health: A theory of syndemic production among urban gay men. In R. Wolitski, R. Stall, & R. Valdiserri (Eds.), *Unequal opportunity: Health disparities affecting gay and bisexual men in the United States* (pp. 251–274). New York: Oxford University Press.

Stall, R., Mills, T., Williamson, J., & Hart, T. (2003). Association of co-occurring psychosocial health problems and increased vulnerability to HIV/AIDS among urban men who have sex with men. *American Journal of Public Health, 93*, 939–942.

Steeves, S. (2008). *Combined viruses cause more deadly disease in pigs, researchers discover* (Press Release). Purdue University. Retrieved March 20, 2008, from http://news.uns.purdue.edu/x/2008a/080213Roman Pigvirus.html.

Stein, J., Golding, J., Siegel, J., Burnam, M., & Sorenson, S. (1988). Long-term psychological sequelae of child sexual abuse: The Los Angeles Epidemiologic Catchment Area study. In G. Wyatt & G. Powell (Eds.), *Lasting effects of child sexual abuse* (pp. 135–154). Thousand Oaks, CA: Sage.

Stein, R. (2008, April 4). Report cites abuse of 91,000 babies under 1. *Washington Post*, p. A02.

Sterne, M., Schaefer, S., & Evans, S. (1983). Women's sexuality and alcoholism. In P. Golding (Ed.), *Alcoholism: Analysis of a world-wide problem* (pp. 421–425). Lancaster, England: MTP Press.

Stevenson, C., Forouhi, N., Roglic, G., Williams, B., & Lauer, J. (2007). DM and tuberculosis: The impact of the DM epidemic on tuberculosis incidence. *BMC Public Health, 7*, 234.

Stewart, S., & Israeli, A. (2002). Substance abuse and co-occurring psychiatric disorders in victims of intimate violence. In C. Wekerle & A. Wall (Eds.), *The violence and addiction equation* (pp. 98–122). New York: Brunner-Routledge.

Stoll, N. (1962). On endemic hookworm, where do we stand today? *Experimental Parasitology, 12*(4), 241–252.

Struck, D. (2006, May 5). Climate change drives disease to new territory. *Washington Post*, p. A16.

Stueve, A., O'Donnell, L., Duran, R., San Doval, A., Geier, J., & the Community Intervention Trial for Youth Study Team. (2002). Being high and taking sexual risks: Findings from a multisite survey of urban young men who have sex with men. *AIDS Education and Prevention, 14*, 482–495.

Suk, W., & Collman, G. (1998). Genes and the environment: Their impact on children's health. *Environmental Health Perspectives, 106*(Suppl. 3), 817–820.

Summers, J. (1989). *Soho: A history of London's most colourful neighborhood*. London: Bloomsbury.

Suzuki, K., Takeda, A., & Matsushita, S. (1995). Coprevalence of bulimia with alcohol abuse and smoking among Japanese male and female high school students. *Addiction, 90*, 971–975.

Swaminath, S., & Narendr, G. (2008). HIV and tuberculosis in India. *Journal of Biosciences, 33*, 527–537.

Swedlund, A., & Donta, A. (2003). Scarlet fever epidemics of the nineteenth century: A Case of evolved pathogenic virulence. In D. Herring & A. Swedlund (Eds.), *Human biologists in the archives* (pp. 159–177). New York: Cambridge University Press.

Sykes, A., Mallia, P., & Johnson, S. (2007). Diagnosis of pathogens in exacerbations of chronic obstructive pulmonary disease. *Proceedings of the American Thoracic Society, 4*, 642–646.

Syndemics Prevention Network. (2005a). *Exploring foundations*. Retrieved June 5, 2006, from http://www.cdc.gov/syndemics/foundations.htm.

Syndemics Prevention Network. (2005b). *Syndemics overview: Definition: What is a syndemic?* Retrieved June 12, 2006, from http://www.cdc.gov/syndemics/definition.htm.

Syndemics Prevention Network. (2005c). *Syndemics overview: Furthering scientific and social change*. Retrieved January 8, 2006, from http://www.cdc.gov/syndemics/overview-furtherchange.htm.

Syndemics Prevention Network. (2005d). *Syndemics overview: What principles characterize a syndemic orientation?* Retrieved January 8, 2006, from http://www.cdc.gov/syndemics/overview-principles.htm.

Syndemics Prevention Network. (2008a). *Spotlight on syndemics*. Retrieved December 2, 2008, from http://www.cdc.gov/syndemics.

Syndemics Prevention Network. (2008b). *Syndemics overview: What procedures are available for planning and evaluating initiatives to prevent syndemics?* (Revised). Retrieved May 2, 2008, from http://www.cdc.gov/syndemics/overview-planeval.htm.

Talwar, G. (2005). A destiny to fulfill. *Journal of Bioscience, 30*, 435–447.

Tamayo, J. (2001, August 18). *Thriving heroin culture alarms Colombian, U.S. authorities*. Miami Herald, p. A1.

Tamura, T., & Goldenberg, R. (1996). Zinc nutriture and pregnancy outcome. *Nutrition Research, 16*, 139–181.

Tang, A., Graham, N., Chandra, R., & Saah, A. (1997). Low serum vitamin B-12 concentrations are associated with faster human immunodeficiency virus type 1 (HIV-1) disease progression. *Journal of Nutrition, 127*, 345–351.

Tarleton, J., Haque, R., Mondal, D., Shu, J., Farr, B., & Petri, W. (2006). Cognitive effects of diarrhea, malnutrition, and *Entamoeba histolytica* infection on school age children in Dhaka, Bangladesh. *American Journal of Tropical Medicine and Hygiene, 74*, 475–481.

Tasali, E., Mokhlesi, B., & Van Cauter, E. (2008). Obstructive sleep apnea and type 2 diabetes: Interacting epidemics. *Chest, 133*, 496–506.

Taubenberger, J., & Morens, D. (2006). 1918 influenza: The mother of all pandemics. *Emerging Infectious Diseases, 12*. Retrieved November 3, 2007, from http://www.cdc.gov/ncidod/EID/vol12no01/05-0979.htm.

Taylor, C., Bryson, S., Altman, T., Abascal, L., Celio, A., Cunning, D., et al. (2003). Risk factors for the onset of eating disorders in adolescent girls: Results of the McKnight Longitudinal Risk Factor Study. *American Journal of Psychiatry, 160*, 248–254.

Taylor, M. (2003). *Wolbachia* in the inflammatory pathogenesis of human filariasis. *Annals of the New York Academy of Sciences, 990*, 444–449.

Tell, G., Hylander, B., Craven, T., & Burkart, J. (1996). Racial differences in the incidence of end-stage renal disease. *Ethnicity and Health, 1*(1), 21–31.

Terris, M. (1979). The epidemiologic tradition. *Public Health Reports, 94*(3), 203–209.

Tesh, S. (1988). *Hidden arguments: Political ideology and disease prevention policy.* New Brunswick, NJ: Rutgers University Press.

Teusch, R. (2001). Substance abuse as a symptom of childhood sexual abuse. *Psychiatric Services, 52*, 1530–1532.

Thio, C., Seaberg, E., Skolasky, R., Phair, J., Visscher, B., Munoz, A., & the Multicenter AIDS Cohort Study. (2002). HIV-1, hepatitis B virus, and risk of liver-related mortality in the Multicenter Cohort Study (MACS). *Lancet, 14*, 1921–1926.

Thompson, S., & Hammond, K. (2003). Beauty is as beauty does: Body image and self-esteem of pageant contestants. *Eating and Weight Disorders, 8*, 231–237.

Thompson, W., Shay, D., Weintraub, E., Brammer, L., Cox, N., Anderson, L., et al. (2003). Mortality associated with influenza and respiratory syncytial virus in the United States. *JAMA, 289*, 179–186.

Tice, D. (1997, March 10). Flu deaths rivaled, ran alongside World War I. *St. Paul Pioneer Planet*, p. 1E.

Tillmann, H., Heiken, H., Knapik-Botor, A., Heringlake, S., Ockenga, J., Wilber, J., et al. (2001). Infection with GB virus C and reduced mortality among HIV-infected patients. *New England Journal of Medicine, 345*, 715–724.

Tjaden, P., & Thoennes, N. (2000). *Extent, nature, and consequences of intimate partner violence: Findings of the National Violence Against Women Survey.* Atlanta: Centers for Disease Control and Prevention.

Tolstoy, L. (1998). *War and peace.* New York: Oxford University Press. (Original work published 1865–1869)

Toosi, Z., Wu, M., Islam, N., Teixeira-Johnson, L., Hejal, R., & Aung, H. (2004). Transactivation of human immunodeficiency virus-1 in T-cells by *Mycobacterium tuberculosis*-infected mononuclear phagocytes. *Journal of Laboratory and Clinical Medicine, 144*, 108–115.

Treisman, G., Angelino, A., & Hutton, H. (2001). Psychiatric issues in the management of patients with HIV infection. *JAMA, 286*, 2857–2864.

Troy, C., Derossi, D., Prochiantz, A., Greene, L., & Shelanski, M. (1996). Downregulation of Cu/Zn superoxide dismutase leads to cell death via the nitric oxide-peroxynitrite pathway. *Journal of Neuroscience, 16*, 253–261.

Tschanz, J., Corcoran C., Skoog, I., Khachaturian, A., Herrick, J., Hayden, K., et al., & the Cache County Study Group. (2004). Dementia: The leading predictor of death in a defined elderly population: The Cache County Study. *Neurology, 62*, 1156–1162.

Tsutsumi, A., Izutsu, T., Poudyal, A., Kato, S., & Marui, E. (2008). Mental health of female survivors of human trafficking in Nepal. *Social Science & Medicine, 66*, 1841–1847.

Tull, E., & Chambers, E. (2001). Internalized racism is associated with glucose intolerance among black Americans in the U.S. Virgin Islands. *Diabetes Care, 24*, 1498.

Tull, E., Wickramasuriya, T., Taylor, J., Smith-Burns, V., Brown, M., Champagnie, G., et al. (1999). Relationship of internalized racism to abdominal obesity and blood pressure in Afro-Caribbean women. *Journal of the National Medical Association, 9*, 447–451.

Turco, S. (1999). Adversarial relationship between the leishmania lipophosphoglycan and protein kinase C of host macrophages. *Parasite Immunology, 21*, 597–600.

Tyagi, B., Yadav, S., Sachdev, R., & Dam, P. (2001). Malaria outbreak in the Indira Gandhi Nahar Pariyojna command area in Jaisalmer district, Thar desert, India. *Journal of Communicable Diseases, 33*(2), 88–95.

UNAIDS. (2004). *HIV/AIDS estimates, Egypt.* Geneva: World Health Organization.

UNAIDS & World Health Organization. (2007). *AIDS epidemic update.* Geneva: UNAIDS.

UNICEF. (2006). *Childhood interrupted in Darfur's refugee camps.* Retrieved January 5, 2009, from http://www .unicef.org/sowc/index_30568.html.

United Nations Administrative Committee on Coordination, Sub-Committee on Nutrition. (2000). *Fourth report on the world nutrition situation: Nutrition throughout the life cycle.* Geneva: Author.

United Nations Development Programme. (2008). *Fighting climate change: Human solidarity in a divided world* (Human Development Report 2007/2008). New York: Author.

United States Renal Data System. (2000). *Annual data report.* Bethesda, MD: National Institutes of Health, National Institute of Diabetes and Digestive and Kidney Diseases.

Unklesday, N. (1992). *World food and you.* Binghamton, NY: Food Products Press.

U.S. Department of Agriculture and Agricultural Research Service. (2006). *Eradicating hog cholera.* Agricultural Research Service Timeline. Retrieved March 18, 2008, from http://www.ars.usda.gov/is/timeline/cholera.htm.

U.S. Department of Health and Human Services. (1979). *Healthy people: The surgeon general's report on health promotion and disease prevention.* Washington, DC: U.S. Government Printing Office.

U.S. Department of Health and Human Services. (1990). *Healthy people 2000: National health promotion and disease prevention objectives.* Washington, DC: U.S. Government Printing Office.

U.S. Department of Health and Human Services. (2000). *Healthy people 2010: Understanding and improving health* (conference ed.). Retrieved January 31. 2009, from http://www.eric.ed.gov/ERICDocs/data/ ericdocs2sql/content_storage_01/0000019b/80/16/5b/7c.pdf.

U.S. Department of Health and Human Services. (2006). *The health consequences of involuntary exposure to tobacco smoke: A report of the Surgeon General.* Rockville, MD: Author.

U.S. Department of Health and Human Services, Children's Bureau. (2001). *Child maltreatment 1999.* Washington, DC: U.S. Government Printing Office.

U.S. Department of Health and Human Services, Children's Bureau. (2007). *Child maltreatment 2005.* Washington, DC: U.S. Government Printing Office.

Vadheim, C., Greenberg, D., Bordenave, N., Ziontz, L., Christenson, P., Waterman, S., et al. (1992). Risk factors for invasive *Haemophilus influenzae* type B in Los Angeles County children 18–60 months of age. *American Journal of Epidemiology, 136*, 221–235.

Valdez, A., Kaplan, C., & Curtis, R. (2007). Aggressive crime, alcohol and drug use, and concentrated poverty in 24 U.S. urban areas. *American Journal of Drug and Alcohol Abuse, 33*, 595–603.

Valent, F., Little, D., Bertollini, R., Nemer, L., Barbone, F., & Tamburlini, G. (2004). Burden of disease attributable to selected environmental factors and injury among children and adolescents in Europe. *Lancet, 363*, 2032–2039.

van der Kuyl, A., & Cornelissen, M. (2007). Identifying HIV-1 dual infections. *Retrovirology, 4*, 67.

van Eeuwijk, P. (2000). Health care from the perspectives of Minahasa villagers, Indonesia. In L. Whiteford & L. Manderson (Eds.), *Global health policy, local realities: The fallacy of the level playing field* (pp. 79–101). Boulder, CO: Lynne Rienner.

Van Geen, A., Ahmed, K., & Graziano, J. (2005, July 30). Bangladesh's deadly wells. *New York Times*, p. 8.

Van geertruyden, J., & D'Alessandro, U. (2007). Malaria and HIV: A silent alliance. *Trends in Parasitology, 23*, 465–467.

van Kooyk, Y., Appelmelk, B., & Geijtenbeek, T. (2003). A fatal attraction: *Mycobacterium tuberculosis* and HIV-1 target DC-SIGN to escape immune surveillance. *Trends in Molecular Medicine, 9*, 153–159.

van Lettow, M., Fawzi, W., & Semba, R. (2003). Triple trouble: The role of malnutrition in tuberculosis and human immunodeficiency virus co-infection. *Nutrition Reviews, 61*(3), 81–90.

Vanholder, R., Massy, Z., Argiles, A., Spasovski, G., Verbeke, F., Lameire, N., & the European Uremic Toxin Work Group. (2005). Chronic kidney disease as cause of cardiovascular morbidity and mortality. *Nephrology, Dialysis, Transplantation, 20*, 1048–1056.

Vermund, S., & Yamamoto, N. (2007). Co-infection with human immunodeficiency virus and tuberculosis in Asia. *Tuberculosis, 87*(Suppl. 1), S18–S25.

Viana, S., Paraná, R., Moreira, R., Compri, A., & Macedo, V. (2005). High prevalence of hepatitis B virus and hepatitis D virus in the western Brazilian Amazon. *American Journal of Tropical Medicine and Hygiene, 73*, 808–814.

Vijaykrishna, D., Smith, G., Zhang, J., Peiris, J., Chen, H., & Guan, Y. (2007). Evolutionary insights into the ecology of coronaviruses. *Journal of Virology, 81*, 4012–4020.

Villacian, J., Tan, G., Teo, L., & Paton, N. (2005). The effect of infection with Mycobacterium tuberculosis on T-cell activation and proliferation in patients with and without HIV co-infection. *Journal of Infection, 51*, 408–412.

Viney, M., Brown, M., Omoding, N., Bailey, J., Gardner, M., Roberts, E., et al. (2004). Why does HIV infection not lead to disseminated strongyloidiasis? *Journal of Infectious Diseases, 190*, 2175–2180.

Viravaidya, M. (1993). The economic impact of AIDS on Thailand. In D. Bloom & J. Lyons (Eds.), *Economic implications of AIDS in Asia* (pp. 23–34). Hanoi: United Nations Development Program.

Voisin, D., Salazar, L., Crosby, R., Diclemente, R., Yarber, W., & Staples-Horne, M. (2007). Witnessing community violence and health-risk behaviors among detained adolescents. *American Journal of Orthopsychiatry, 77*, 506–513.

Volkova, N., McClellan, W., Klein, M., Flanders, D., Kleinbaum, D., Soucie, M., et al. (2008). Neighborhood poverty and racial differences in ESRD incidence. *Journal of the American Society of Nephrology, 19*, 356–364.

Wacquant, L. (2004). Response to Farmer's *An Anthropology of Structural Violence. Current Anthropology, 45*, 322.

Waitzkin, H. (2006). One and a half centuries of forgetting and rediscovering: Virchow's lasting contributions to social medicine. *Social Medicine 1*(1), 5–10.

Waldram, J., Herring, D., & Young, T. (2006). *Aboriginal health in Canada: Historical, cultural, and epidemiological perspectives.* Toronto: University of Toronto Press.

Wall, A. (2009). Including persons with Alzheimer disease in research on comorbid conditions. *IRB: Ethics & Human Research, 31*, 1–6.

Wallace, D., & Wallace, R. (1998). *A plague on your houses: How New York was burned down and national public health crumbled.* New York: Verso.

Wallace, R. (1988). A synergism of plagues: "Planned shrinkage," contagious housing destruction, and AIDS in the Bronx. *Environmental Research, 47*, 1–33.

Wallace, R. (1990). Urban desertification, public health and public order: "Planned shrinkage," violent death, substance abuse and AIDS in the Bronx. *Social Science & Medicine, 31*, 801–813.

Walters, R., & Parke, R. (1964). Social motivation, dependency, and susceptibility to social influence. In L. Berkowitz (Ed.), *Advances in experimental social psychology* (Vol. 1, pp. 231–276). New York: Academic Press.

Waterston, A. (1993). *Street addicts in the political economy.* Philadelphia: Temple University Press.

Watt, G., Jongsakul, K., & Suttinot, C. (2003). Possible scrub typhus coinfections in Thai agricultural workers hospitalized with leptospirosis. *American Journal of Tropical Medicine and Hygiene, 66*, 89–91.

Weinberg, S. (1992). *Dreams of a final theory: The search for the fundamental laws of nature.* New York: Pantheon Books.

Weiss, H., Buve, A., Robinson, N., Van Dyck, E., Kahindo, M., Anagonou, S., et al. (2001). The epidemiology of HSV-2 infection and its association with HIV infection in four urban African populations. *AIDS, 15*(Suppl. 4), S97–S108.

Wekerle, C., & Wolfe, D. (1998). The role of child maltreatment and attachment style in adolescent relationship violence. *Developmental Psychopathology, 10*, 571–586.

Whitehead, M., & Dahlgren, G. (2006). *Levelling up (part 1): A discussion paper on concepts and principles for tackling social inequities in health.* Copenhagen: WHO Regional Office for Europe.

Whitrow, M. (1990). Wagner-Jauregg and fever therapy. *Medical History, 34*, 294–310.

Whitworth, J., Morgan, D., Quigley, M., Smith, A., Mayanja, B., Eotu, H., et al. (2000). Effect of HIV-1 and increasing immunosuppression on malaria parasitaemia and clinical episodes in adults in rural Uganda: A cohort study. *Lancet, 356*, 1051–1056.

Widom, C. (1989). Does violence beget violence? A critical examination of the literature. *Psychological Bulletin, 106*(1), 3–28.

Wilce, J. (Ed.). (2003). *Social and cultural lives of immune systems*. New York: Routledge.

Williams, B., Waters, D., & Parker, K. (1999). Evaluation and treatment of weight loss in adults with HIV disease. *American Family Physician, 60*, 843–860.

Wines, M. (2007, January 28). Virulent TB in South Africa may imperil millions. *New York Times*. Retrieved April 22, 2008, from http://www.nytimes.com/2007/01/28/world/africa/28tuberculosis.html?pagewanted=1&_r=1.

Wintergerst, E., Maggini, S., & Hornig, D. (2007). Contribution of selected vitamins and trace elements to immune function. *Annals of Nutrition and Metabolism, 51*, 301–323.

Winterton, W. (1980, March/April). The Soho cholera epidemic 1854. *History of Medicine*, pp. 11–17.

Wolday, D., Berhe, N., Akuffo, H., & Britton, S. (1999). Leishmania–HIV-interaction: Immunopathogenic mechanisms. *Parasitology Today, 15*, 182–187.

Wolfgang, M., & Ferracuti, F. (1967). *The subculture of violence: Towards an integrated theory in criminology*. London: Tavistock.

Wong, W., Chen, T., Yang, S., Wang, F., Cheng, N., Kuo, B., et al. (2003). Clinical characteristics of fatal patients with severe acute respiratory syndrome in a medical center in Taipei. *Journal of the Chinese Medical Association, 66*, 323–327.

Wongsrichanalai, C., Murray, C., Gray, M., Miller, R., McDaniel. P., Liao, W., et al. (2003). Co-infection with malaria and leptospirosis. *American Journal of Tropical Medicine and Hygiene, 68*, 583–585.

Woodham-Smith, C. (1992). *The great hunger: Ireland 1845–1849*. New York: Penguin Books.

Woods, C., Karpati, A., Grein, T., McCarthy, N., Khan, A., Swanepoel, R., et al., & the World Health Organization Hemorrhagic Fever Task Force. (2002). An outbreak of Rift Valley fever in northeastern Kenya, 1997–98. *Emerging Infectious Diseases, 8*, 138–144.

World Health Organization. (1995). *Physical status: The use of and interpretation of anthropometry*. Geneva: Author.

World Health Organization. (1998). *Rift Valley fever*. Retrieved June, 5, 2007, from http://www.who.int/mediacentre/factsheets/fs207/en.

World Health Organization. (1999). Leishmania/HIV co-infection, South-western Europe, 1990–1998. *Weekly Epidemiological Record, 74*, 365–375.

World Health Organization. (2000). *Lymphatic filariasis* (Fact Sheet 102). Retrieved June 2, 2007, from www.who.int/mediacentre/factsheets/fs102/en.

World Health Organization. (2001). *Water-related diseases* (Prepared for World Water Day 2001). Retrieved May 16, 2008, from http://www.who.int/water_sanitation_health/diseases/malnutrition/en.

World Health Organization. (2002a). Urbanization: An increasing risk for leishmaniasis. *Weekly Epidemiological Record, 77*, 365–372.

World Health Organization. (2002b). *The world health report 2002: Reducing risks, promoting healthy life*. Geneva: Author.

World Health Organization. (2002c). *World report on violence and health*. Geneva: Author.

World Health Organization. (2003). *Severe acute respiratory syndrome (SARS): Status of the outbreak and lessons for the immediate future*. Geneva: World Health Organization, CDS Information Resource Centre.

World Health Organization. (2004a). *Diabetes*. Retrieved February 4, 2004, from http://www.who.int/hpr/NPH/docs/gs_diabetes.pdf.

World Health Organization. (2004b, January 21). *WHO pushing to rapidly scale-up measures to fight TB and HIV* (Press Release). Geneva: Author.

World Health Organization. (2006a). *Children's environmental health*. Geneva: Author.

World Health Organization. (2006b). *Obesity and overweight* (Fact Sheet). Geneva: Author.

World Health Organization. (2007). *A safer future: Global public health security in the 21st century*. Geneva: Author.

World Health Organization. (2008a). *Communicable disease risk assessment and interventions: Cyclone Nargis: Myanmar*. Myanmar: World Health Organization Regional Office for South-East Asia.

World Health Organization. (2008b). *Enterovirus in China*. Retrieved May 2, 2008, from http://www.who.int/csr/don/2008_05_01/en/index.html.

World Health Organization. (2008c). *Leishmaniasis: Background information*. Retrieved April 6, 2008, from http://www.who.int/leishmaniasis/en.

World Health Organization. (2008d). *Tuberculosis* (Fact Sheet). Retrieved April 22, 2008, from http://www.who.int/mediacentre/factsheets/fs104/en/index.html.

Wright, R., Hanrahan, J., Tager, I., & Speizer, F. (1997). Effect of the exposure to violence on the occurrence and severity of childhood asthma in an inner-city population. *American Journal of Respiratory and Critical Care Medicine, 155*, A972.

Wright, R., & Steinbach, S. (2001). Violence: An unrecognized environmental exposure that may contribute to greater asthma morbidity in high-risk inner-city populations. *Environmental Health Perspectives, 109*, 1085–1089.

Wyatt, C., Rosenstiel, P., & Klotman, P. (2008). HIV-associated nephropathy. *Contributions to Nephrology, 159*, 151–161.

Wynne, B. (1996). May the sheep graze safely: A reflective view of the expert–lay knowledge divide. In S. Lash, B. Szerszynski, & B. Wynne (Eds.), *Risk, environment and modernity: Towards a new ecology* (pp. 44–83). Thousand Oaks, CA: Sage.

Yamada, S., & Palmer, W. (2007). An ecosocial approach to the epidemic of cholera in the Marshall Islands. *Social Medicine 2*(2), 79–86.

Yang, J., Feng, Y., Yuan, M., Yuan, S., Fu, H., Wu, B., et al. (2006). Plasma glucose levels and diabetes are independent predictors for mortality and morbidity in patients with SARS. *Diabetic Medicine, 23*, 623–628.

Yanovski, S. (2003). Sugar and fat: Cravings and aversions. *Journal of Nutrition, 133*(Suppl.), 835S–837S.

Yarborough, K. (1999). *Understanding body image*. Retrieved April 3, 2008, from http://menwithed.healthyplace2.com/page29.html.

Zamrini, E., Parrish, J., Parsons, D., & Harrell, L. (2004). Medical comorbidity in black and white patients with Alzheimer's disease. *Southern Medical Journal, 97*, 2–6.

Zhao, J., Takamura, M., Yamaoka, A., Odajima, Y., & Iikura, Y. (2002). Altered eosinophil levels as a result of viral infection in asthma exacerbation in childhood. *Pediatric Allergy and Immunology, 13*(1), 47–50.

Zink, A., Sola, C., Reischl, U., Grabner, W., Rastogi, N., Wolf, H., et al. (2003). Characterization of Mycobacterium tuberculosis complex DNAs from Egyptian mummies by spoligotyping. *Journal of Clinical Microbiology, 41*, 359–367.

Zinsser, H. (1936). Biographical memoir of Theobald Smith, 1859–1934. In *Biographical Memoirs* (Vol. 17). New York: National Academy of Science.

Zinsser, H. (2000). *Rats, lice, and history*. New York: Penguin Books. (Original work published 1935)

INDEX

Page references followed by *t* indicate a table.